Springer Japan KK

N. Tamaki, U. Batzdorf
T. Nagashima (Eds.)

Syringomyelia

Current Concepts in Pathogenesis and Management

With 148 Figures, Including 1 in Color

Springer

Norihiko Tamaki, M.D., Ph.D.
Professor and Chairman, Department of Neurosurgery, Kobe University, Graduate School of Medicine, 7-5-1 Kusunoki-cho, Chuo-ku, Kobe 650-0017, Japan

Ulrich Batzdorf, M.D.
Professor and Director of Spine Surgery, Division of Neurosurgery, UCLA Medical Center, 10833 Le Conte Avenue, Los Angeles, CA 90095, USA

Tatsuya Nagashima, M.D., Ph.D.
Lecturer, Department of Neurosurgery, Kobe University, Graduate School of Medicine, 7-5-1 Kusunoki-cho, Chuo-ku, Kobe 650-0017, Japan
As of June 2001:
Chief, Department of Neurosurgery, Hyogo Prefectural Kobe Children's Hospital, 1-1-1 Takakura-dai, Suma-ku, Kobe 654-0081, Japan

ISBN 978-4-431-70305-1

Library of Congress Cataloging-in-Publication Data

Syringomyelia : current concept in pathogenesis and management / N. Tamaki, U. Batzdorf, T. Nagashima (eds.).
p. ; cm.
Includes bibliographical references and index.
ISBN 978-4-431-70305-1 **ISBN 978-4-431-67893-9 (eBook)**
DOI 10.1007/978-4-431-67893-9
1. Syringomyelia—Congresses. I. Tamaki, Norihiko. II. Batzdorf, Ulrich, 1928- III. Nagashima, T. (Tatsuya), 1952-
[DNLM: 1. Syringomyelia—therapy—Congresses. 2. Syringomyelia—etiology—Congresses. WL 400 S9948 2001]
RC406.S9 S965 2001
616.8'3—dc21

2001032082

Printed on acid-free paper

Typesetting: Best-set Typesetter Ltd., Hong Kong

SPIN: 10786462

Preface

Surgical skill and imaging technology in the field of neurosurgery have developed remarkably during the past decade. Magnetic resonance imaging (MRI), with high-contrast resolution and multiplanar capabilities, allows for accurate preoperative localization and postoperative assessment of syringomyelia. Recent advances in dynamic MRI techniques have made it possible to evaluate normal and abnormal cerebrospinal fluid (CSF) flow at the foramen magnum, within the syrinx, and in the spinal subarachnoid space, without invasion of the closed CSF system. These developments have yielded substantial information concerning various aspects of syringomyelia. However, many issues related to the pathophysiology and treatment of syringomyelia remain controversial.

This book contains the scientific contributions presented at the international symposium "Syringomyelia 2000," held in Kobe, Japan, June 16–17, 2000. The purpose of the symposium was to bring together experts in the fields of neurosurgery, neurology, and neuropathology, in order to enhance the level and scope of their knowledge by making them more aware of work done in complementary fields. The contributions also report on clinical and basic studies pertinent to the topic of the symposium. This volume thus represents a comprehensive description of the state of the art regarding this disease in the hope that it may help to define comprehensively what is already known and to find new ways toward a better understanding of the pathophysiology, diagnosis, and treatment of syringomyelia.

The symposium was made possible with the generous support of the Japanese Ministry of Education, Science, Sports and Culture; the Osaka Pharmaceutical Manufacturers Association; the Kobe Convention and Visitors Association; and the Tsutomu Nakauchi Foundation.

We express our thanks to the contributors for their participation and cooperation, and to Springer-Verlag for their assistance in publishing this book. We sincerely hope that this volume will contribute to an improvement in the treatment outcome of patients suffering from syringomyelia.

The Editors

Contents

3. Pathophysiology of Syringomyelia

4. Syringomyelia Associated with Abnormalities of the Craniocervical Junction

Contributors

Abe, T. 154, 180, 194
Asada, S. 62
Barua, K.K. 253
Batzdorf, U. 3, 121
Bhatt, P. 113
Bhattacharjee, A.K. 90, 253
Chang, H.S. 69
Davis, C. 113
DeVroom, H.L. 75
Ehara, K. 90
Fox, A. 10
Fujii, K. 56
Gao, Y.-Z. 147
Gunawardena, W. 113
Hadden, A.G. 233
Hashizume, Y. 31, 49
Heiss, J.D. 75
Hida, K. 164
Hida, T. 154, 180, 194
Hirano, Y. 188
Ide, K. 175
Imae, S. 169
Isobe, M. 49
Isoshima, A. 180, 194
Itakura, T. 169
Itoh, Y. 188
Iwasaki, Y. 164
Iyer, V. 113
Kanno, T. 97
Kitamura, J. 102
Knierim, D.S. 233
Kuno, S. 97
Kuwahara, N. 188
LaMarca, F. 203
McLone, D.G. 203
Menezes, A.H. 136
Milhorat, T.H. 10
Mizoi, K. 188
Mizuno, J. 49
Nagahisa, S. 97
Nagashima, H. 180
Nagashima, T. 43, 62, 90, 102, 253
Nakagawa, H. 49, 69
Nakamura, M. 62, 102, 253
Nishimura, Y. 169
Nishizawa, T. 159
Okada, Y. 175
Okuda, Y. 154, 180, 194
Oldfield, E.H. 75
Sasajima, T. 188
Sato, H. 218
Sato, N. 218
Sato, S. 107
Senoo, M. 175
Shirane, R. 249
Shoda, M. 97
Suzuki, A. 188
Tachibana, S. 56, 107
Tada, Y. 62
Takahashi, A. 43, 62
Takahashi, H. 175
Takayasu, M. 159
Tamaki, N. 43, 62, 90, 102, 253
Tamura, S. 62, 102, 253
Tanaka, N. 175
Tani, S. 154, 180, 194

1. Classification and Pathology of Syringomyelia

A Brief History of Syringomyelia

Ulrich Batzdorf

Summary. The history of syringomyelia is considered from the original observation of the entity, the theories of pathogenesis, and the history of the development of treatment modalities.

Key words. Syringomyelia, Chiari malformation

Description of the Entity

As far as we know today, Estienne [1], a French anatomist, first observed cavitation within the spinal cord in a cadaver in the 16th century, although an earlier report in 1545 by Stephanus [2] has been cited. These two publications are very similar and appear to refer to the same observation, Stephanus writing in Latin and Estienne, a year later, in French. In 1688, Brunner [3] reported an infant with hydrocephalus and a liquor-filled cavity within the spinal cord. The term syringomyelia was coined by Ollivier d'Angers [4] in 1824, who defined it as a tubular dilatation within the spinal cord communicating with the fourth ventricle and believed the cyst to represent a dilated central canal. It was later suggested by Schüppel [5] that persistence and dilatation of the fetal central canal should be termed hydromyelia and that the term syringomyelia be reserved for cysts not connected to the central canal [6]. The distinction between these two conditions was also believed to be based on differences in the lining cells of these cavities. Hydromyelic cavities were believed to be lined by ependymal cells, whereas syringomyelic cavities were believed to be lined by glial cells [7].

The relationship between hindbrain descent and spinal cord cysts became clearly established through the work of Cleland [8] and Chiari [9]. In 1880, Strümpell [10] described what might have been the first instance of syringomyelia related to spine trauma.

In later years, the theoretical distinction between hydromyelia and syringomyelia became less clear. Several important observations have contributed to this development, including evidence that communication between the fourth ventricle and the spinal cord cyst is demonstrable in only about 10% of patients with syringomyelia

Division of Neurosurgery, UCLA Medical Center, Los Angeles, CA 90095-6901, USA

[11]; that the differentiation based on the cell type of lining cells is not consistent [12]; and that rupture of traumatic cysts into the regions of the central canal may occur and overdistension of an ependyma-lined cyst may result in identification of only islands of ependyma in a glial-lined cavity.

The common terminology today is to designate as syringomyelia all forms of clinical conditions with spinal cord cysts containing fluid identical with or closely resembling cerebrospinal fluid. Although spinal cord tumors may be associated with true syringomyelic cavities, tumor cysts, which often contain proteinaceous fluid, should not be included under the term syringomyelia. Slitlike residual foci of the central canal of the cord, of doubtful clinical significance, have been observed with modern magnetic resonance technology, and these also should not be designated as syringomyelia.

The terms communicating and noncommunicating syringomyelia, at one time thought to distinguish between hindbrain-related and primary spinal forms of the disorder, have become meaningless in their original intent for reasons already noted. Hindbrain-related forms most commonly do not communicate with the fourth ventricle; on the other hand, posttraumatic cavities may secondarily rupture into the subarachnoid space.

Recognition of the Clinical Syndrome

Weakness accompanying the presence of a spinal cord cyst was described in 1804 by Portal [13]. Schultze [14] detailed the combination of motor and sensory deficits in 1882, but credit for the description of the clinical picture of dissociated sensory loss in capelike distribution with syringomyelia belongs to Gowers [15].

Many additional summaries of the clinical picture associated with syringomyelia have appeared subsequently. Some of these do not distinguish clearly between symptoms due to hindbrain descent with brainstem compression and stretching of cranial nerve roots from symptoms caused by the cystic cavity; similarly, it is sometimes not easy to differentiate symptoms caused by the initial spinal cord injury from those due to the subsequently formed syrinx cavity. Barnett and Jousse [16] called attention to the importance of progression of spinal cord symptoms after a lengthy period of neurological stability following an injury. A recent, very comprehensive catalogue of symptoms associated with hindbrain-related syringomyelia has been contributed by Milhorat et al. [17].

Development of Theories of Pathogenesis

The earliest concept of pathogenesis of hindbrain-related syringomyelia assumed that a patent communication existed between the fourth ventricle and the syrinx cavity. Such a relationship was demonstrated in the neonatal cases described by Cleland [8] and by Chiari [9]. The concept did not convincingly change until the introduction of magnetic resonance imaging, when it became clear that a communication at the obex existed in only a small percentage of patients. Thus in 1959, when Gardner [18,19] expounded his waterhammer theory, it was based on the assumption that cerebrospinal fluid was driven from the ventricular system into the spinal cord cavity through an opening at the obex of the fourth ventricle, reinforcing the concept of a developmental malformation.

A new phase in our thinking of the pathogenesis of syringomyelia began with the work of Williams [20]. He developed a theory of craniospinal pressure dissociation at the level of the foramen magnum as the basis for the development of hindbrain- (i.e., Chiari-) related syringomyelia. Williams theorized that venous distension with coughing and straining forces the cerebellar tonsils against the foramen magnum, but that a ball valve mechanism prevented pressure equalization and transiently higher pressures in the spinal subarachnoid space resulted in fluid entering into the spinal cord.

Oldfield et al. [21] postulated that in hindbrain-related syringomyelia systolic pressure waves impart a piston-like action to the wedged cerebellar tonsils, forcing cerebrospinal fluid through the perivascular spaces of the spinal cord. Transparenchymally migrating fluid travels toward the central canal, aided, in part, by arterial pulsations [22]. Factors such as the distensibility of the spinal subarachnoid space may also play a role.

Magnetic resonance imaging also changed our concepts of the pathogenesis of primary spinal syringomyelia, originally thought to be a sequel to traumatic hematomyelia. Such foci of hemorrhage are not seen as frequently as one would anticipate, whereas restriction of cerebrospinal fluid flow in the subarachnoid space seems to underlie almost all cases of primary spinal syringomyelia, whether posttraumatic or postinflammatory in origin. The observation that syringomyelia may develop following relatively minor spinal trauma [23,24], not accompanied by clinical evidence of cord injury or hematomyelia, but followed by gradual development of a subarachnoid scar, suggests this concept. It is not clear whether such scar tissue dampens the normal cerebrospinal fluid pulsations, or sets up a pressure differential at the level of scar, favoring intrusion of fluid into the cord parenchyma.

Russell and Donald [25] established the association of spina bifida with syringomyelia in 1935. Fischer, Welch, and Shillito [26] reported the association of syringomyelia with lumboureteral shunting in 1977. A relationship between lumbar cerebrospinal fluid shunting and syringomyelia is now considered to be quite common [26a].

Development of Treatment

Concepts of surgical treatment have, to some degree, developed in parallel with the evolution of concepts of pathogenesis of both syringomyelia and the pathological alterations underlying this condition. However, some of the earliest treatment efforts were directed at the spinal cord cyst as such, rather than the underlying pathology. Drainage of the cyst by aspiration [27], myelotomy, i.e., syringostomy [28], and placement of a stent into the cyst cavity [29] represent some of the first attempts to treat syringomyelia. These concepts led quite naturally to the development of modern shunting techniques when biocompatible synthetic materials became available. Syrinx cavity shunting into the peritoneal cavity was introduced by Edgar [30], shunting into the subarachnoid space by Tator et al. [31] and the Sapporo group [32], and cyst shunting into the pleural cavity by Williams [33]. The use of microsurgical techniques then allowed further refinements of these techniques [34].

Better understanding of the pathophysiology of syringomyelia and the relatively high shunt failure rate reported by some [35,36] established a trend that favored the use of surgical techniques directed at what, at a given time, was understood to be the basic abnormality. As an outgrowth of the concept that hydrocephalus was the abnormality leading to the development of syringomyelia, it was natural that shunting of the ventricular system would be tried. However, the early efforts of Benini and Krayenbühl [37] were abandoned. Quite recently, the concept of diverting cerebrospinal fluid "ahead of" the syrinx has been applied to primary spinal syringomyelia in the form of the so-called thecoperitoneal shunt [38].

Penfield and Coburn [39] performed a suboccipital craniectomy for Chiari malformation in 1938, but this patient did not have a syringomyelic cavity, although she had previously been operated on for a thoracic meningocele. When Gardner [40] postulated that syrinx cavities fill from above through an opening at the obex associated with outlet obstruction of the fourth ventricle, he recommended plugging the opening at the obex. This procedure obviously necessitated a suboccipital craniectomy, so that even in retrospect, it is not clear whether the obex plugging procedure per se added any benefit.

The modern era of treatment of syringomyelia followed the work of Williams [20] and his theory of craniospinal pressure dissociation. He developed a rationale for posterior fossa decompression, which he sometimes referred to as "inactivation of the filling mechanism" of the syrinx. The newer techniques of treating hindbrain-related syringomyelia have generally consisted of relief of subarachnoid space compression at the level of the foramen magnum by posterior or anterior decompression or both; techniques for treatment of primary spinal syringomyelia have aimed at relief of spinal subarachnoid flow impairment by lysis of adhesions with posterior decompression of the subarachnoid space, anterior correction of spinal kyphosis, or both.

Additionally, the introduction of the concept that the posterior fossa is disproportionately small in patients with the so-called Chiari I malformation has been reflected in current approaches to surgical therapy [41–43]. With the exception of anterior decompression by odontoid resection for the treatment of craniocervical junction abnormalities with associated hindbrain descent introduced by Menezes et al. [44], most surgical procedures advocated today fall into two categories:

1. Enlarging the posterior fossa, with the expectation that the cerebellar tonsils will recede and cerebrospinal fluid circulation at the craniocervical junction will improve
2. Restoring better cerebrospinal fluid circulation at the craniocervical junction (a smaller craniectomy) by means of an expansile duraplasty often accompanied by active reduction of the cerebellar tonsils

Enlarging the posterior fossa has been achieved with a large craniectomy and without or with posterior fossa reconstruction, as advocated by Sahuquillo et al. [45] and by Milhorat (personal communication, 1999). The arachnoid and often the dura are sometimes left, at least partially, intact [46].

Craniectomies were performed together with reduction of the cerebellar tonsils by Bertrand [47], Williams [48], and, by a simplified technique, by Halamandaris and Batzdorf [49]. A smaller craniectomy is often used because this technique does not emphasize enlarging the entire posterior fossa. Williams did not reconstruct the posterior fossa dura, but many other surgeons did [50].

Reconstruction of the spinal subarachnoid space has evolved as an alternative to shunting of posttraumatic syringomyelic cavities. Williams [51], who avoided dural reconstruction, described posterior decompression with resection of scar tissue. Klekamp et al. [52] recommended scar resection and duraplasty. Anterior subarachnoid decompression in patients with a posttraumatic kyphotic spinal deformity has been advocated by Holly et al. [53].

References

1. Estienne C (1546) La dissection du corps humain. Simon de Colines, Paris
2. Stephanus C (1545) De dissectione partium corporis humani. Colinaeum, Paris
3. Brunner (1700) Bonet's sepulchretum, 2nd edn, book 1. Geneva, p 394 [cited in Schlesinger (1895) Die Syringomyelie. Franz Deuticke, Leipzig und Wien]
4. Ollivier d'Angers CP (1827) Traite de la moelle epiniere et de ses maladies. Crevot, Paris, pp 178–183
5. Schüppel O (1865) Über Hydromyelus. Arch Heilkd 6:289–315
6. Simon T (1875) Über Syringomyelie und Geschwulstbildung im Rückenmark. Arch Psychiatr Nervenkr 5:120–163
7. Kahler O, Pick A (1879) Beitrag zur Lehre von der Syringo-und Hydromyelie. Vjschr Prakt Heilkd 142:20–41
8. Cleland J (1883) Contribution to the study of spina bifida, encephalocele and anencephalus. J Anat Physiol 17:257–291
9. Chiari H (1891) Ueber Veränderungen des Kleinhirns infolge von Hydrocephalie des Grosshirns. Dtsch Med Wochenschr 42:1172–1175
10. Strümpell A (1880) Beiträge zur Pathologie des Rückenmarks. Arch Psychiatr Nervenkr 10:676
11. West RJ, William B (1980) Radiographic studies of the ventricles in syringomyelia. Neuroradiology 20:5–16
12. Vinters HV (1991) Neuropathology of syringomyelia. In: Batzdorf U (ed) Syringomyelia: current concepts in diagnosis and treatment. Williams & Wilkins, Baltimore, pp 35–58
13. Portal A (1804) Cours d'anatomie médicale, vol 4. Baudouin, Paris, pp 111–120
14. Schultze F (1882) Über Spalt-, Höhlen-und Gliombildung im Rückenmark und in der Medulla oblongata. Virchows Arch Pathol Anat 87:510–540
15. Gowers WR (1886) A manual of diseases of the nervous system, vol 1. Churchill, London, pp 433–443
16. Barnett HJM, Jousse AT (1973) Syringomyelia as a late sequel to traumatic paraplegia and quadriplegia. In: Barnett HJM, Foster JB, Hudgson P (eds) Syringomyelia. Saunders, London, pp 129–513
17. Milhorat TH, Chou MW, Trinidad EM, et al (1999) Chiari I malformation redefined: clinical and radiographic findings for 364 symptomatic patients. Neurosurgery 44(5): 1005–1017
18. Gardner WJ, Angel J (1959) The mechanism of syringomyelia and its surgical correction. Clin Neurosurg 6:131–140
19. Gardner WJ, Abdullah AF, McCormack LJ (1957) The varying expressions of embryonal atresia of the 4th ventricle in adults: Arnold-Chiari malformation, Dandy-Walker Syndrome, "arachnoid" cyst of the cerebellum, and syringomyelia. J Neurosurg 14: 591–605
20. Williams B (1986) Progress in syringomyelia. Neurol Res 8:130–145

21. Oldfield EH, Muraszko K, Shawker TH, et al (1994) Pathophysiology of syringomyelia associated with Chiari I malformation of the cerebellar tonsils. Implications for diagnosis and treatment. J Neurosurg 80:3–15
22. Stoodley MA, Jones NR, Brown CJ (1996) Evidence for rapid fluid flow from the subarachnoid space into the spinal cord central canal in the rat. Brain Res 707:155–164
23. Barnett HJM (1973) Syringomyelia consequent on minor to moderate trauma. In: Barnett HJM, Foster JB, Hudgson P (eds) Syringomyelia. Saunders, London, pp 174–178
24. La Haye PA, Batzdorf U (1988) Posttraumatic syringomyelia. West J Med 148(6): 657–663
25. Russell DS, Donald C (1935) The mechanism of internal hydrocephalus in spina bifida. Brain 58:203–215
26. Fischer EG, Welch K, Shillito J Jr (1977) Syringomyelia following lumboureteral shunting for communicating hydrocephalus. J Neurosurg 47:96–100
26a. Chumas PD, Kulkarni AV, Drake JM, Hoffman HJ, Humphreys RP, Rutka JP (1993) Lumboperitoneal shunting: A retrospective study in the pediatric population. Neurosurgery 32:376–383
27. Abbe R, Coley WB (1892) Syringomyelia; operation, exploration of the cord; withdrawal of fluid. J Nerv Ment Dis 19:512–520
28. Elsberg CA (1921) Surgery of intramedullary affections of the spinal cord: anatomic basis and technic with report of cases. JAMA 59:1532–536
29. Frazier CH, Rowe SN (1936) The surgical treatment of syringomyelia. Ann Surg 103: 481–497
30. Edgar RE (1976) Surgical management of spinal cord cysts. Paraplegia 14:21–27
31. Tator CH, Meguro K, Rowed DW (1982) Favorable results with syringosubarachnoid shunts for treatment of syringomyelia. J Neurosurg 56(4):517–523
32. Isu T, Iwasaki Y, Akino M, et al (1990) Syringo-subarachnoid shunt for syringomyelia associated with Chiari malformation (type 1). Acta Neurochir (Wien) 107:152–160
33. Williams B, Page N (1987) Surgical treatment of syringomyelia with syringo-pleural shunting. Br J Neurosurg 1:63–80
34. Iwasaki Y, Koyanagi I, Hida K, et al (1999) Syringo-subarachnoid shunt syringomyelia using partial hemilaminectomy. Br J Neurosurg 13(1):41–45
35. Sgouros S, Williams B (1995) A critical appraisal of drainage in syringomyelia. J Neurosurg 82(1):1–10
36. Batzdorf U, Klekamp J, Johnson JP (1998) A critical appraisal of syrinx cavity shunting procedures. J Neurosurg 89:382–388
37. Benini A, Krayenbühl H (1969) Ein neuer chirurgischer Weg zur Behandlung der Hydro-und Syringomyelie. Schweiz Med Wochenschr 99:1137–1142
38. Vengsarkar U, Panchal VG, Tripathi PD, et al (1991) Percutaneous thecoperitoneal shunt for syringomyelia. J Neurosurg 74:827–831
39. Penfield W, Coburn DF (1938) Arnold–Chiari malformation and its operative treatment. Arch Neurol Psychiatry 40:328–336
40. Gardner JW, Angel J (1958) The cause of syringomyelia and its surgical treatment. Clevel Clin Q 25:4–8
41. Marin-Padilla M, Marin-Padilla TM (1981) Morphogenesis of experimentally induced Arnold-Chiari malformation. J Neurol Sci 50:29–53
42. Badie B, Mendoza D, Batzdorf U (1995) Posterior fossa volume and response to suboccipital decompression in patients with Chiari I malformation. Neurosurgery 37:214–218
43. Nishikawa M, Sakamoto H, Hakuba A (1997) Pathogenesis of Chiari malformation: a morphometric study of the posterior cranial fossa. J Neurosurg 86:40–47
44. Menezes AH, VanGilder JC, Graf CJ, et al (1980) Craniocervical abnormalities. J Neurosurg 53:444–455

45. Sahuquillo J, Rubio E, Poca M, et al (1994) Posterior fossa reconstruction: a surgical technique for the treatment of Chiari I malformation and Chiari I/syringomyelia complex: preliminary results and magnetic resonance imaging quantitative assessment of hindbrain migration. Neurosurgery 35(5):874–884
46. Isu T, Sasaki H, Takamura H, et al (1993) Foramen magnum decompression with removal of the outer layer of the dura as treatment for syringomyelia occurring with Chiari I malformation. Neurosurgery 33:845–850
47. Bertrand G (1973) Dynamic factors in the evolution of syringomyelia and syringobulbia. In: Clinical neurosurgery, vol 20. Waverly, Baltimore, pp 322–333
48. Williams B (1993) Surgery for hindbrain related syringomyelia. Adv Tech Stand Neurosurg 20:107–164
49. Halamandaris CG, Batzdorf U (1989) Adult Chiari malformation. Contemp Neurosurg 11(26):1–6
50. Batzdorf U (1988) Chiari I malformation with syringomyelia: evaluation of surgical therapy by magnetic resonance imaging. J Neurosurg 68(5):726–730
51. Williams B (1990) Syringomyelia. Neurosurg Clin N Am 1:653–685
52. Klekamp J, Batzdorf U, Samii M, et al (1997) Treatment of syringomyelia associated with arachnoid scarring caused by arachnoiditis or trauma. J Neurosurg 86:233–240
53. Holly LT, Johnson JP, Maciopinto JE, et al (2000) The treatment of posttraumatic syringomyelia with extradural decompression. Neurosurg Focus 8(3): Article 8, 1–6, March 2000

Pathology, Classification, and Treatment of Syringomyelia

Thomas H. Milhorat, Andrew Fox, and D. Roxanne Todor

Summary. Syringomyelia poses unique challenges for the clinician because of its complex symptomatology, varied pathology, and multiple options for treatment. The purpose of this chapter is to review current knowledge concerning the pathology and pathophysiology of syringomyelia as a foundation for diagnosis and treatment. Conclusions are based on pathological findings in 175 patients coming to autopsy in the years 1955–1993, clinical and magnetic resonance imaging (MRI) findings in a database of 1245 patients (1993–2000), and operative findings in 387 patients undergoing surgical treatment between the years 1994 and 2000. The use of a pathology-based classification of syringomyelia provides a scientific basis for diagnosis and treatment.

Key words. Syringomyelia, Chiari malformation, Posttraumatic syringomyelia, Hydrocephalus, Basilar invagination

Introduction

The clinical management of syringomyelia has been significantly influenced by prevailing concepts of pathogenesis. Until recent years, the most widely accepted view was that spinal cord cavitation was caused by the forceful diversion of cerebrospinal fluid (CSF) from the fourth ventricle into the central canal of the spinal cord, either as a consequence of a caudally directed CSF pulse wave [1] or the development of the CSF pressure gradient at the level of the foramen magnum [2]. This hypothesis helped to shape modern surgical treatment and led to the development of specific operative approaches such as posterior fossa decompression, shunting of the fourth ventricle, and "plugging of the obex" [3–6]. However, with the advent of magnetic resonance (MR) imaging, it became evident that only a minority of syrinxes communicate directly with the fourth ventricle [5–7]. Some cavities were found in the absence of a hindbrain abnormality, and most arose below a long syrinx-free segment of spinal cord [7]. These and other observations, including the remarkable variety

Department of Neurosurgery, State University of New York Health Science Center at Brooklyn, Kings County Hospital Center, and The Long Island College Hospital, Brooklyn, NY, USA

of cavitary patterns, etiological factors, and neurological findings in syringomyelia, have suggested that spinal cord cavitation cannot be explained by a single unifying hypothesis [8–11].

Pathology and Clinicopathological Correlations

Autopsy Data

Between the years 1955 and 1993, autopsies were performed in 175 individuals with tubular cavitations of the spinal cord, 94 males and 81 females who had ranged in age from 1 day to 87 years (mean age, 41.6 years). In all cases, a standard complete autopsy was performed. After opening the cranial cavity, the upper end of the spinal cord was divided at the foramen magnum and removed with the brain side of the specimen. The remainder of the spinal cord was removed via the abdominal and thoracic cavities, as described elsewhere [11]. The review of histological material was facilitated by an institutional policy requiring that original slides and paraffin blocks be retained with the permanent autopsy file. Old and new paraffin blocks were cut serially to a thickness of 6 μm mounted on glass slides and stained with hematoxylin and eosin. Supplemental stains included Luxol fast blue, Weil stain, Gomori's stain, Bodian's stain, periodic-acid-Schiff, phosphotungstic acid hematoxylin, and glial fibrillary acidic protein. Histological sections were viewed through a microscope at magnifications ranging from ×10 to ×1000. Final diagnoses were as follows: nonneoplastic syringomyelia (105 cases), syringomyelia ex vacuo (52 cases), and neoplastic cysts (18 cases). The pathological findings in 105 cases of nonneoplastic syringomyelia have been previously reported [8].

Clinical Data

Between the years 1999 and 2000, 1245 patients with cavitary lesions of the spinal cord were evaluated at our institution, 863 female and 382 male patients who ranged in age from 8 months to 82 years (mean age, 38.2 years). Each patient underwent a detailed neurological examination and at least one MR imaging scan of the spinal cord that included the area of cavitation and the cervicomedullary junction. In many cases, additional information was provided by the whole neuraxis MRI, cine-MRI, computerized tomography (CT) myelography, somatosensory evoked potentials (SSEPs), and other neurodiagnostic tests. The protocol for diagnostic workup and the specific techniques of neuroimaging have been previously published [9].

Tubular enlargements of the spinal cord that were not caused by intramedullary tumors were classified as follows on the basis of pathological findings [8]: (1) dilations of the central canal that are anatomically continuous with the fourth ventricle (communicating syringomyelia); (2) dilations of the central canal that do not communicate with the fourth ventricle (noncommunicating syringomyelia); and (3) extracanalicular syrinxes that originate in the spinal cord parenchyma and do not communicate with the central canal or fourth ventricle (primary parenchymal cavitations). These lesions are distinguished from two other types of spinal cord cavitation: (1) atrophic syrinxes, occurring with myelomalacia (syringomyelia ex vacuo); and (2) neoplastic cysts [8–10].

Communicating Central Canal Dilations

Communicating syrinxes are caused by an obstruction of the CSF pathways distal to the outlets of the fourth ventricle (Fig. 1). In typical cases, there is generalized enlargement of the cerebral ventricles, and the central canal participates in the hydrocephalic process like a "fifth ventricle." Causative factors include postmeningitic and posthemorrhagic hydrocephalus, complex hindbrain malformations such as Chiari II malformation and encephalocele, and Dandy–Walker cysts. An experimental model of communicating syringomyelia can be produced by injecting kaolin into the cisterna magna [12].

On histological examination, communicating syrinxes appear as simple dilations of the central canal, lined wholly or partially by ependyma (Fig. 1B). In acquired

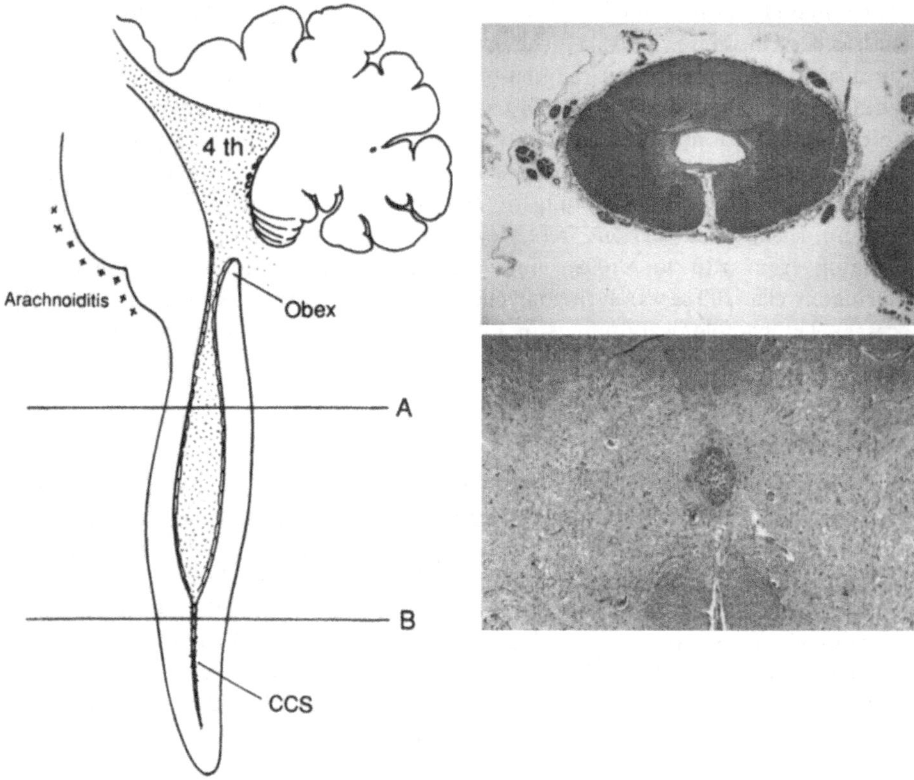

A B C

FIG. 1A–C. Communicating syringomyelia. **A** Pathological findings in a 49-year-old man with postmeningitic hydrocephalus, basilar arachnoiditis, and syringomyelia. The syrinx is anatomically continuous with the fourth ventricle, and its length has been determined by central canal stenosis (*CCS*). **B** In same patient, axial section through spinal cord at C5 (*section A* on diagram, **A**) shows a symmetrically enlarged central cavity that is lined by ependyma. Hematoxylin and eosin. ×10. **C** In same patient, axial section through spinal cord at T10 (*section B* on diagram, **A**) shows occlusion of the central canal. Hematoxylin and eosin. ×40. (From [8], with permission)

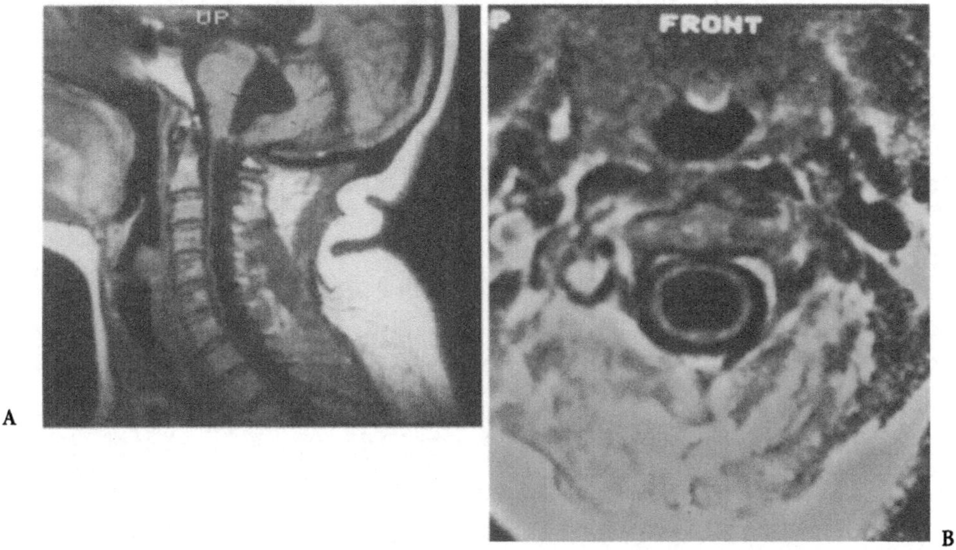

FIG. 2A,B. Communicating syringomyelia. Magnetic resonance images in 58-year-old man with posthemorrhagic hydrocephalus and syringomyelia. **A** Sagittal image of cervical spine demonstrates that the syrinx is continuous with the fourth ventricle. **B** Axial image at C2 shows symmetrically enlarged central cavity. (From [18], with permission)

examples, the length of the cavity is defined caudally by gliosis of the central canal (Fig. 1C). Central canal stenosis is an age-related phenomenon affecting the majority of normal individuals by the early years of adult life [11]. Holocord enlargements are most often of congenital origin and may be anatomically continuous with caudal lesions such as myelomeningocele. With distension of the central canal, the ependymal epithelium becomes stretched and denuded. Nevertheless, despite the large size of some communciating syrinxes, these lesions are much less prone to rupture paracentrally than noncommunicating syrinxes, and this may explain why a significant number of communciating syrinxes remain asymptomatic throughout life or are associated with only minor neurological findings [8,9]. Figure 2 illustrates the MRI correlates of communicating syringomyelia.

Noncommunicating Central Canal Dilations

Dilations of the central canal that do not communicate with the fourth ventricle are associated with obstructions of the CSF pathways at or below the foramen magnum. Causative factors include the Chiari I malformation (CMI), basilar invagination, spinal arachnoiditis, extramedullary compressions, tethered cord, and acquired tonsillar herniation. There is accumulating evidence that noncommunicating syrinxes fill from the spinal subarachnoid space as a consequence of a pressure gradient that drives CSF through anatomically continuous perivascular and interstitial spaces of the spinal cord [13–16]. An experimental model of noncommunciating syringomyelia can be

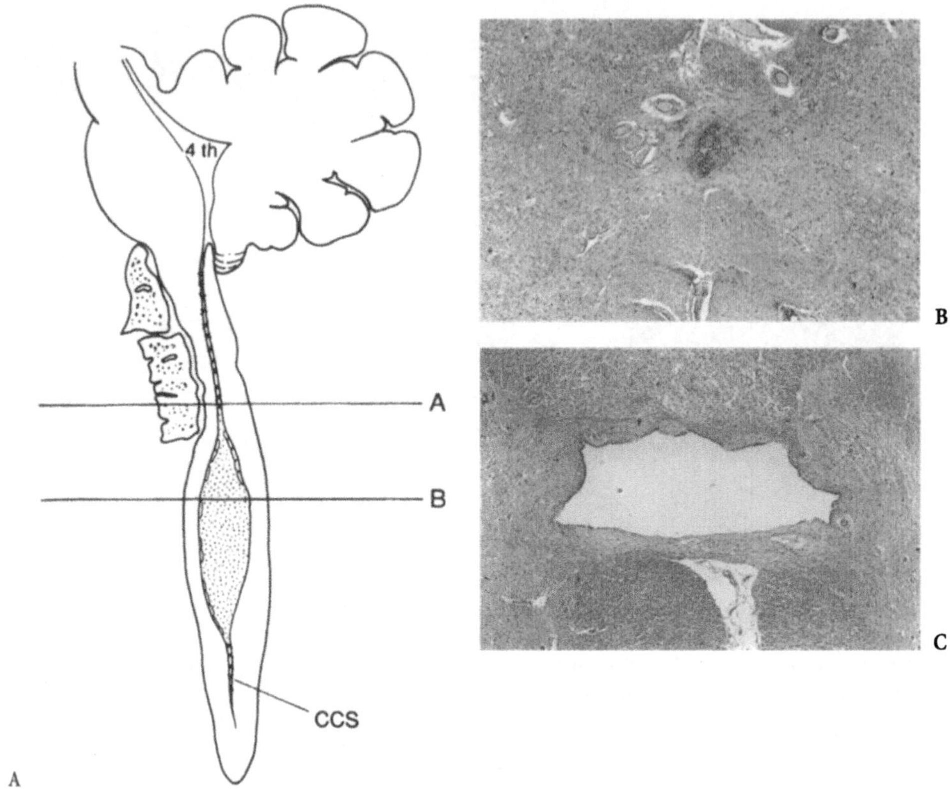

FIG. 3A–C. Noncommunicating syringomyelia. **A** Pathological findings in a 66-year-old man with syringomyelia occurring in association with basilar invagination and a Klippel Feil anomaly. The syrinx is defined rostrally and caudally by central canal stenosis (*CCS*) and was asymptomatic during life. **B** In same patient, axial section through spinal cord at C5 (*section A* on diagram, **A**) shows occlusion of the central canal. Hematoxylin and eosin. ×40. **C** In same patient, axial section through syrinx at T3 (*section B* on diagram, **A**) demonstrates a symmetrically enlarged central canal with some denuding of the ependyma. Hematoxylin and eosin. ×40. (From [8], with permission)

produced by injecting kaolin into the dorsal horns of the cervical spinal cord [17], which results in segmental occlusion of the central canal and regional obstruction of the subarachnoid space due to arachnoiditis.

On histological examination, noncommunicating syrinxes appear as isolated cavities that are defined rostrally and caudally by central canal stenosis (Fig. 3). These syrinxes tend to be complex lesions and are characterized histologically by extensive areas of ependymal denuding, paracentral dissection, and the formation of intracanalicular septae [8]. In contrast to communicating syrinxes, which rarely rupture paracentrally, noncommunicating syrinxes exhibit a propensity for dissecting into the spinal cord parenchyma (Fig. 4). Parenchymal dissections occur preferentially into the dorsolateral quadrant of the spinal cord and may extend through the pial surface to

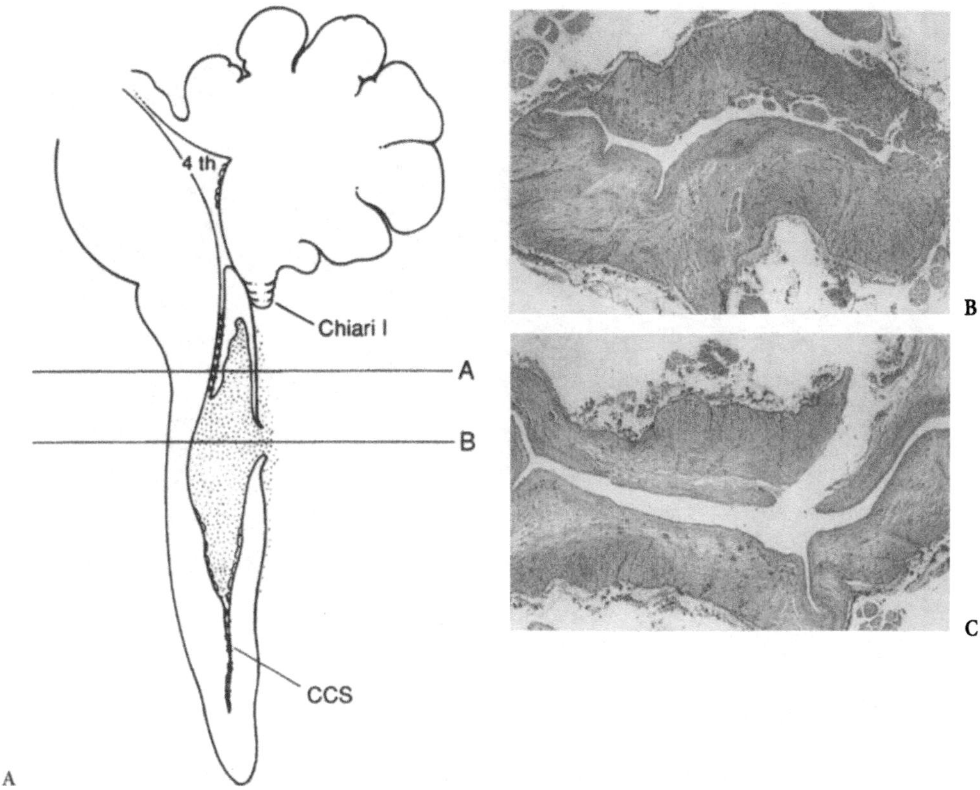

Fig. 4A–C. Noncommunicating syringomyelia. **A** Pathological findings in a 62-year-old woman with a Chiari I malformation and syringomyelia. The syrinx is defined rostrally and caudally by central canal stenosis (*CCS*). At C7, the syrinx has ruptured into the dorsal white matter columns and dissected rostrally. Clinical findings had included numbness and clawing of the left hand, impaired position sense, and spastic weakness of the legs. **B** In the same patient, axial section through the spinal cord at C4 (*section A* on diagram, **A**) shows an extracanalicular cavitation of the dorsal white matter columns; the central canal is stenotic. Hematoxylin and eosin. ×40. **C** In the same patient, axial sections through the syrinx at C7 (*section B* on diagram, **A**) reveal an ependyma-lined cavity that has ruptured through the dorsal root entry zone on the left (symptomatic side) to communicate with the subarachnoid space. Hematoxylin and eosin. ×40. (From [8], with permission)

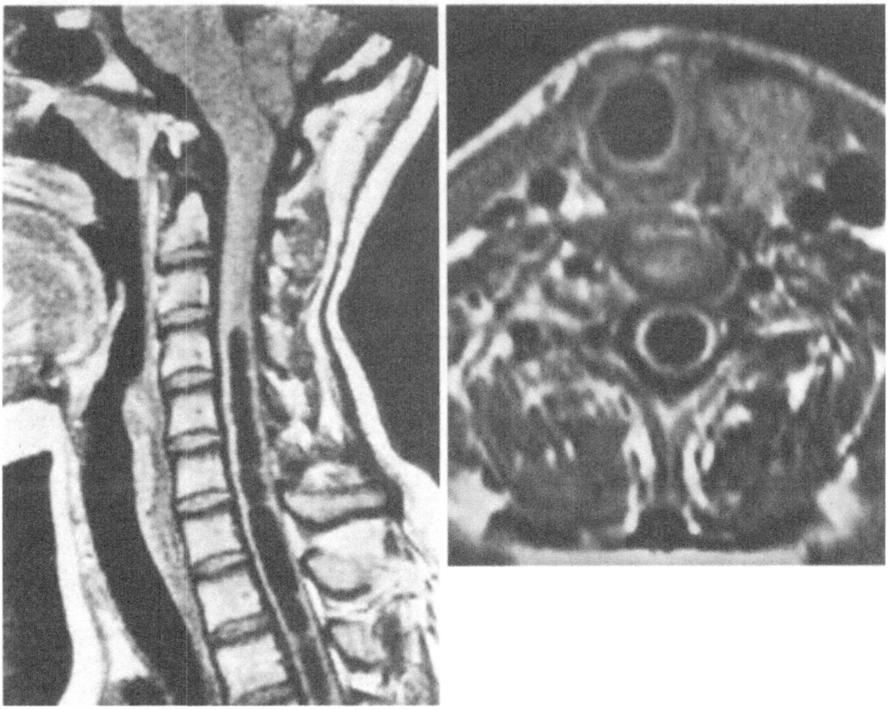

FIG. 5A,B. Noncommunicating syringomyelia. Magnetic resonance images in a 42-year-old woman with a Chiari I malformation and syringomyelia. Clinical findings were limited to fatiguable weakness of the extremities and hyperreflexia. **A** Sagittal image of cervical spine reveals that the syrinx is separated from the fourth ventricle by a long, syrinx-free segment of the spinal cord. **B** Axial image at T1 demonstrates a symmetrically enlarged central cavity

communicate with the subarachnoid space. Neurological findings can often be correlated with the anatomy of cavitation as demonstrated by MR imaging (Figs. 5, 6).

Primary Parenchymal Cavitations

These lesions consist of tubular cavitations of the spinal cord that originate in the parenchyma and do not communicate with the central canal or fourth ventricle (Fig. 7). A distinguishing feature of this type of syringomyelia is its association with conditions that injure spinal cord tissue. Common causative factors include trauma, infection, ischemia/infarction, and spontaneous intramedullary hemorrhage. Although the mechanism by which parenchymal cavities fill and distend is incompletely understood, current evidence suggests that arachnoiditis occurring at the time of injury produces a regional CSF block that forces fluid from the subarachnoid space into the interstitial spaces of the spinal cord [16].

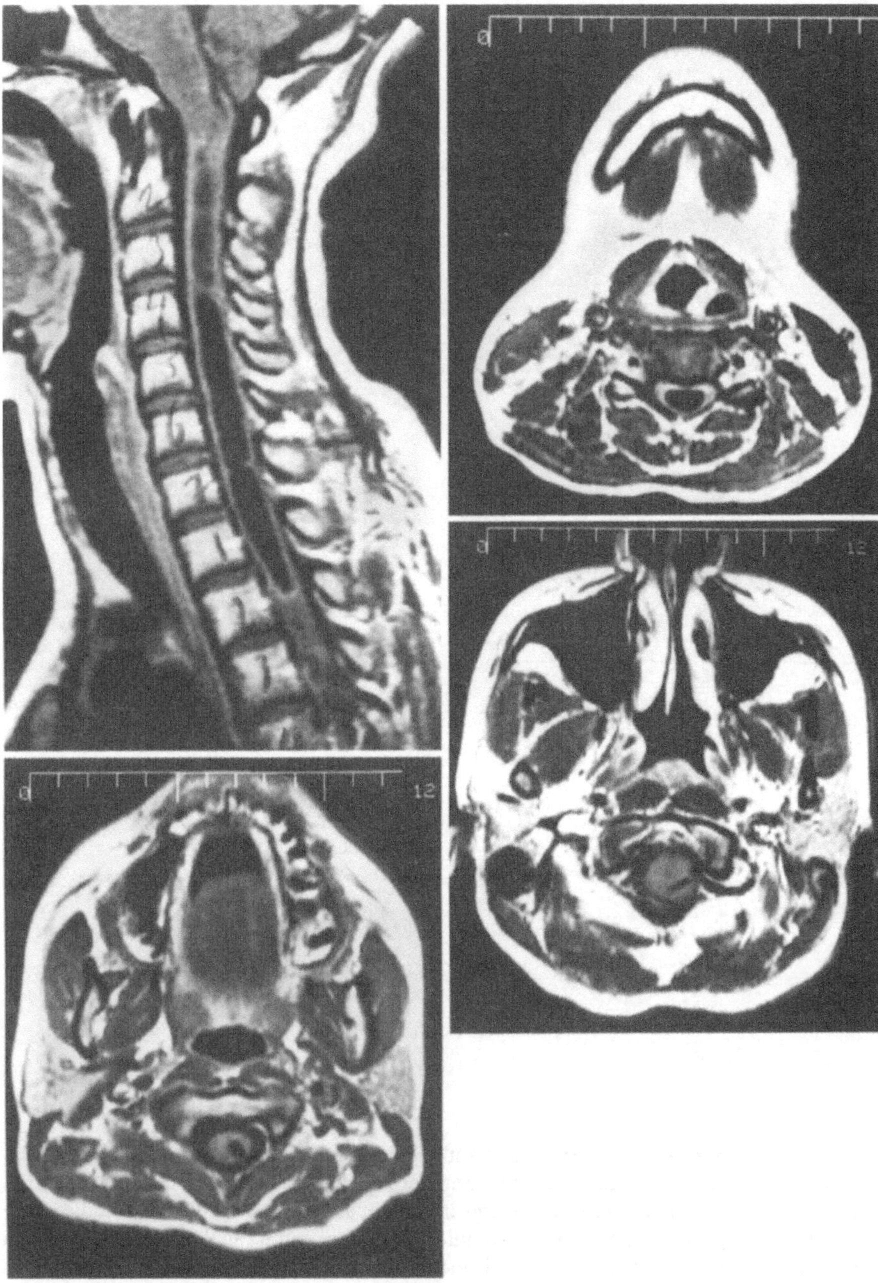

B

A

D

C

Fig. 6A–D. Noncommunicating syringobulbia. Magnetic resonance images in a 24-year-old woman with a Chiari I malformation and syringomyelia. Neurological findings included a decreased corneal reflex on the left, impaired pain and temperature sensation involving all three divisions of the left trigeminal nerve, weakness of the left arm and leg, patchy analgesia of the left arm, and impaired pain and temperature sensation below T2 on the right. **A** Sagittal image of cervical spine reveals a noncommunicating syrinx from C1 to T2 in association with Chiari I malformation. **B** Axial image at C5 shows a symmetrically enlarged central cavity. **C** Axial image at C3 reveals that the syrinx has expanded into the left dorsolateral quadrant of the spinal cord and has dissected rostrally to enter the medulla on the left side (**D**). (From [9], with permission)

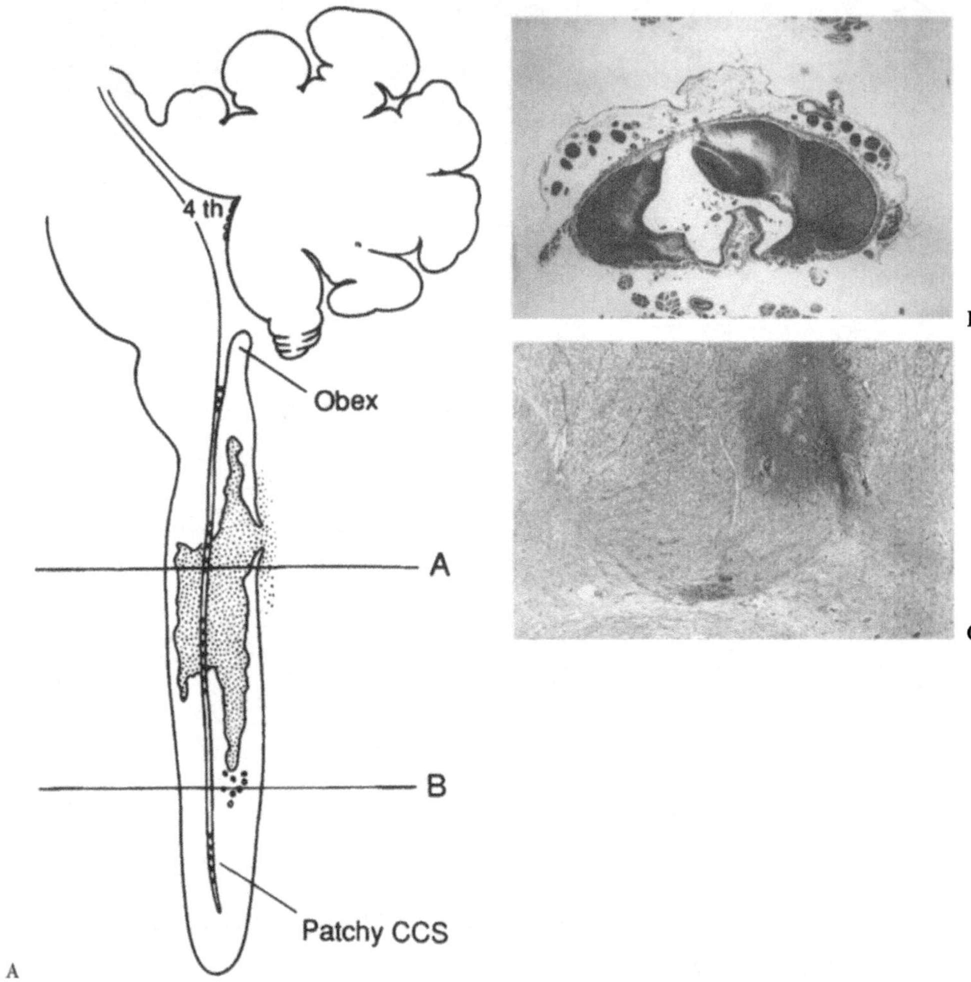

Fig. 7A–C. Posttraumatic syringomyelia. **A** Pathological findings in a 62-year-old woman who had been paraplegic for 23 years following a motor vehicle accident. **B** In same patient, axial section (*A*) through syrinx at T2 shows a large irregular parenchymal cavity that occupies three quadrants of the spinal cord, does not communicate with the central canal, and extends through the dorsal root entry zone to reach the pial surface. The central canal is stenotic. Hematoxylin and eosin. ×40. **C** In same patient, axial section of the spinal cord through original injury site at T8 (*section B* on diagram, **A**) demonstrates a glial scar with hemosiderin-laden macrophages. The central canal is stenotic. Hematoxylin and eosin. ×40. (From [8], with permission)

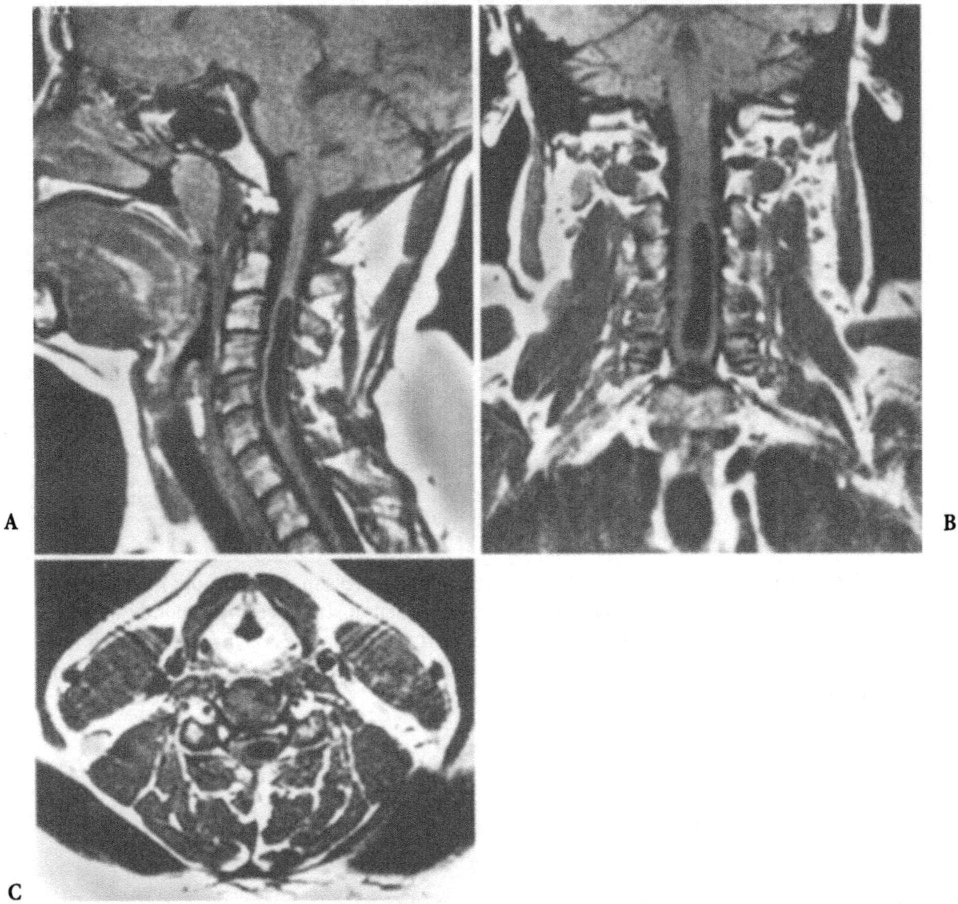

FIG. 8A–C. Posttraumatic syringomyelia. Magnetic resonance images in a 42-year-old woman with history of cervical spine trauma and burning dysesthesias of the left arm and upper chest. Neurological findings included weakness of the left arm and leg, areflexia of the left arm, and impaired sensation with trophic changes from C5 to T4 on the left side. **A** Sagittal image of cervical spine demonstrates congenital stenosis of cervical canal in association with a noncommunicating syrinx that extends from C3 to C7. **B** Horizontal image shows lateralization of the syrinx to the left hemicord. **C** Axial image at C5 demonstrates that the syrinx occupies the left dorsolateral quadrant of the spinal cord. (From [9], with permission)

Primary parenchymal cavitations typically arise in the watershed area of the spinal cord, dorsal and lateral to the central canal. Similarly to the paracentral dissections of central canal dilations, these lesions are lined by glia or fibroglial tissue, and are characterized histologically by varying degrees of necrosis, neuronophagia, and Wallerian degeneration [8]. A particularly common histological finding is the presence of hemosiderin-laden macrophages in the walls of cavities caused by trauma or hemorrhage. Figure 8 illustrates the MR imaging correlates of this type of syringomyelia.

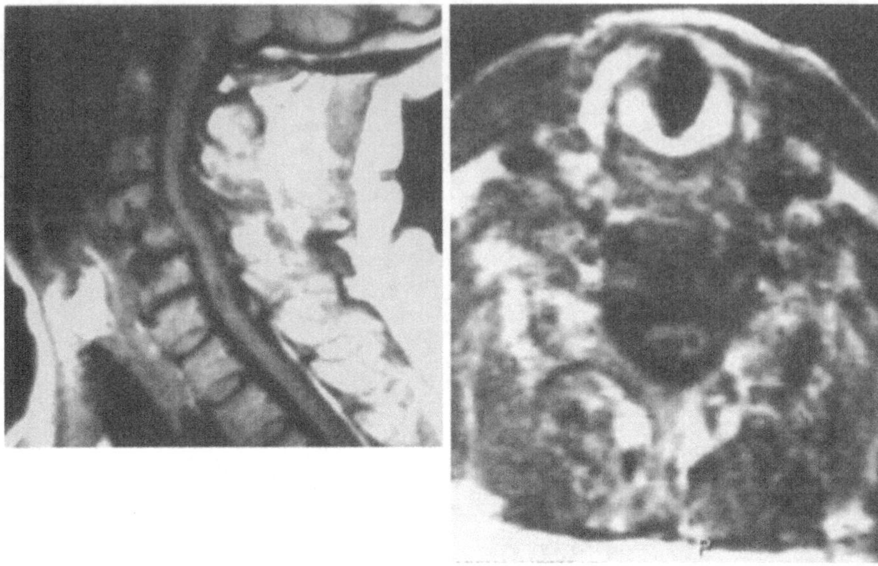

A

B

Fig. 9A,B. Syringomyelia ex vacuo. Magnetic resonance images in a 76-year-old man with progressive myelopathy. **A** Sagittal image of cervical spine demonstrates cervical spondylosis, focal spinal cord atrophy, and a small intramedullary cleft within an area of myelomalacia. **B** Axial image shows a transversely collapsed intramedullary cavity in association with spinal cord atrophy. (From [18], with permission)

Atrophic Cavitations (Syringomyelia Ex Vacuo)

Degenerative changes occurring in conjunction with spinal cord atrophy can lead to the formation of microcysts, intramedullary clefts, and localized dilations of the central spinal canal. Atrophic cavitations do not propagate, presumably because of the absence of a CSF filling mechanism, and are caused by the loss of parenchymal tissue (syringomyelia ex vacuo). On MR imaging, these lesions appear as nondistended cavities confined to an area of myelomalacia (Fig. 9).

Neoplastic Cavitations

Syrinx-like cavities can be formed by the cystic degeneration of intramedullary tumors such as astrocytomas, ependymomas, hemangioblastomas, and other less common neoplasms. The necrotic process begins centrally and tends to extend rostrally or caudally from the poles of the tumor. Neoplastic cysts contain yellowish proteinaceous fluid that is quite different from CSF, and the walls of the cyst are lined by tumor or tightly packed glial tissue around a mural nodule. The diagnosis is established by performing contrast-enhanced MR imaging (Fig. 10).

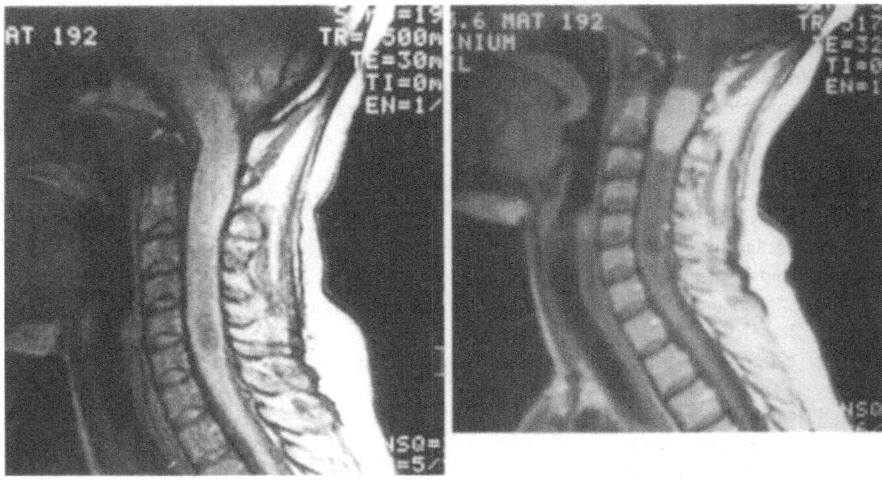

A B

FIG. 10A,B. Neoplastic cyst. Magnetic resonance images in a 21-year-old woman with a cystic intramedullary ependymoma. **A** Sagittal image of cervical spine shows cystic lesion from C3 to C6. The tumor is difficult to see on noncontrast-enhanced scan. **B** Tumor enhances brilliantly after administration of gadolinium. (From [18], with permission)

Classification of Syringomyelia

Table 1 provides a classification of syringomyelia that is based on pathological findings and MRI-confirmed clinicopathological correlates [10]. It is appropriate to point out that autopsy studies tend to report a disproportionate number of neonatal and pediatric deaths attributable to hydrocephalus, myelodysplasia, and intraventricular hemorrhage of the newborn; this can skew the incidence of communciating syringomyelia in pathological reports to 40% or more of all cases [8]. In contrast, only 76 patients in our current database of 1245 cases (6%) were found to have MR evidence of a communication between the syrinx cavity and fourth ventricle.

The separation of syrinxes into communicating, noncommunicating, and atrophic types imputes the different mechanisms of pathogenesis. Causative factors have been summarized according to standard nomenclature. The inclusion of neoplastic cavitations in this classification is meant to emphasize their importance in the differential diagnosis of syringomyelia rather than to suggest any pathological similarities.

Pathogenesis and Pathophysiology

Communicating Syringomyelia

A distinguishing feature of communicating syringomyelia is its association with hydrocephalus. This relationship is most direct in cases of hydrocephalus attributable to diffuse obstructions of the subarachnoid space (e.g., postmeningitic and posttraumatic

TABLE 1. Classification of syringomyelia

I.	Communicating syringomyelia
	Central canal dilations
	1. Communicating hydrocephalus (e.g., posthemorrhagic, postmeningitic)
	2. Complex hindbrain malformations (e.g., Chiari II, encephalocele)
	3. Dandy–Walker cyst
II.	Noncommunicating syringomyelia
	A. Central canal/paracentral syrinxes
	1. Chiari malformations
	2. Basilar invagination
	3. Spinal arachnoiditis (posttraumatic, postmeningitic)
	4. Extramedullary compressions (e.g., spondylosis, tumors, cysts)
	5. Tethered cord
	6. Acquired tonsillar herniation (e.g., hydrocephalus, intracranial mass lesions, craniosynostosis)
	B. Primary parenchymal cavitations
	1. Spinal cord trauma
	2. Ischemia/infarction
	3. Intramedullary hemorrhage
III.	Atrophic cavitations (syringomyelia ex vacuo)
IV.	Neoplastic cavitations

arachnoiditis) in which there is generalized enlargement of the cerebral ventricles and the communicating segment of the central canal [8,9]. In patients with Chiari II malformations, the relationship is more complex. Because the aqueduct of Sylvius is typically obstructed, the fourth ventricle does not communicate with the cerebral ventricles, and caudally displaced outlets may be occluded by cerebellar impaction into the foramen magnum. The result is a "double compartment" type of hydrocephalus in which the fourth ventricle and the upper end of the central canal communicate directly [8]. A similar relationship is present in cases of syringomyelia occurring with Dandy–Walker cysts and other complex hindbrain malformations [8,10].

Noncommunicating Syringomyelia

The majority of the syrinx cavities encountered clinically do not communicate with the fourth ventricle (noncommunicating syringomyelia). Common etiological factors include Chiari malformations, basilar invagination, arachnoiditis, cervical spondylosis, intraspinal cysts and tumors, and spinal cord tethering [8–10,18,19]. Current evidence suggests that noncommunicating syringomyelia is caused by an obstruction of the CSF circulation at or below the foramen magnum. To explain how syringomyelia develops in patients with Chiari malformations, Oldfield et al. [13] proposed that obstruction of the CSF circulation at the foramen magnum increases the pulsatile systolic pulse wave in the spinal subarachnoid space and exaggerates the piston-like action of the cerebellar tonsils, which drives CSF into the spinal cord. This important hypothesis reconciles the systolic pulse wave theory of Gardner [1] and the proposition that syrinx cavities fill from the subarachnoid space through expanded Virchow–Robin spaces [20] or the dorsal roots [21], but it does not apply to all types of syringomyelia.

How syringomyelia develops in the absence of foramen magnum impaction is less clear. Stoodley et al. [16], in a study of experimental noncommunicating syringomyelia induced by injecting kaolin into the dorsal horns of the spinal cord, have shown that syrinx formation is related to arachnoiditis and the development of a partial block of CSF flow at the level of kaolin injection. The authors observed that when horseradish peroxidase (HRP) was injected into CSF, the marker passed rapidly from the cervical subarachnoid space into Virchow–Robin spaces and the perivascular spaces of the neuropil to reach the central canal. Findings were limited to light microscopic observations. The authors concluded that the most likely cause of syrinx formation was an increase in pulse pressure above the block that accentuated arterial pulsation-dependent CSF flow [15] into the perivascular spaces of the spinal cord.

In a recently completed study [22], the fine structure of the intramedullary pathway for filling noncommuniating syrinx cavities has been described. Using the same experimental model [17] employed by Stoodley et al. [16], it was shown that when HRP is injected into the cisterna magna, it enters the spinal cord at all points along the pial surface through Virchow–Robin spaces and the ubiquitous extracellular spaces of the marginal glia. These latter spaces are open channels [23–25] that are patent for molecules as large as ferritin and HRP (molecular weight, 40 000; diameter, 50–60 Å). From the pial surface, the marker distributed widely through a series of interconnecting extracellular spaces having an average width of 150–200 Å [25] to reach the subependyma. Thereafter, the marker passed with relative ease through the intercellular clefts and apical gap junctions of adjacent ependymal cells to enter the syrinx cavity. Figure 11 illustrates the transmedullary movement of CSF in experimental noncommunicating syringomyelia.

To investigate the possibility that the rapid movement of HRP from the spinal subarachnoid space into syrinx cavities occurs by bulk flow, agar gel experiments were performed in which cylinders of gel conforming to the dimensions of rat spinal cord were immersed in HRP at varying intervals at 37°C. Agar gel has a water space of 98% and is a standard medium for calculating diffusion coefficients [26]. In these experiments, the diffusional movement of HRP in agar gel was 0.34 ± 0.02 mm (SD) at 14 days. This result compares with a transmedullary movement of at least 3.0 mm at 60–120 min in experimental syringomyelia. Although the comparison does not

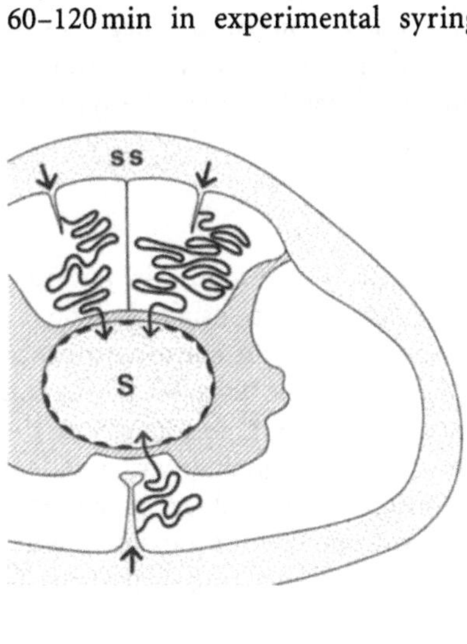

FIG. 11. Transmedullary bulk flow pathway for CSF filling of noncommunicating syringomyelia. The pathway extends from the spinal subarachnoid space (*SS*) through anatomically continuous extracellular spaces of neuropil into syrinx cavity (*S*)

account for CSF pulsations, the vast difference in the rates of movement of the marker is strong evidence that syrinx filling in this experimental model occurs by bulk flow and not diffusion [22]. These findings support the proposition that noncommunicating syringomyelia is caused by an obstruction of CSF flow caudal to the cervicomedullary junction and provide evidence of a transmedullary bulk flow pathway that extends from the spinal subarachnoid space through anatomically continuous extracellular spaces of the neuropil into the syrinx cavity.

Atrophic Syringomyelia

Atrophic cavitations of the spinal cord are caused by the injury and loss of parenchymal tissue [18]. What distinguishes these lesions from examples of syringomyelia occurring with trauma, infection, or inflammatory arachnoiditis is the absence of a CSF filling mechanism. In such cases, the spinal cord is small (less than 70% of the transverse interpedicular diameter) and the cavity represents an ex vacuo space that is nondistended and under no tension.

Diagnosis and Treatment

The use of a pathology-based classification of syringomyelia facilitates diagnosis and the interpretation of MR imaging findings (see Table 1). As illustrated in Figs. 3–8, it is often possible to establish precise clinicopathological correlations. The ability of MR imaging to distinguish between communicating, noncommuniating, and atrophic syrinxes has important treatment implications. For example, communicating syrinxes are generally treated by ventricular shunt. In the case of noncommunicating syrinxes, the goal of surgery is to relieve the CSF obstruction, and shunt placement is reserved as a treatment of last resort. Atrophic syrinxes are obviously not treated surgically.

Communicating Syringomyelia

This diagnosis can usually be established on the basis of MRI scans of the brain and spinal cord. In exceptional instances, it may be desirable to confirm the diagnosis by CT myelography or ventriculography. The preferred treatment of communicating syringomyelia is a valve-regulated ventriculoperitoneal shunt. Failure of the syrinx to collapse is evidence of shunt failure or misdiagnosis.

Noncommunicating Syringomyelia

Table 1 emphasizes the wide variety of etiological factors responsible for noncommunicating syringomyelia. The correct diagnosis can usually be established on the basis of conventional MRI, but it is important to obtain scans of the entire neuraxis to rule out unexpected factors such as tethered cord and acquired tonsillar herniation occurring with hydrocephalus and intracranial mass lesions. An important goal of the diagnostic workup is to localize the level of the CSF block. Although this may be evident in patients with Chiari malformations, basilar invagination, and extramedullary compressions, it is often obscure in cases of posttraumatic or postmeningitic syringomyelia. Because the preferred treatment of noncommunciating syringomyelia is to restore CSF dynamics in the spinal subarachnoid space, it is advisable to define the block to the extent possible by cine-MRI or CT myelography.

Chiari I Malformation

The diagnostic criteria for this disorder have been recently revised [19]. Although the correct diagnosis can usually be established by an MRI scan of the cervical spine, the following workup is strongly recommended: (1) an MRI scan of the brain to rule out hydrocephalus and other causes of acquired tonsillar herniation; (2) an MRI scan of the thoracolumbar spine to rule out spinal cord tethering; and (3) cine-MRI to assess CSF velocity/flow at the cervicomedullary junction. Approximately one-third of patients with CMI will be found to have anterior encroachment of the foramen magnum by a retroflexed odontoid process or basilar invagination [19]. Thus, before formulating a surgical plan for such patients, a decision needs to be made whether posterior decompression, anterior decompression, or both is the optimal treatment.

Operative strategies for treating CMI and syringomyelia have yet to be fully standardized. The traditional approach is to perform a posterior fossa decompression consisting of a suboccipital craniectomy, upper cervical laminectomy, and duraplasty. Unfortunately, specific details such as the size of the craniectomy, the extent of the laminectomy, and the preferred integument for duraplasty (e.g., cadavaric dura, pericranium, bovine pericardium, or synthetic material) are rarely discussed. Also controversial are additional steps such as lysis of adhesions, plugging of the obex, terminal ventriculostomy, drainage of the fourth ventricle, leaving the dura open, and resection or shrinkage of the cerebellar tonsils [3–7,18,27,28]. No one procedure has been uniformly successful, and it is estimated that a significant improvement in preoperative symptoms and a reduction in syrinx size occurs in only 40%–60% of patients [4–6].

At our institution, the preferred technique for treating Chiari-related syringomyelia is as follows: (1) a moderate to large craniectomy that increases the volume of the undersized posterior fossa; (2) an expansile duraplasty employing cadaveric dura; and (3) reconstruction of the bony defect with a titanium mesh/acrylic cranioplasty. A laminectomy is not performed unless the cerebellar tonsils extend below C1 (approximately 10 mm herniation). If the cerebellar tonsils are impacted or deeply herniated through the foramen magnum, it is common practice to lyse adhesions and shrink the tonsillar tips with bipolar coagulation. These and other surgical decisions are guided intraoperatively by the use of ultrasound, somatosensory evoked potentials, and color doppler imaging that has been modified for measurement of CSF flow and velocity.

The most common complications of Chiari surgery are a failure to stabilize or reverse symptoms, intractable pain, pseudomeningocele formation, cranial settling, and cervical spine instability. Osseous complications appear to be related in most instances to the extent of the laminectomy. Table 2 summarizes the indications for reoperation in 147 patients who were referred to our institution for treatment for failed Chiari surgery between the years 1995 and 1999. Reoperation was not performed unless the patient met one or more of the following criteria: (1) evidence of neurological deterioration; (2) intractable and disabling symptoms; or (3) MRI evi-

TABLE 2. Failed Chiari surgery (147 patients; 1995–2000)

Variable	Total
Intractable or progressive symptoms	147
Persistent or enlarging syrinx	71 (of 90)
Pseudomeningocele	53
Cranial settling/basilar invagination	28
Cervical spine instability	27
Hydrocephalus	5

dence of syrinx propagation. The standard preoperative protocol included updated MRI scans, cine-MRI, flexion/extension MRI or roentgenograms of the cervical spine, and CT reconstruction of the posterior fossa. Although reoperations typically involved more than one variable, the basic surgical steps were the same as those described for primary operations. Additional procedures were usually required in patients with cranial settling, swan neck deformity, and cervical spine instability and consisted of complex cervical or craniovertebral fusions, sometimes in combination with a transoral odontoidectomy.

Basilar Invagination/Retroflexed Odontoid

Anterior encroachment of the foramen magnum by basilar invagination or retroflexion of the odontoid process is a recognized cause of primary syringomyelia. However, because odontoid abnormalities are common in patients with CMI, the pathogenesis of syringomyelia in such cases may be difficult to establish when both lesions are present. It is the policy at our institution not to perform a posterior fossa decompression until the role of the anterior lesion has been considered. The workup consists of a detailed neurological examination supplemented by the following studies: CT reconstruction of the foramen magnum, cine-MRI, flexion/extension MRI, motor evoked potentials (MEPs), sleep apnea monitoring, Holter monitoring, and vestibular function tests. If there is evidence of clinically significant anterior compression, the odontoid abnormality is handled first. Reducible lesions are managed by a posterior cervical or craniovertebral fusion, whereas irreducible lesions usually require a transoral odontoidectomy followed by a staged posterior fusion. Anterior decompression may result in syrinx resolution despite persistent tonsillar ectopia (see the chapter by A. Menezes in this volume).

Arachnoiditis

Inflammations of the leptomeninges occurring as a consequence of hemorrhage and infection are an important cause of syringomyelia. In patients with posttraumatic or postmeningitic syringomyelia, the diagnostic goal is to establish the level and extent of the CSF block. This image is rarely possible with conventional MRI and it is appropriate in most cases to obtain a CT myelogram or cine-MRI of the entire spinal cord.

The preferred treatment for syringomyelia occurring with arachnoiditis is a direct operation on the CSF block consisting of a lysis of adhesions and an expansile duraplasty [29]. Intraoperative decisions are sometimes facilitated by the use of color doppler imaging or the intrathecal injection of indigo carmine [30]. When direct operations fail, or when preoperative studies provide evidence of extensive leptomeningeal scarring, a syrinx shunting procedure may be required.

Extramedullary Compressions

Extramedullary lesions such as arachnoid cysts, tumors, spondylosis, and disk herniations are an occasional cause of syringomyelia [18]. Spinal cord cavitation may occur at almost any level at or below the obstruction. It is important to establish that the extramedullary lesion is not a coincidental finding, and the neuroradiological workup should include MRI scans of the whole neuraxis. Preferred treatment consists of excising the extramedullary compression. If syringomyelia persists, a syrinx shunting procedure may be required.

Tethered Spinal Cord

Spinal cord tethering attributable to myelodysplasia, shortening of the filum terminale, and traumatic or iatrogenic scarring is a recognized cause of syringomyelia. In adult patients, syrinx formation tends to be related to a CSF block at the level of the lesion, whereas in children continuing somatic growth can result in acquired tonsillar herniation with obstruction of CSF flow at the level of the foramen magnum. Preferred treatment consists of spinal cord untethering. If syringomyelia persists, a syrinx shunting procedure may be required.

Acquired Tonsillar Herniation

Although herniation of the cerebellar tonsils is a characteristic feature of Chiari malformations, it may also occur in association with a wide variety of other disorders [19] including hydrocephalus, infratentorial cysts and tumors, supratentorial tumors, subdural hematoma, craniosynostosis, achondroplasia, and spinal cord tethering. Errors in diagnosis are likely to occur if MR imaging is limited to the cervicomedullary junction. Surgical treatment of acquired tonsillar herniation is directed at the causal lesion, and it is rarely necessary to specifically decompress the foramen magnum.

Idiopathic Syringomyelia

Syringomyelia of unknown origin is an increasingly rare diagnosis. However, examples are still encountered in which the precise mechanism of spinal cord cavitation is unclear. It is advisable in such cases to perform an exhaustive neuroradiologic workup that focuses on the detection of an occult CSF block. Cine-MRI and CT myelography are often helpful in this regard. In pediatric patients, it is important to obtain an MRI scan of the thoracolumbar spine to rule out spinal cord tethering. Iskander et al. [31] have reported that children with idiopathic syringomyelia may benefit from a posterior fossa decompression (the so-called Chiari 0 malformation). A more recent follow-up of this series [32] suggests that "Chiari 0" patients do in fact have a compromised posterior fossa and caudal displacement of the brainstem that fulfill the criteria for a "borderline" malformation [19].

TABLE 3. Syrinx shunting procedures

(1) Syringosubarachnoid shunt
(2) Syringopleural shunt
(3) Syringoperitoneal shunt

Syrinx Shunting Procedures

The role of shunting procedures in the treatment of syringomyelia is currently under review. Whereas syrinx shunting has been performed with considerable success in the primary treatment of noncommunicating lesions [33–36], the long-term results of these procedures tend to be poor, and the incidence of shunt failure tends to increase the longer a series is followed. For these and other reasons (such as the risk of spinal cord injury at the time of shunt implantation), there is a growing trend to perform a direct operation on the causal lesion and to reserve syrinx shunting as a procedure of last resort [30].

Current indications for syrinx shunting procedures are limited to the following: (1) cases of idiopathic syringomyelia in which the causal lesion cannot be identified; (2) cases of posttraumatic or postmeningitic syringomyelia in which the arachnoidal block is so severe or widespread that it prohibits surgical reconstruction of the spinal subarachnoid space; and (3) cases of noncommunciating syringomyelia in which direct operations on the obstructing lesion have failed.

Table 3 summarizes the most commonly employed syrinx shunting procedures. Syringosubarachnoid shunts that divert CSF from the syrinx cavity into the spinal subarachnoid space are generally preferred over extraspinal shunts because they are more physiological, less affected by somatic growth, and do not require a valve [37]. An absolute requirement of subarachnoid shunts is that the CSF pathways rostral to the syrinx be patent. At our institution, it is standard practice to implant the proximal end of the shunt through the posterior longitudinal sulcus rather than the dorsal root entry zone to minimize the incidence of postoperative dysesthetic pain [37,38]. The distal end of the the shunt is directed anteriorly into the ventral subarachnoid space, which is more capacious than its dorsal counterpart, and drains rostrally toward the basilar cisterns [39]. In cases in which the cervical theca is obstructed, effective treatment can often be achieved by shunting the syrinx to the cisterna magna or cerebellopontine angle cistern (syringocisternostomy) [38].

The principal alternative to subarachnoid shunting is an extraspinal shunt to the pleural or peritoneal cavity. The former is easier to perform and has the advantage of the hydrostatic constancy and negative pressure of the pleural compartment. Lumboperitoneal shunts are not generally recommended because of the significant incidence of complications including acquired tonsillar herniation [40].

References

1. Gardner WJ, Goodall RJ (1950) The surgical treatment of Arnold-Chiari malformation in adults. An explanation of its mechanism and importance of encephalography in diagnosis. J Neurosurg 7:199–206

2. Williams B (1980) On the pathogenesis of syringomyelia: a review. J R Soc Med 73:798–806
3. Levy WJ, Mason L, Hahn JF (1983) Chiari malformation presenting in adults: a surgical experience in 127 cases. Neurosurgery 12:377–390
4. Rhoton AL Jr (1976) Microsurgery of Arnold-Chiari malformation in adults with and without hydromyelia. J Neurosurg 45:473–483
5. Dyste GN, Menezes AH, VanGilder JC (1989) Symptomatic Chiari malformations. An analysis of presentation, management and long-term outcome. J Neurosurg 71:159–168
6. Pillay PK, Awan IA, Little JR, Hahn JF (1991) Symptomatic Chiari malformation in adults: a new classification based on magnetic resonance imaging with clinical and prognostic significance. Neurosurgery 28:639–645
7. Park TS, Cail WS, Broaddus WC, et al (1989) Lumboperitoneal shunt combined with myelotomy for treatment of syringomyelia. J Neurosurg 70:721–727
8. Milhorat TH, Capocelli AL Jr, Anzil AP, et al (1995) Pathological basis of spinal cord cavitation in syringomyelia: analysis of 105 autopsy cases. J Neurosurg 82:802–812
9. Milhorat TH, Johnson RW, Milhorat RH, et al (1995) Clinicopathological correlations using axial magnetic resonance imaging. Neurosurgery 37:206–213
10. Milhorat TH (2000) Classification of syringomyelia. Neurosurg Focus 8(3):1
11. Milhorat TH, Kotzen RM, Anzil AP (1994) Stenosis of central canal of spinal cord in man: incidence and pathological findings in 232 autopsy cases. J Neurosurg 80:716–722
12. Eisenberg HM, McLennan JE, Welch K (1974) Ventricular perfusion in cats with kaolin-induced hydrocephalus. J Neurosurg 41:20–28
13. Oldfield EH, Muraszko K, Shawker TH, et al (1994) Pathophysiology of syringomyelia associated with Chiari I malformation of the cerebellar tonsils. Implications for diagnosis and treatment. J Neurosurg 80:3–15
14. Heiss JD, Patronas N, DeVroom HJ, et al (1999) Elucidating the pathophysiology of syringomyelia. J Neurosurg 91:553–562
15. Stoodley MA, Brown SA, Brown CJ, et al (1997) Arterial pulsation-dependent perivascular cerebrospinal fluid flow into the central canal in the sheep spinal cord. J Neurosurg 86:686–693
16. Stoodley MA, Gutschmitz B, Jones NR (1999) Cerebrospinal fluid flow in an animal model of noncommunicating syringomyelia. Neurosurgery 44:1065–1076
17. Milhorat TH, Nobandegani F, Miller JI, et al (1993) Noncommunicating syringomyelia following occlusion of central canal in rats. Experimental model and histological findings. J Neurosurg 78:274–279
18. Milhorat TH, Johnson WD, Miller JI, et al (1992) Surgical treatment of syringomyelia based on magnetic resonance imaging criteria. Neurosurgery 31:231–245
19. Milhorat TH, Chou MW, Trinidad EM, et al (1999) Chiari I malformation redefined. Clinical and radiographic findings in 364 symptomatic patients. Neurosurgery 44:1005–1017
20. Ball MJ, Dayan AD (1972) Pathogenesis of syringomyelia. Lancet 2:799–801
21. Aboulker J (1979) La syringomyélie et les liquides intra-rachidiens. Neurochirurgie 25(suppl 1):1–44
22. Milhorat TH, Girgis PS, Pan J, et al (2001) Bulk flow pathway for cerebrospinal fluid filling of noncommunicating syrinx cavities: an ultrastructural study in rats. J Neurosurg (in press)
23. Brightman MW (1965) The distribution within the brain of ferritin injected into cerebrospinal fluid compartments. 1. Ependymal distribution. J Cell Biol 26:99–123
24. Brightman WM (1965) The distribution within the brain of ferritin injected into cerebrospinal fluid compartments. 2. Parenchymal distribution. Am J Anat 117:193–220
25. Brightman MW (1968) The intracerebral movement of proteins injected into blood and cerebrospinal fluid of mice. Prog Brain Res 29:19–37

26. Fenstermacher JD, Bradbury MWB, duBoulay G, et al (1980) The distribution of ^{125}J-metrizamide and ^{125}I-diatrizoate between blood, brain and cerebrospinal fluid in the rabbit. Neuroradiology 19:171–180
27. Williams B (1986) Progress in syringomyelia: a review. Neurol Res 8:139–145
28. Batzdorf U (1988) Chiari I malformation with syringomyelia: evaluation of surgical therapy by magnetic resonance imaging. J Neurosurg 68:726–730
29. Klekamp J, Batzdorf U, Samii M, et al (1997) Treatment of syringomyelia associated with arachnoid scarring caused by arachnoiditis or trauma. J Neurosurg 86:233–240
30. Batzdorf U (1000) Primary spinal syringomyelia: a personal perspective. Neurosurg Focus 8(3):7
31. Iskander BJ, Hedlund GL, Grabb PA, et al (1998) The resolution of syringohydromyelia wihtout hindbrain herniation after posterior fossa decompression. J Neurosurg 89:212–216
32. Tubbs RS, Elton S, Grabb P, et al (2001) Analysis of the posterior fossa in children with the Chiari O malformation. Neurosurgery (in press)
33. Barbaro NM, Wilson CB, Gutin PH, et al (1984) Surgical treatment of syringomyelia: favorable results with syringoperitoneal shunting. J Neurosurg 61:531–538
34. Peerless SJ, Durward QJ (1982) Management of syringomyelia: a pathophysiological approach. Clin Neurosurg 30:531–576
35. Wisoff JH, Epstein F (1989) Management of hydromyelia. Neurosurgery 25:562–571
36. Tator CH, Megura K, Rowed DW (1982) Favorable results with syringosubarachnoid shunts for treatment of syringomyelia. J Neurosurg 56:517–523
37. Milhorat TH, Johnson WD, Miller JI (1992) Syrinx shunt to posterior fossa cisterns (syringocisternostomy) for bypassing obstructions of the upper cervical theca. J Neurosurg 77:871–874
38. Milhorat TH, Kotzen RM, Mu HTM, et al (1996) Dysesthetic pain in patients with syringomyelia. J Neurosurg 38:940–947
39. Milhorat TH (1972) Hydrocephalus and the cerebrospinal fluid. Williams and Wilkins, Baltimore, pp 1–35
40. Scott RM (1996) Shunt complications In: Wilkins RH, Rengachary SS (eds) Neurosurgery, vol III. McGraw Hill, New York, pp 3655–3664

Age-Related Morphological Change of the Central Canal of the Human Spinal Cord and the Mechanism of Syrinx Formation in Syringomyelia and Hydromyelia

Yoshio Hashizume[1], Keizo Yasui[2], and Mari Yoshida[1]

Summary. To elucidate the physiological and pathogenetic role of the human central spinal canal in acquired syringomyelia, we analyzed age-related morphological changes of the normal human central canal of the spinal cord and discussed the mechanism of syrinx formation in syringomyelia and hydromyelia. The subjects included 158 cases ranging in age from 1 day post gestation to 116 years. Autopsy cases of syringomyelia and hydromyelia were also examined. Microscopic images of the central canal were classified as patent or occluded at each level for each age decade. The patency rate under 1 year of age was 100% in almost all segments, which markedly decreased in the second decade, and the canals were occluded in all segments with advancing age. The occlusion of the central canal started at T6 and L5 to S2 levels. In cases of acquired syringomyelia, there was no communication between the central canal and the syrinx, in contrast to hydromyelia. From these observations, we suggest that the central canal does not function after infancy because of its occlusion and that it is not involved in the development of syringomyelia in adult patients.

Key words. Spinal central canal, Aging, Histology, Syringomyelia, Spinal cord

Introduction

In humans, it is generally accepted that the lumen of the central canal of the spinal cord is patent in most autopsy cases in newborn or younger children, whereas it often closes in adult cases [1–3]. The central canal in rats allows the flow of cerebrospinal fluid (CSF) in a rostral direction and functions in the removal of waste matter. The function of the central canal in adult humans, however, is not well understood [4]. On the other hand, syringomyelia of the spinal cord frequently involves the central canal. It remains obscure whether the central canal of spinal cord is related to syringomyelia. In this study, we analyzed age-related morphological changes of the normal human

[1] Institute for Medical Science of Aging, Aichi Medical University, Nagakute-cho, Aichi-gun, Aichi 480-1195, Japan
[2] Department of Neurology, Nagoya Daini Red Cross Hospital, Myoken-cho, Showa-ku, Nagoya 466-8650, Japan

Table 1. Summary of the 158 cases examined

Age	No. of cases	Male	Female
Less than 1 year old	6	4	2
1 to 5 years old	12	8	4
6 to 9 years old	8	6	2
2nd decade	12	7	5
3rd decade	11	9	2
4th decade	11	7	4
5th decade	13	7	6
6th decade	14	8	6
7th decade	13	7	6
8th decade	13	8	5
9th decade	17	11	6
10th decade	12	6	6
More than 100 years old	16	1	15
Total	158	89	69

central canal of the spinal cord. We would like to make these results important basic data in considering the pathogenesis of acquired syringomyelia.

Materials and Methods

This study included 158 autopsy cases, ranging in age from 1 week postnatal to 116 years of age. The cases were classified on the basis of each successive decade (Table 1). Whole fixed spinal cords were cut in segmenets from the C3 to S3 levels in the axial plane, and histological change in the central canal was investigated. Occlusion of the central canal with aging and its rostral-caudal distribution in the axial segmenets were also studied. In addition, we investigated the prevalence of a patent canal at each level in each decade. Four syringomyelia cases and four hydromyelia cases obtained from autopsy were also histologically examined to consider the mechanism of syrinx formation.

Results

Histological Changes in the Central Canal

The central canal of the human spinal cord was classified morphologically into the patent type and the occluded type. The central canal of the patent type showed a tubule perfectly lined by ependymal cells (Fig. 1A) or a tubule with a zone of ependymal breakage. The central canal of the occluded type showed an irregular arrangement of ependymal cells without formation of a tubule (Fig. 1B).

Occlusion of the Central Canal with Aging

The patency rate in terms of decade is shown in Fig. 2. In those under 1 year of age and in the 1- to 5-year-old group, canals were fully patent at many segment levels, but even in infants under 1 year, some occluded canals existed. In the 6- to 9-year-old

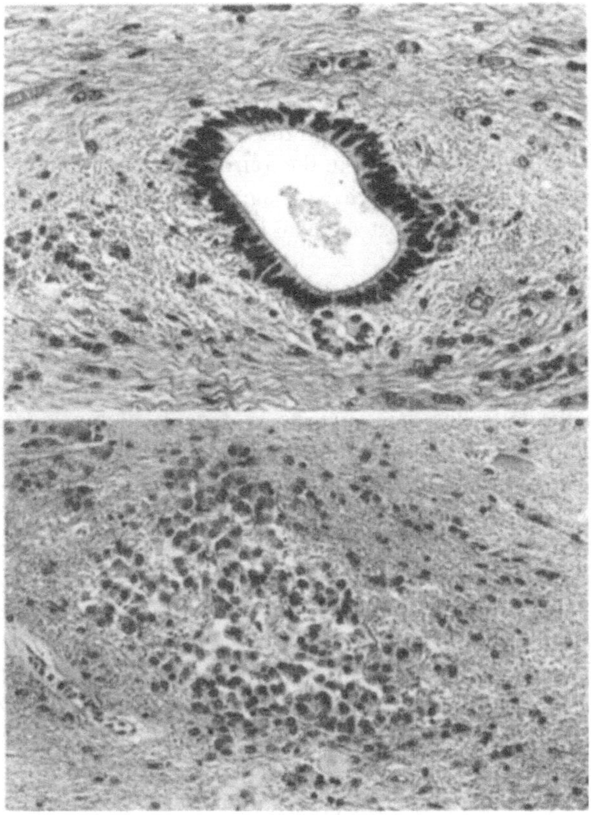

A

B

FIG. 1A,B. Patent and occluded type of central canal. **A** Patent type of central canal: a tubule is perfectly lined by ependymal cells. **B** Occluded type of central canal: irregular arrangment of ependymal cells without formation of tubule. H&E. ×100

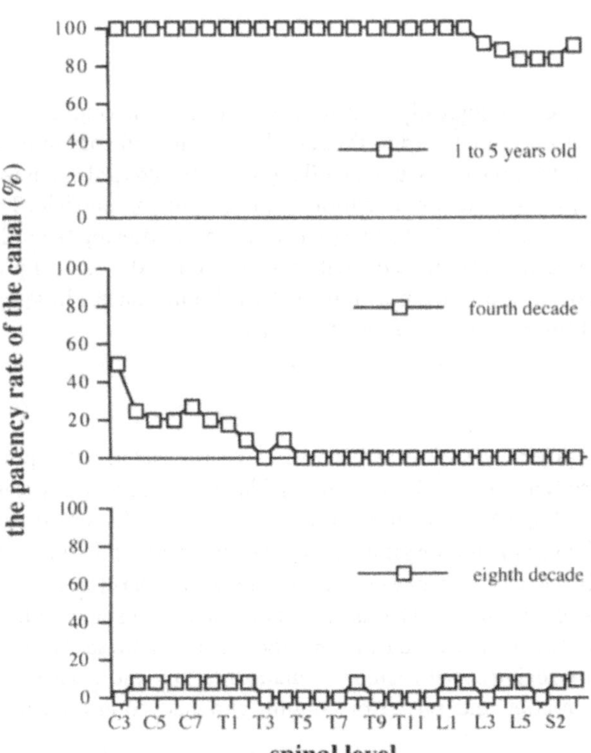

FIG. 2. Patency rate according to decade. In specimens in the 1- to 5-year-old group, the canals were fully patent at many levels. Although the patency rate in the cervical cord remained high in the fourth to sixth decades, the other levels showed occlusion by the fourth decade. In the majority of levels, the patency rate was 0% in the eighth decade

group, the patency rate was 100% at three segment levels and 75% or more at all other segment levels. The patency rate decreased abruptly in the second decade. Finally, all cases had occlusions in at least one segment level in the fourth decade. Although the patency rate in the cervical cord remained high with aging, the other levels had become occluded by the fourth decade. In most segment levels, the patency rate was 0% after the seventh decade.

Occlusion of the Central Canal in Longitudinal Axis and Aging

According to the occlusion pattern of the central canal in the longitudinal axis, we classified the subjects into the following three groups: in type 1, all canals were patent; in type 2, patent and occluded levels were present simultaneously; and in type 3, all canal were occluded (Fig. 3). Of 20 cases of type 1, 19 were in the groups comprising individuals of less than 10 years of age; no type 1 cases were seen after the third decade. Type 3 specimens were found in some cases in the second decade, and their prevalence increased gradually with aging, becoming more than 50% in the fourth decade. Type 2 specimens existed in almost all decades but were less frequent in children and the aged. Because the type 2 specimens were thought to be in the process of occluding, the earliest and latest occluding levels can be identified from these cases. The patency rate of the type 2 cases with respect to the segments in the longitudinal axis (Fig. 4) was lower at T6 and the L5 to S2 levels and higher at the upper cervical levels. This finding indicated that T6 and L5 to S2 levels were the earliest segments to occlude and the upper cervical levels were the last segments to occlude.

Hydromyelia

Four cases of hydromyelia were histologically examined. In one case, the central canal was dilated in all segments of the spinal cord to the sacral cord and had communication with the fourth ventricle. In three cases, partial dilatation of the central canal was observed at some segments, without communication with the fourth ventricle. The dilated cavity of hydromyelia was totally lined by ependymal cells, differing from the cavity of syringomyelia (Fig. 5A,B). The dilated cavity was located at the central part of the spinal cord and had no communication with the subarachnoid space. There was no parenchymal necrosis in the spinal cord of hydromyelia.

Syringomyelia

Secondary acquired syringomyelia was observed in two cases associated with spinal cord tumor (Fig. 6A,B, astrocytoma; Fig. 7A,B, hemangiblastoma) and in one case with adhesive arachnoiditis (Fig. 8A,B). In these cases, the cavity of the syrinx was located mainly at the dorsal column and dorsal horn and had no communication with the central canal. The syrinx cavity was always continuous with necrotic areas or tumor tissue (Fig. 9). In two cases, the cavity was continuous with the subarachnoid space. Proliferation of glial tissue was noted around the cavity in these cases. In the case of syringomyelia associated with Chiari I malformation, the syrinx was located at the central gray matter and posterior column and had communication

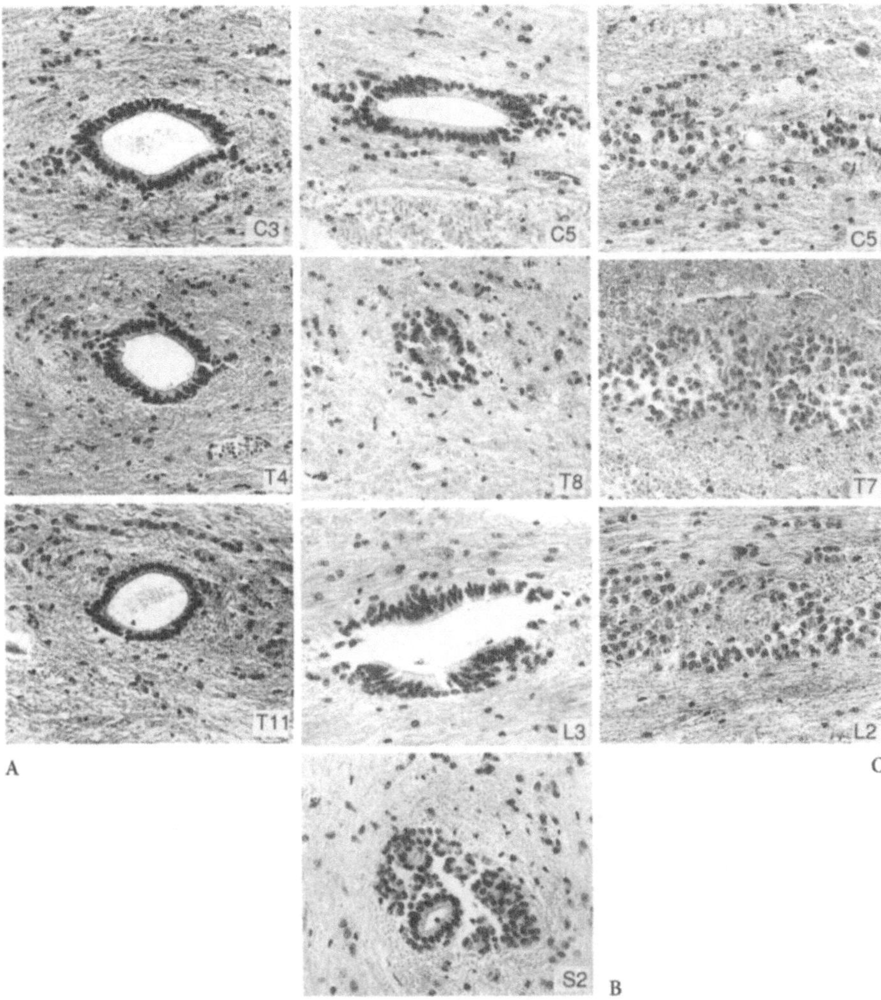

FIG. 3A–C. Occlusion pattern of the central canal in the longitudinal axis. **A** Type 1: all canals were patent. **B** Type 2: patent and occluded levels were present simultaneously. **C** Type 3: all canals were occluded. H&E. ×100

with the central canal at some segments. Ependymal cells were observed only in some parts of the syrinx.

Discussion

The present study demonstrated the detailed three-dimensional and age-dependent progression of occlusion of the human central canal at all spinal levels [5]. Some central canals were occluded at the midthoracic level even in those specimens under

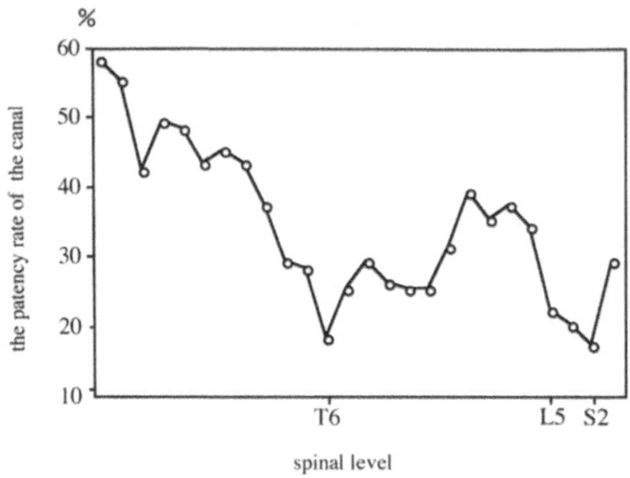

FIG. 4. Patency rate in cases with patent and occluded canals occurring simultaneously. T6 and L5 to S2 levels occluded earlier; the upper cervical levels occluded later

A

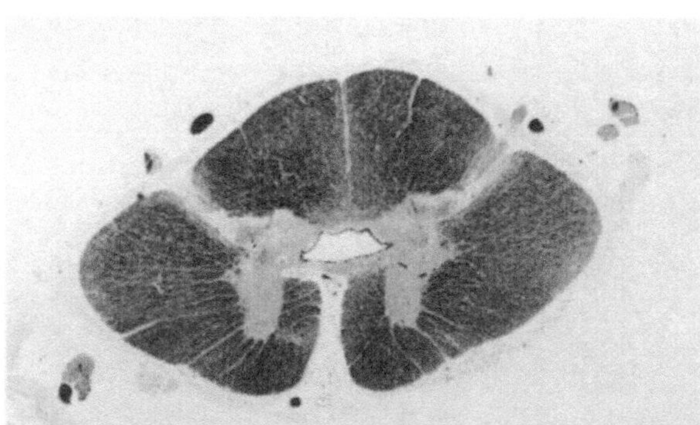

B

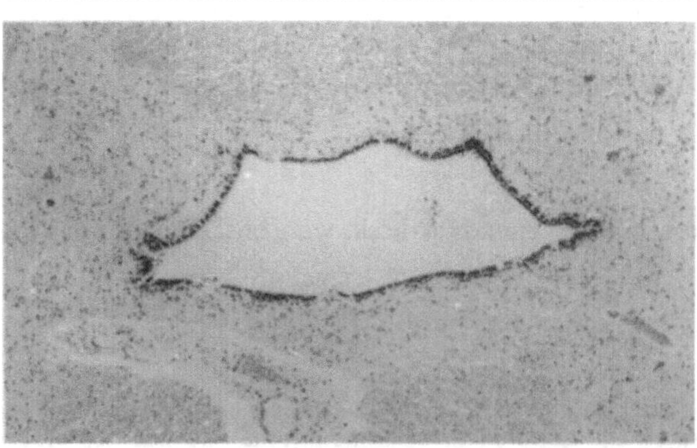

FIG. 5A,B. In hydromyelia, the dilated cavity was totally lined by ependymal cells. **A** T9 segment. Kluver-Barrera. ×10. **B** H&E. ×25

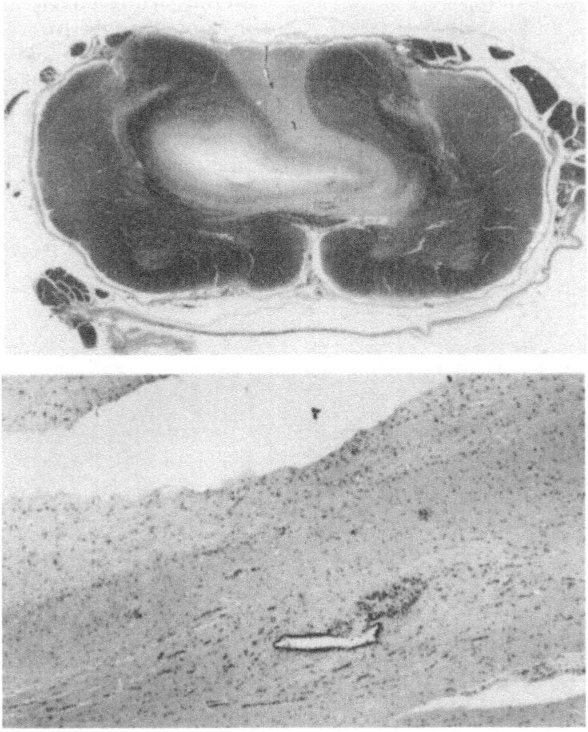

A

B

FIG. 6A,B. Syringomyelia with associated astrocytoma. **A** Syrinx in ventral part of the posterior column of C7 segment. Kluver-Barrera. ×7.1. **B** No communication between syrinx and central canal. H&E. ×25

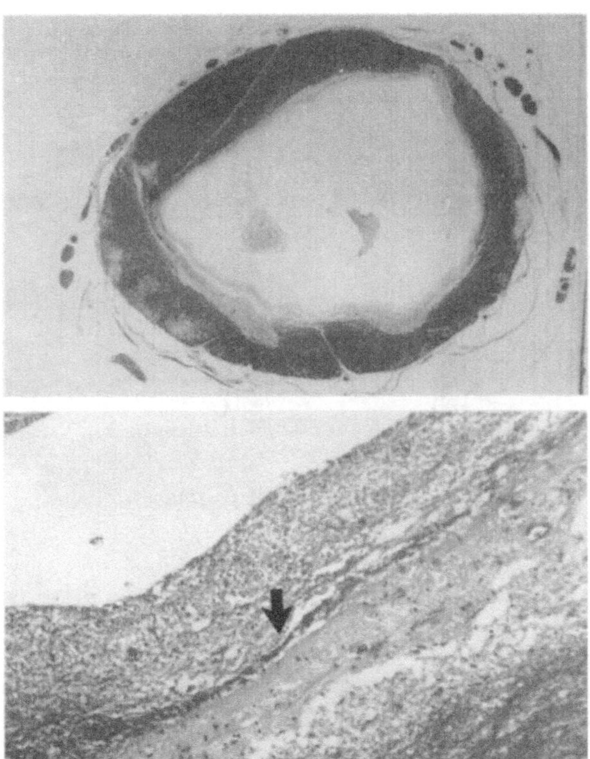

A

B

FIG. 7A,B. Syringomyelia with associated hemangioblastoma. **A** Cross section of T8 segment shows marked dilatation of cystic cavity in the posterior horn. Kluver-Barrera. ×6.7. **B** *Arrow* shows occluded central canal. H&E. ×25

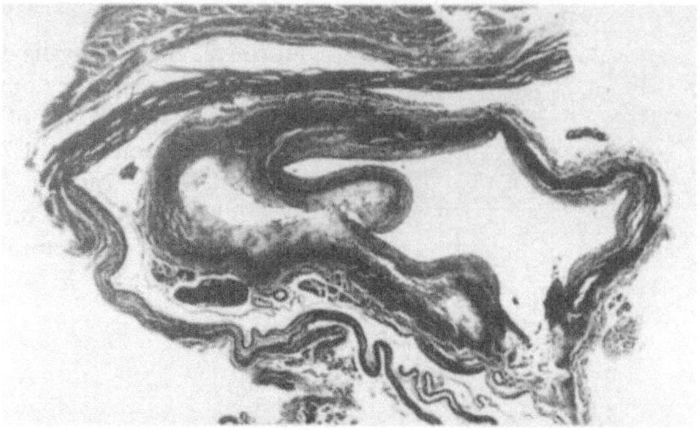

A

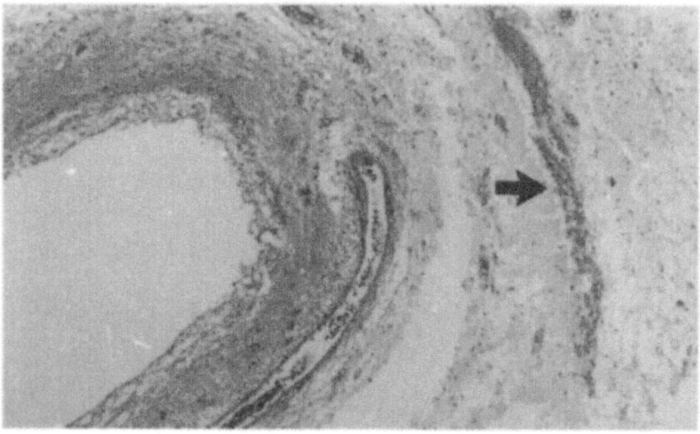

B

FIG. 8A,B. Syringomyelia with associated adhesive arachnoiditis. **A** Syrinx and parenchymal necrosis in the thoracic cord. Azan. ×10. **B** *Arrow* shows occluded central canal. H&E. ×25

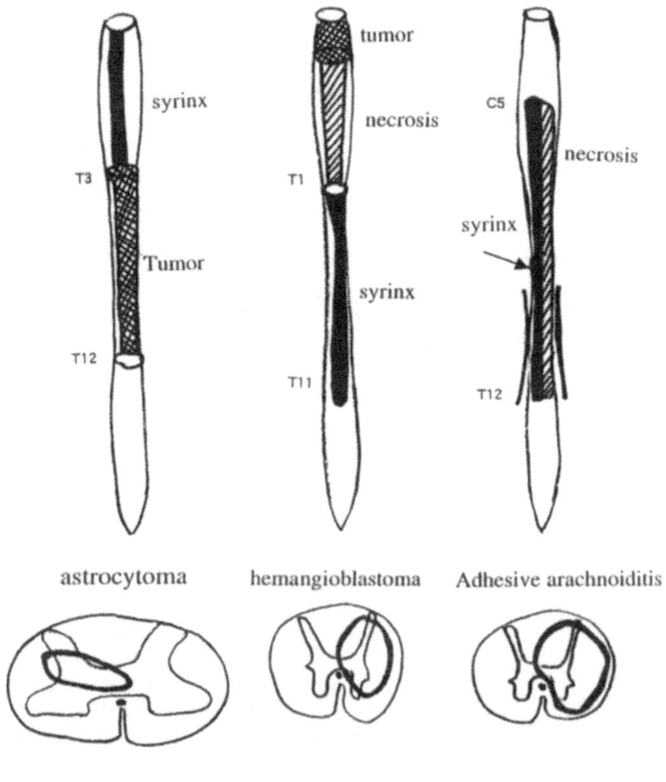

FIG. 9. Schematic representation of tumor, necrosis, and syrinx. The syrinx was often located in the posterior column or posterior horn and did not communicate with the fourth ventricle and central canal; it was always continuous with the necrotic area or tumor tissue

1 year of age. Over the age of 10 years, the canal was occluded at many more levels. Eventually, it closes at all levels. Once the canal closes, it seems impossible for it to reopen because of the proliferation of ependymal cells and astrocytes. Consequently, we do not think that adult syringomyelia with or without Chiari I malformation results from central canal enlargement. The present study showed that the obstructive change of the human central canal occurs in early infancy, suggesting that the hydrodynamic theory does not satisfactory explain the development of syringomyelia after infancy. The hydrodynamic theory also cannot explain syrinxes with an occluded canal at the upper cervical level or syrinxes localized in the thoracic or lumbar levels [6,7]. Hydromyelia is defined as the cystic dilatation of the central canal lined by ependymal cells and is classified into two types according to the existence of communication between the fourth ventricle and the dilated central canal. In communicating hydromyelia, the cavity is formed by continuous dilatation of the central canal by hydrodynamic pressure. In noncommunicating hydromyelia, the part of the central canal that remained open seemed to dilate even after occlusion of the central canal by aging processes had occurred in other segments.

References

1. Kasantikul V, Netsky MG, James AE Jr (1979) Relation of age and cerebral ventricle size to central canal in man. Morphological analysis. J Neurosurg 51:85–93
2. Milhorat TH, Kotzen RM, Anzil AP (1994) Stenosis of central canal of spinal cord in man: incidence and pathological findings in 232 autopsy cases. J Neurosurg 80:716–722
3. Netsky MG (1953) Syringomyelia. A clinicopathological study. Arch Neurol Psychiatry 70:741–777
4. Milhorat TH, Nobandegani F, Miller JI, et al (1993) Noncommunicating syringomyelia following occlusion of central canal in rat. Experimental model and histological findings. J Neurosurg 78:274–279
5. Yasui K, Hashizume Y, Yoshida M, et al (1999) Age-related morphologic changes of central canal of the human spinal cord. Acta Neuropathol 97:253–259
6. Gardner WJ (1965) Hydrodynamic mechanism of syringomyelia: its relationship to myelocele. J Neurol Neurosurg Psychiatry 28:247–259
7. Williams B (1986) Progress in syringomyelia. Neurol Res 8:130–145

2. Experimental Studies

Histological and MRI Study on Experimental Syringomyelia

Kazuki Yamamoto, Norihiko Tamaki, Tatsuya Nagashima, and Ayumi Takahashi

Summary. To clarify the pathogenesis of syringomyelia, we examined MRI and histological changes in experimental syringomyelia in progress. Syringomyelia was induced in 19 rabbits by intracisternal injection of a kaolin solution. MRI was performed at 3, 7, 14, or 21 days after the injection. The rabbits were killed immediately after the last MRI and histological examinations were then performed. MRI showed two types of syrinx: hydromyelia accompanied by ventriculomegaly, and cervical cord cavitation in the posterior horn without ventriculomegaly. All changes observed on MRI findings were verified by histological examination. The first type of syrinx had enlarged central canals that were lined with ependyma, but there was no marked presence of spongy tissue around the central canal. The obex was completely filled with kaolin solution. The second type featured small central canals and sponginess or cavities of gray matter in the upper or middle spinal cords. Kaolin was observed around the obex but it was not completely filled. Fourteen days after kaolin injection, the shapes of syrinxes had remained almost the same. MRI showed the chronological changes very clearly, and histological differences of the syrinx correlated with the degree to which the obex was filled with kaolin.

Key words. Experimental syringomyelia, Magnetic resonance imaging, Histology, Early phase, Syrinx formation

Introduction

Syringomyelia is a relatively rare spinal cord disease that is associated with anomalies at the craniovertebral junction, spinal tumors, trauma, and arachnoiditis. To clarify the pathogenesis of syringomyelia, we examined MRI and histological changes of the spinal cord in the early phase of experimental syringomyelia.

Department of Neurosurgery, Kobe University, Graduate School of Medicine, 7-5-1 Kusunoki-cho, Chuo-ku, Kobe 650-0017, Japan

Materials and Methods

Twenty-three adult Japanese white rabbits, weighing 2.5–3.0 kg, were anesthetized with an intravenous injection of pentobarbital sodium (30 mg/kg). Under anesthesia, syringomyelia was induced into 21 rabbits by percutaneous injection, with a 23 gauge needle, of 2.5% kaolin solution suspension in 1.0 ml normal saline into the cisterna magna. To equalize each kaolin location, and to prevent severe direct compression of the brain stem, each solution of kaolin suspension was injected at a constant rate to avoid a change in the intracranial pressure. Two rabbits received 1.0 ml of normal saline injected into the cisterna magna as a control.

Magnetic resonance (MR) examinations (1.0 T, SMT100A; Shimadzu, Kyoto, Japan) of the craniocervical junction and the cervical spinal cord were performed on day 3 on four rabbits, on day 7 on six rabbits, on day 14 on four, and on day 21 on five rabbits under general anesthesia as already described. Imaging parameters included a 256 × 192, 256 × 240, or 256 × 256 imaging matrix; a 15–20 cm field of view; and a 1.0–2.6 mm section thickness. Sagittal spin echo (SE) images were obtained at 500–800/20–40/2 (TR/TE/excitations) and 2000–3000/30–40, and axial SE images at 500–800/20–40/2.

Immediately after the MR examination, the rabbits were killed with an intravenous injection of an overdose of pentobarbital, and their spinal cords were removed immediately. The specimens were divided into blocks and embedded in paraffin after 1 or 2 weeks fixation in 10% formaldehyde solution. The lower brain stem and upper cervical spinal cord were cut serially and stained with hematoxylin and eosin (H&E).

The experiments were conducted according to the Guidelines for Animal Experiments of Kobe University School of Medicine.

Results

Physical and Neurological Findings

Nineteen of the 21 kaolin-injected rabbits showed syringomyelia on MR images. The 2 rabbits that did not were active immediately after awaking from the anesthesia and showed no physical or neurological abnormalities during the experiment. Seventeen of the rabbits with MRI-verified syringomyelia showed no remarkable physical or neurological signs for the first 1 or 2 days after kaolin injection, but after that they developed ataxic gait or spastic paraparesis. Special care was taken to maintain good nutrition during the experimental period, when the kaolin-injected animals tended to become weak and anorexic. Five or 7 days after kaolin injection, the rabbits showed improvement in their general appearance and ataxic gait and were able to feed themselves, although they continued to show spastic paraparesis.

MR Imaging Findings

The two control rabbits did not show syrinx or hydrocephalus on MR images, whereas the 2 kaolin-injected rabbits without abnormal physical or neurological findings did not show syringomyelia. In 17 kaolin-injected rabbits, intramedullary lesions in the

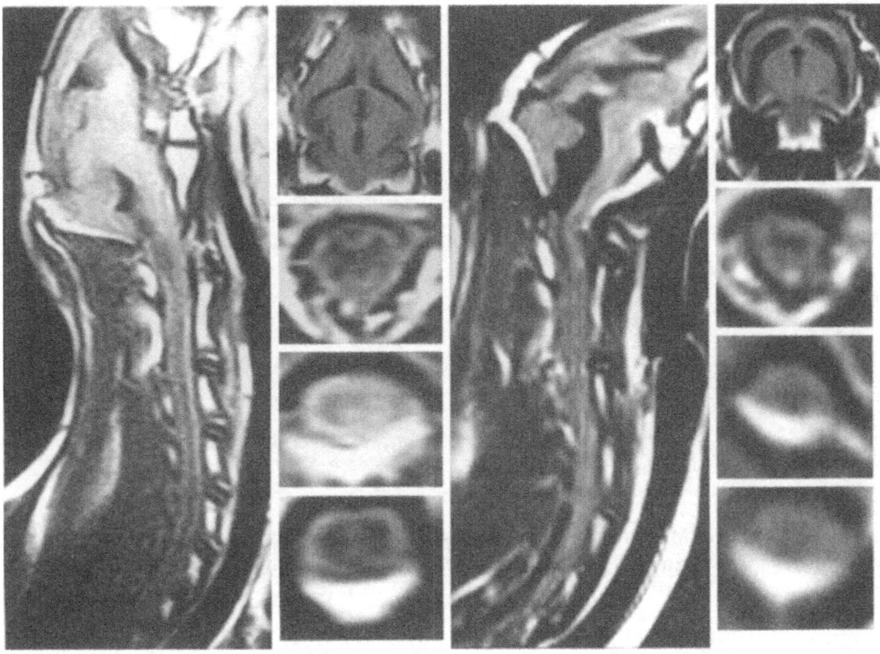

FIG. 1. T_1-weighted MR images show two types of syrinxes. *Left*: no ventriculomegaly or syrinx is present in the posterior horn of the spinal cord. *Right*: ventriculomegaly and syrinx are present within the center of the spinal cord

upper and middle cervical cord were seen, with low signal intensity on T_1-weighted MR images and high signal intensity on T_2-weighted images. It was difficult, however, to discriminate between syringomyelia and degeneration or edematous changes of the spinal cord on MR images.

There were two types of syrinx formation (Fig. 1): syringomyelia with ventriculomegaly and syringomyelia without ventriculomegaly. Six of the 10 rabbits that were studied on days 3 and 7 (Fig. 2) after kaolin injection showed both ventriculomegaly and syringomyelia. All syrinxes were round and located in the center of the spinal cord. They gradually increased in size and extent from the upper to the middle of the cervical spinal cord. Four of the 10 rabbits, which did not show ventriculomegaly in spite of the presence of syringomyelia, had irregularly shaped syrinxes located in the dorsal part of the spinal cord. The syrinx formations were dominant in the upper cervical spinal cord during the first 3 days, but had extended to the middle and lower cervical spinal cord by day 7 (Fig. 3).

Seven of the nine rabbits that were examined on days 14 and 21 after kaolin injection showed both ventriculomegaly and syringomyelia, and the remaining two showed no syringomyelia on day 21. Their syrinxes were located in the dorsal part of the upper and middle cervical spinal cord and at the center of the lower cervical spinal cord.

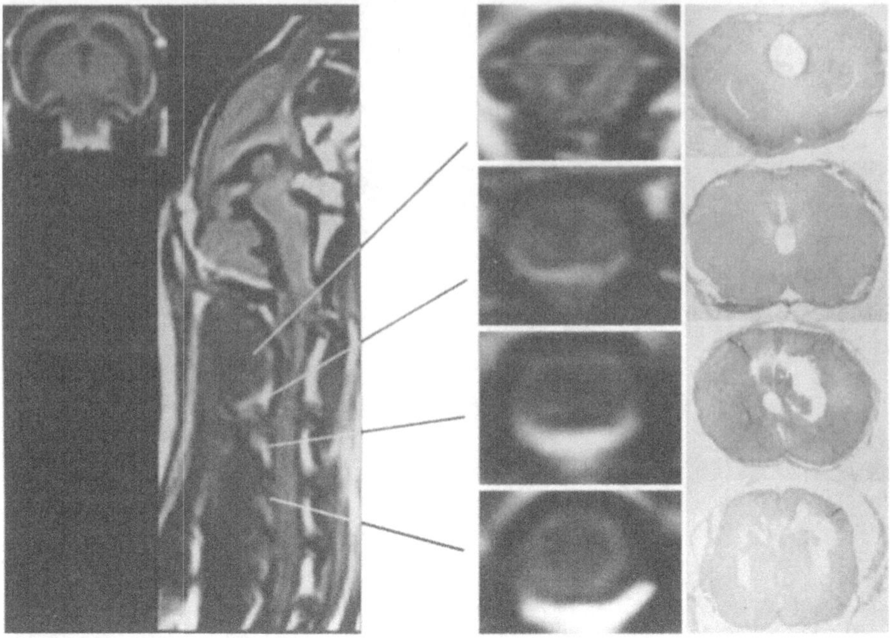

FIG. 2. T_1-weighted MR images and histological findings showing ventriculomegaly and syringomyelia. The syrinx has gradually enlarged and extends from the upper to the middle cervical spinal cord

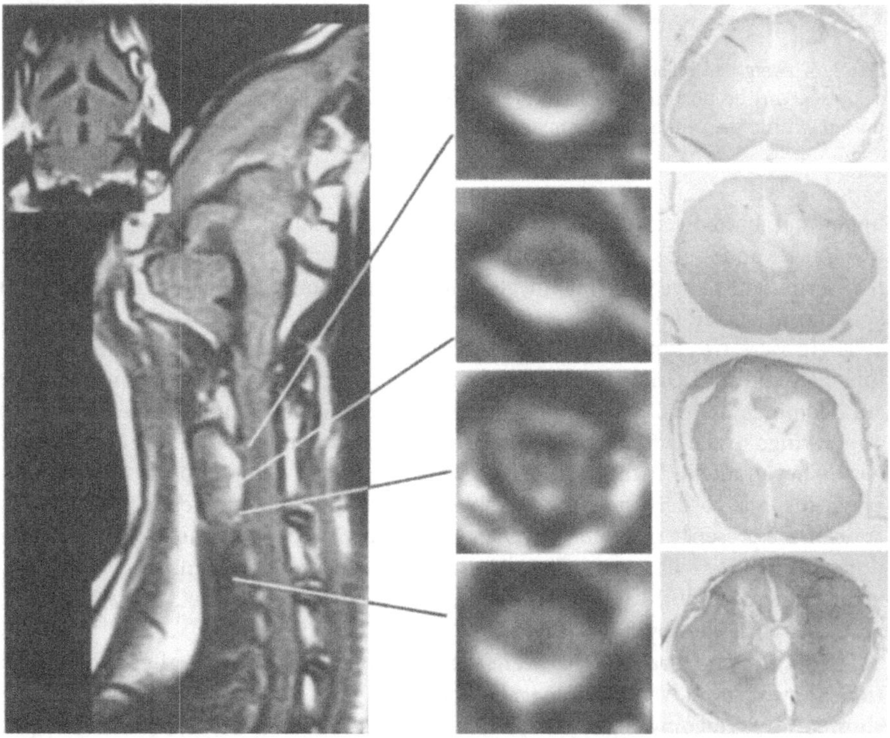

FIG. 3. T_1-weighted MR images and histological findings showing syrinx without ventriculomegaly. The syrinx extended to the middle and lower cervical spinal cord

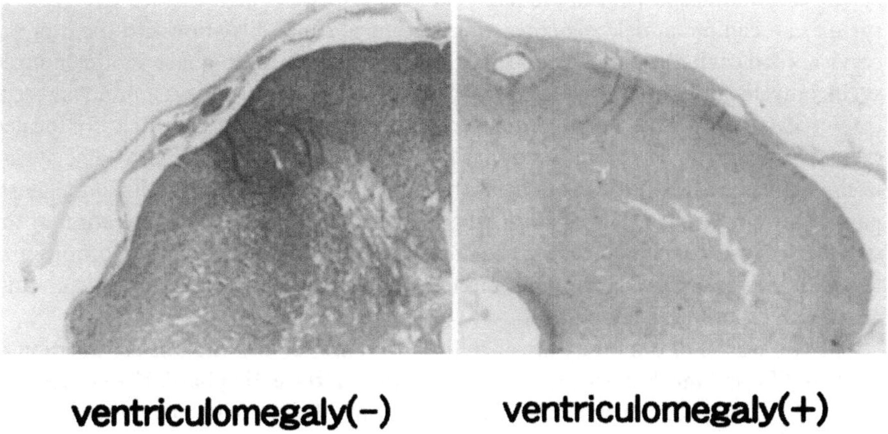

FIG. 4. Photomicrographs. *Left*: rabbit without ventriculomegaly. The central canal is not enlarged, but there was spongy change in the dorsal part of the spinal cord. *Right*: rabbit with ventriculomegaly. There is no remarkable histological abnormality in the intramedullary tissue, and the central canal is dilated without destruction of the ependymal layers

Histological Findings

Ventriculomegaly was demonstrated in thirteen rabbits. Subarachnoid kaolin accumulated around the obex and blocked the flow of cerebrospinal fluid (CSF) to the cerebellomedullary cistern. On day 3 (Fig. 4), no remarkable histological abnormalities were seen in the intramedullary tissue. The central canal was dilated from the upper to the middle cervical cord, but without any destruction of the ependymal layers. On day 7 (see Fig. 2), the central canal had become enlarged and had ruptured as far as the posterior horn in the middle of the cervical spinal cord, and the gray matter adjacent to the point of rupture had become spongy. This sponginess was especially marked in the cranial gray matter. After 14 days, the central canal showed further slow enlargement, and the intramedullary syrinx extended from the point of rupture to the upper part of the cervical spinal cord.

The rabbits without ventriculomegaly showed no enlargement of the central canal, but sponginess occurred in the dorsal part of the spinal cord (see Fig. 4). This sponginess developed in the upper part and then extended to the middle of the cervical cord (see Fig. 3). The obex was not completely filled with accumulated kaolin, and a substantial amount of kaolin remained at the craniocervical junction or the upper cervical subarachnoid space.

Discussion

Many investigators have reported on histopathological and morphological studies of kaolin-induced syringomyelia [1–5]. Chakrabortty et al. studied a chronic kaolin model and described the syrinx as a rupture of the enlarged central canal [1]. They also studied more chronic-phase (6 or 12 months) MR images and showed that the syrinx communicated with the fourth ventricle. Yamada et al. identified two types of syrinx in a canine model, one consisting of central canal dilatation and the other of cervical cord cavitation [6]. Takahashi et al. [7] studied chronic-phase kaolin-induced syringomyelia and classified syrinxes into two different types; one was round and centrally located from the fourth ventricle, and the other was an eccentrically located syrinx with varying shape in the upper and middle cervical spinal cord. The syrinx in the upper cervical cord was irregularly shaped and extended into the dorsolateral part of the spinal cord. They described the electron microscopic regeneration of the spinal cord and concluded that syringomyelia requires early treatment to minimize tissue injury, especially in the gray matter, where many important synaptic circuits are at risk of irreversible damage.

The two points of our study are as follows. The first point concerns clarification of the two different mechanisms in syrinx formation in the early phase. The syrinx consisted of a continuous dilatation of the central canal from the fourth ventricle in the rabbits with ventriculomegaly. The enlarged central canal then ruptured intramedullarly, and the syrinx progressed up to the cranial spinal cord. On the other hand, in the rabbits without ventriculomegaly, intramedullary degeneration proceeded to central canal enlargement and progressed down to the caudal spinal cord.

The second point is histopathological evidence that the presyrinx state on MR imaging is seen as sponginess of the spinal cord. Levy et al. reported a patient who developed spinal cord edema as an intermediate stage in the development of a syrinx [8]. In our study, the syrinxes identified on MR images showed microscopic sponginess in the dorsal part of the spinal cord within 3 days after kaolin injection. This sponginess may represent support for the concept of a presyrinx state.

References

1. Chakrabortty S, Tamaki N, Ehara K, Ide C (1994) Experimental syringomyelia in the rabbit: an ultra-structural study of the spinal cord tissue. Neurosurgery 35:1112–1120
2. Cho KH, Iwasaki Y, Imamura H, et al (1994) Experimental model of posttraumatic syringomyelia: the role of adhesive arachnoiditis in syrinx formation. J Neurosurg 80:133–139
3. Dohrmann GI (1972) Cervical spinal cord in experimental hydrocephalus. J Neurosurg 37:538–542
4. McLaurin RL, Baily OT, Schurr PH, Ingraham FD (1954) Myelomalacia and multiple cavitations of spinal cord secondary to adhesive arachnoiditis: an experimental study. Arch Pathol 57:138–146
5. Tatara N (1992) Experimental syringomyelia in rabbits and rats after localized spinal arachnoiditis. No To Shinkei 44:1115–1125 (in Japanese)
6. Yamada H, Yokota A, Haratake I, Horie A (1996) Morphological study of experimental syringomyelia with kaolin-induced hydrocephalus in a canine model. J Neurosurg 84:999–1005
7. Takahashi A, Tamaki N, Kurata H, et al (1999) Effect of cerebrospinal fluid shunting on experimental syringomyelia: magnetic resonance imaging and histological findings. Neurol Med Chir (Tokyo) 39:668–679
8. Levy EI, Heiss JD, Kent MS, et al. (2000) Spinal cord swelling preceding syrinx development. J Neurosurg (Spine 1) 92:93–97

Histological Evaluation for the Mechanism of Syrinx Formation in the Rat Experimental Model with Injury and Secondary Adhesive Arachnoiditis

Junichi Mizuno[1], Hiroshi Nakagawa[1], Yoshio Hashizume[2], and Masanori Isobe[3]

Summary. To elucidate the mechanism of cavity formation, histological findings of the spinal cord of the rat experimental model with injury and secondary adhesive arachnoiditis were examined. Twenty-two Wistar rat spinal cords were injured by epidural clipping at the level of T8 (model 1). Among these 22 specimens, 11 rats were injected with kaolin solution into the subarachnoid space of the lower lumbar spine (model 2). Rats were killed 2–16 days after injury. The spine and spinal cord were removed en bloc and sectioned transversely. Both models showed a high rate of syrinx formation (10/12 in model 1; 8/10 in model 2) in the gray matter to the posterior column with no relation to the central canal. In the early stage, parenchymal bleeding occurred, and an intramedullary cavity with surrounding reactive cells was then formed in the later stage. Venous dilatation and occlusion of subarachnoid space were more prominent in model 2. The size of the cavity enlarged chronologically. Syrinx formation in these experimental models indicated that the intramedullary cavity was initially caused by mechanical stress and was enhanced by circulatory disturbance with or without arachnoiditis. We conclude that syringomyelia caused by injury is the result of intramedullary degeneration in association with arachnoiditis, which makes it difficult to treat.

Key words. Syringomyelia, Injury, Arachnoiditis, Mechanism, Histology

Introduction

Posttraumatic syringomyelia is a well-known complication as a sequala of spinal cord injury; however, its pathogenesis remains obscure [1]. Several causative factors such as trauma, intramedullary hemorrhage, infarction, and inflammatory changes have been reported [2–4]. Seemingly, posttraumatic cavity formation is initiated by trauma and associated intramedullary destruction and is aggravated by the secondary adhe-

[1]Department of Neurological Surgery, [2]Institute of Medical Science for Aging, Aichi Medical University, 21 Karimata, Yazako, Nagakute, Aichi-gun, Aichi 480-1195, Japan
[3]Neurosurgery, Teine Keijinkai Hospital, 1-2-355 Maeda, Teine-ku, Sapporo 006-8555, Japan

sive arachnoiditis. Caplan et al. [3] and Williams [2] described the similarity between posttraumatic and postinflammatory syringomyelia. The location of the cavity is in the watershed zone of the spinal cord with no relation to the central canal [1].

To elucidate the pathogenesis of syringomyelia, various experimental models have been reported [5–7]. Syringomyelia produced by kaolin-induced hydrocephalus is the model most widely used for communicating syringomyelia; therefore, syringomyelia without relation to the central canal is rarely observed [6]. Cho et al. [5] reported that animals experimentally treated with kaolin injection into the subarachnoid space and spinal cord injury by weight-drop contusion frequently showed intramedullary cavity formation.

In this chapter, we pay special attention to the morphological changes of the spinal cord after trauma with or without adhesive arachnoiditis and consider the possible mechanism of syrinx formation.

Materials and Methods

Animal Preparation

Twenty-two male Wistar rats, each weighing about 250 g, were used for this study. The rats were anesthetized by diethyl ether inhalation and subsequent intraabdominal injection of pentobarbital sodium. The rats were placed in a prone position on a surgical table, and laminectomy at T8 was performed. Spinal cord injury was created by placing a #53 Sugita clip around the cord epidurally at 70 g for 30 s (model 1). Of these 22 rats, 11 rats received kaolin solution (200 mg/ml/kg) into the subarachnoid space in the lumbar spine at the same time (model 2). The wound was closed and the rats were allowed to recover and survive with special care and housing. All rats showed paraparesis in various degrees after surgery, and were killed at 2 days or at 1, 2, 4, 6, 8, or 16 weeks after operation.

Histological Preparation

The spine and spinal cord were removed en bloc and fixed immediately in 10% formalin. These specimens were sectioned transversely at each segment and stained with hematoxylin and eosin (H&E). Each transverse section was analyzed microscopically.

Results

Occurrence Rate

The occurrence rate of syrinx formation was 83.3% (10 of 12 rats) in model 1 and 80% (8 of 10 rats) in model 2. Both models showed a high occurrence rate.

Pathology of Spinal Cord and Syrinx

Model 1: Injury Only

By 48 h after operation, no cavity formation was observed; however, small parenchymal hemorrhage and spongy or microcystic changes occurred in the posterior

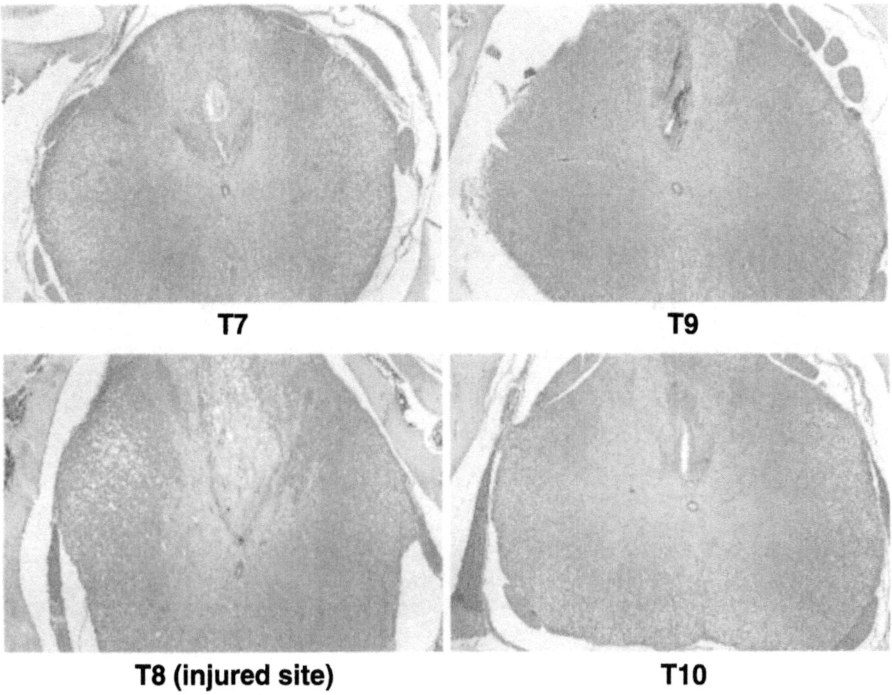

FIG. 1. Photomicrographs of specimens 48 h after operation show small parenchymal hemorrhage, cystic degeneration, and microcavity formation in the several consecutive segments rostrally and caudally from the injured site. Hematoxylin and eosin (H&E). ×40

column in several segments rostally and caudally from the injured site (Fig. 1). At more than 2 weeks after operation, an obvious intramedullary cavity had developed. The cavity was situated in the posterior column to the gray matter without ependymal lining. The cavity was usually oval and separated from the central canal. The margin of the cavity was essentially irregular with the adjacent parenchyma (Fig. 2). In the later stage, defined as longer than 8 weeks after operation, development of cavity formation was more prone to occur both rostrally and caudally. The margin of the cavity was rather regular, and reactive gliosis and macrophages or lymphocytes were observed around the margin of the cystic changes (Fig. 3).

Model 2: Combined Injury and Arachnoiditis

There was no significant difference in the size, extent, and location of the cavity or the parenchymal spongy changes around the cavity between model 1 and model 2. However, the subarachnoid space was largely obstructed or narrow as the result of kaolin-induced granulation. The venous system in granulation became enlarged, indicating venous congestion. The cavity was clearly separated from the central canal (Fig. 4).

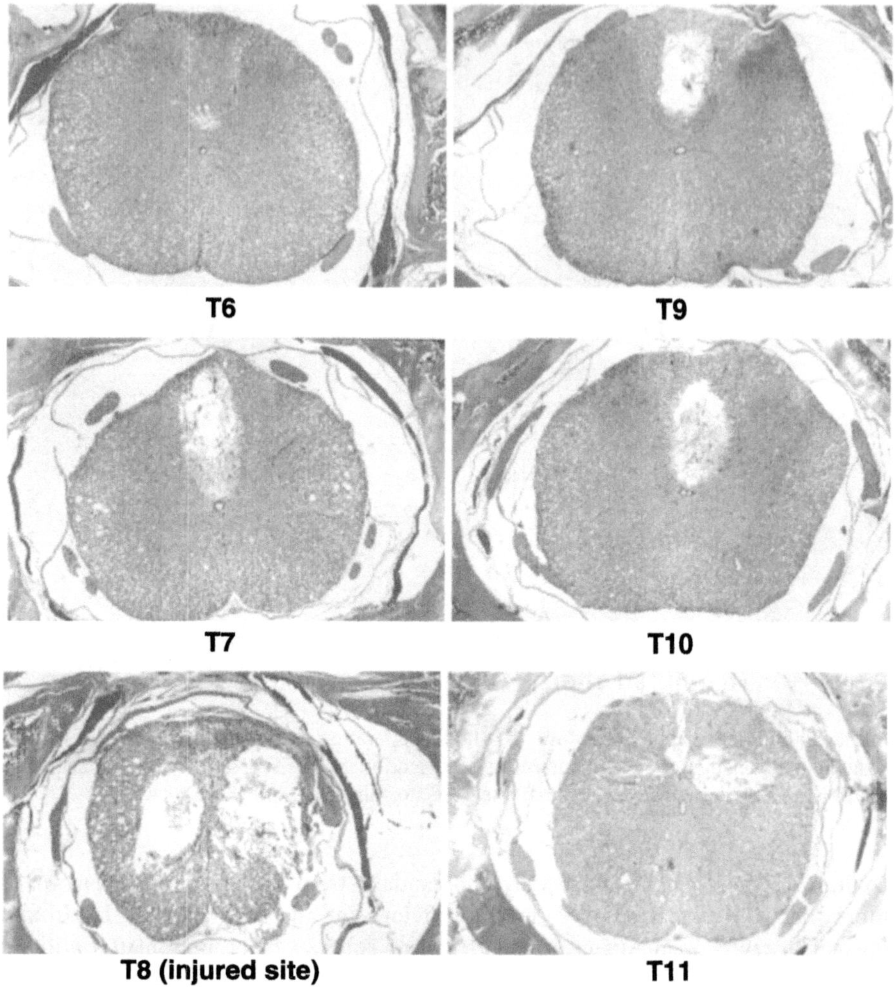

FIG. 2. Photomicrographs of specimens 4 weeks after operation show cavity formation continuously from the injured site rostrally and caudally, several segments in both directions. H&E. ×40

Discussion

Many theories relating to the pathogenesis of syringomyelia have been proposed based on the causative or underlying pathology including Chiari malformation, intramedullary tumor, trauma, or arachnoiditis [2,8–10]. Milhorat et al. [1] classified syrinx into three subtypes on the basis of location in the axial plane, and found that cavity in the posterior column and the gray matter without ependymal lining was prone to develop in trauma and arachnoiditis. This type of syringomyelia is resistant to treatments, and therefore the Japanese Ministry of Health and Welfare organized a multicenter study beginning in 1993.

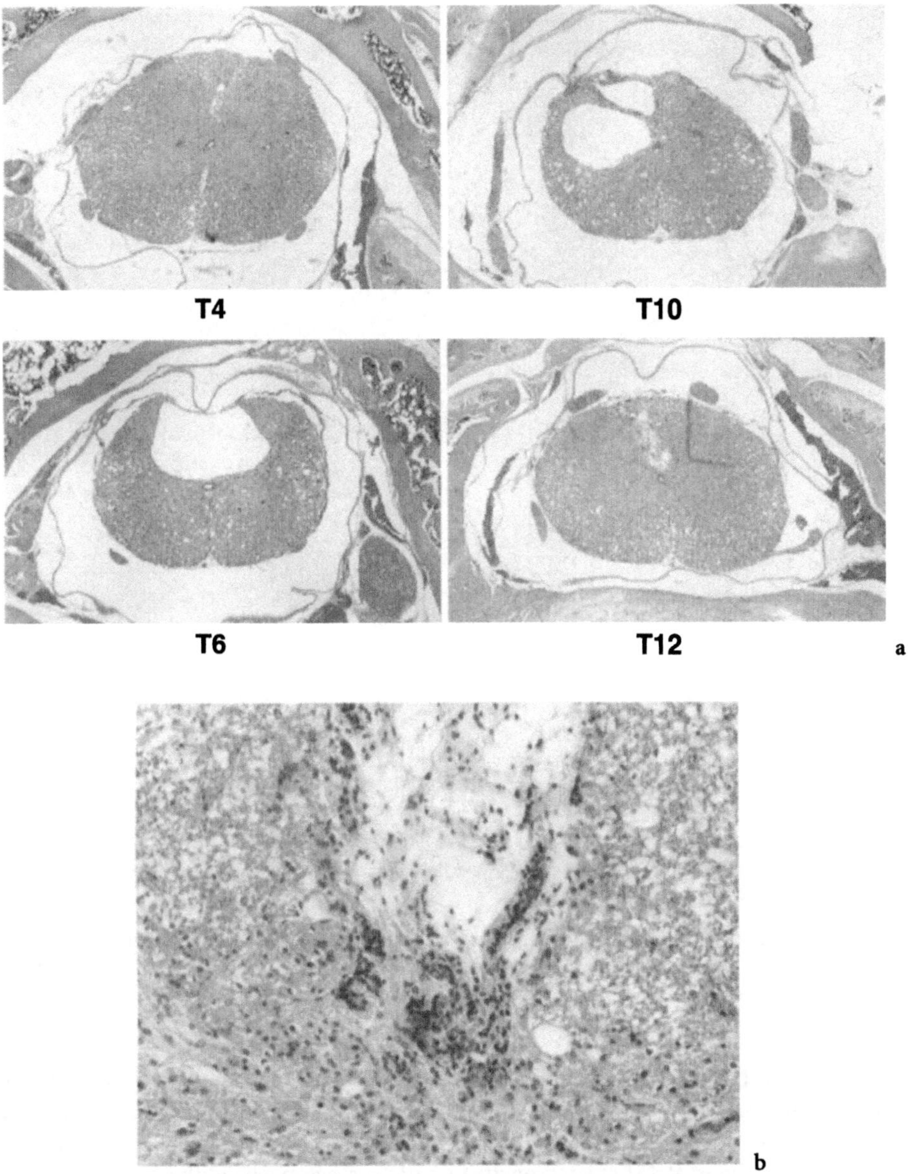

FIG. 3. **a** Photomicrographs of specimens 16 weeks after operation show more extended cavity formation with rather regular margin. H&E. ×40. **b** Higher power of specimen in active portion shows collection of lymphocytes and macrophages around the cavity. H&E. ×100

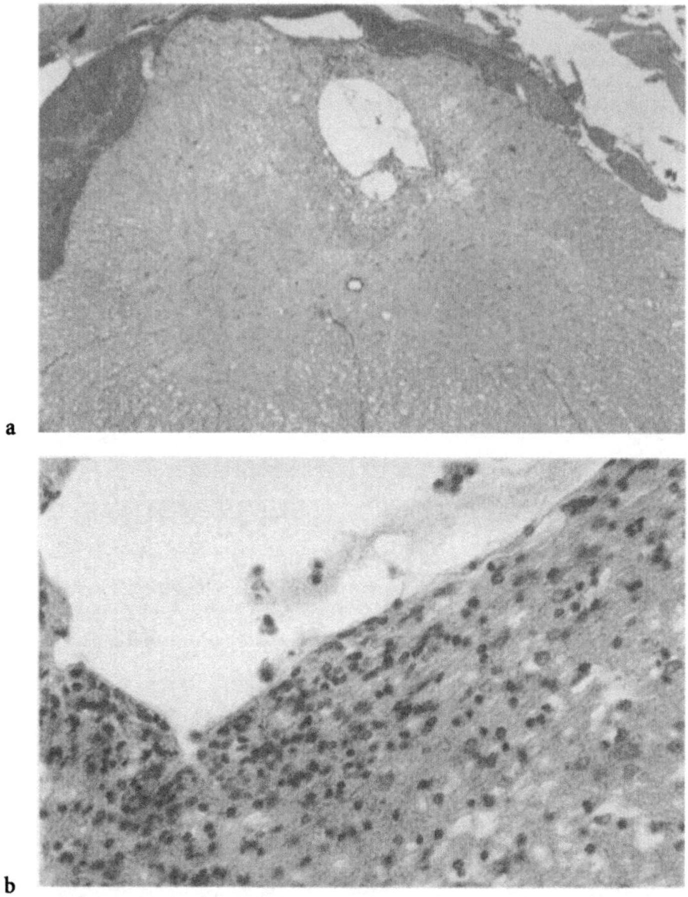

FIG. 4. Photomicrographs of specimens show (**a**) cavity formation in the posterior column and granulation in the subarachnoid space with dilated veins and (**b**) reactive lymphocytes and macrophages in the parenchyma adjacent to the cavity. H&E. ×100 (**a**); ×400 (**b**)

Although the mechanism of posttraumatic syringomyelia is not fully understood, direct mechanical injury together with the secondary insults of the damaged spinal cord such as ischemia, edema, and local arachnoiditis may enhance cavity extension [2,4,11,12]. Cho et al. [5] created posttraumatic syringomyelia with or without arachnoiditis using the rabbit as an experimental model and suggested subarachnoid block secondary to adhesive arachnoiditis was important in initiating extension of the syringomyelia cavity. However, our experimental models did not show a significant difference in occurrence rate or extension of the syrinx between model 1 and model 2. There was no communication between the syrinx and the central canal or the subarachnoid space except for the injured segment. Intramedullary pathological changes including hemorrhage and cystic necrosis in the posterior column in the early stage and cavity formation with proliferation of macrophages and lymphocytes and reactive gliosis in the late stage after trauma in our models indicate that cystic necrosis by trauma increases intrapial pressure, and secondary arachnoiditis encasing the cord then disturbs venous circulation, resulting in progression of cystic changes. Narrowing of the subarachnoid space by reactive granuloma disturbs the normal movement of cerebrospinal fluid (CSF) and promotes the longitudinal extension of syrinx formation.

Although the results obtained in this study show only histological changes, cystic necrosis by trauma and secondary venous infarction and irregular movement of the CSF are considered to play an important role in posttraumatic syringomyelia.

References

1. Milhorat TH, Capocelli AL Jr, Anzil AP, et al (1995) Pathological basis of spinal cord cavitation in syringomyelia: analysis of 105 autopsy cases. J Neurosurg 82:802–812
2. Williams B (1990) Post-traumatic syringomyelia, an update. Paraplegia 28:296–313
3. Caplan LR, Norohna AB, Amico LL (1990) Syringomyelia and arachnoiditis. J Neurol Neurosurg Psychiatry 53:106–113
4. Umbach I, Heilporn A (1981) Post-spinal cord injury syringomyelia. Paraplegia 29: 219–221
5. Cho KH, Iwasaki Y, Imamura H, et al (1994) Experimental model of posttraumatic syringomyelia: the role of adhesive arachnoiditis in syrinx formation. J Neurosurg 80:133–139
6. Yamada H, Yokota A, Haratake J, et al (1996) Morphological study of experimental syringomyelia with kaolin-induced hydrocephalus in a canine model. J Neurosurg 84:999–1005
7. Milhorat TH, Nobandegani F, Miller JI, et al (1993) Noncommunicating syringomyelia following occlusion of central canal in rats. Experimental model and histological findings. J Neurosurg 78:274–279
8. Ball MJ, Dayan AD (1972) Pathogenesis of syringomyelia. Lancet 2:799–801
9. Gardner WJ (1965) Hydrodynamic mechanism of syringomyelia: its relationship to myelocele. J Neurol Neurosurg Psychiatry 28:247–259
10. Taylor AR (1975) Another theory of the aetiology of the syringomyelia cavity. J Neurol Neurosurg Psychiatry 38:825
11. Feigin I, Ogata J, Budzilovich G (1971) Syringomyelia: the role of edema in its pathogenesis. J Neurol Neurosurg Psychiatry 53:106–113
12. Oakley JC, Ojemann GA, Alvord EC Jr (1981) Posttraumatic syringomyelia. Case report. J Neurosurg 55:276–281

Role of Active Cerebrospinal Fluid Transport in Syrinx Formation: An Experimental Study on a Model of Chronic Tonsillar Herniation in Rats

Yoshinori Yamazaki, Shigekuni Tachibana, and Kiyotaka Fujii

Summary. To identify a definite causal relationship between tonsillar herniation and syringomyelia, the dynamics of the cerebrospinal fluid in an animal model of syringomyelia caused by chronic tonsillar herniation was studied. In ten rats of the chronic tonsillar herniation model, 20% wheat germ agglutinin conjugated to horseradish peroxidase (WGA-HRP) solution was continuously injected into the lateral ventricle for 24 h using an osmotic pump. After injection, the rats were killed and electron and light microscopic analysis was performed. Four normal rats were subjected to the same surgical procedures for controls. In six of ten rats, all experimental steps were successfully performed, and tonsillar herniations were observed in two rats. In these two rats, WGA-HRP was found in the luminal space of the dilated central canal, inside the ependymal cells, and in the swollen astrocytic processes in the dorsal gray matter, reaching to the dorsal column. In the control group and four transplanted rats without tonsillar herniations, no WGA-HRP was detected in the spinal cord. It is apparent that, in the rats with tonsillar herniations, cerebrospinal fluid flowed into the central canal and was transported into the astrocytes through the ependymal cells.

Key words. Syringomyelia, Tonsillar herniation, Chiari malformations, Horseradish peroxidase, Pathogenesis

Introduction

We previously developed an experimental model of syringomyelia caused by chronic tonsillar herniation in the rat and reported this elsewhere [1]. In the present study, to clarify the pathogenesis of syrinx formation, the dynamics of cerebrospinal fluid (CSF) flow were studied using this animal model.

Materials and Methods

The experiments were carried out using adult female Fischer strain rats weighing 120–160 g each. The animals were anesthetized with sodium pentobarbital, 1 mg/kg, given intraperitoneally.

Department of Neurosurgery, Kitasato University School of Medicine, 1-15-1 Kitasato, Sagamihara, Kanagawa 228-8555, Japan

Injection of Horseradish Peroxidase-Conjugated Wheat Germ Agglutinin into the Lateral Ventricle of Normal Rat (Control Group)

Four normal rats received stereotaxic tapping of the lateral ventricle under anesthesia; a 20% horseradish peroxidase-conjugated wheat germ agglutinin (WGA-HRP) solution was then continuously injected into the ventricle for 24h (flow rate, 1.0µl/h) using an Alzet osmotic pump (model 1003D; CA, USA). The pump, containing 20% WGA-HRP solution, was implanted into a subcutaneous pocket in the back of the rat. After injection, the animals were reanesthetized and killed by total body perfusion.

Specimens for light microscopy were taken from the brain (at the tapping point of the lateral ventricle) and multiple levels of the spinal cord (C3, C5, T3, T8, T12, and L2 segments). After routine processing, specimens were embedded in paraffin, sectioned, and stained with hematoxylin and eosin as well as luxol fast blue. Tissue samples for electron microscopy were taken as for light microscopy. Specimens were sectioned at 70µm on a Vibratome and stained free floating using diaminobenzidine (DAB) according to the method of Graham and Karnovsky [2].

Injection of WGA-HRP into the Lateral Ventricle of Chronic Tonsillar Herniation Model Rats

In ten rats, to produce chronic tonsillar herniation, a small piece of mammary cancer weighing approximately 3mg was transplanted to the supraoccipital bone under anesthesia (the detailed method to produce the model has been reported elsewhere [1]). In the previous study, tonsillar herniation occurred about 8 weeks after transplantation. Therefore, in this study, the continuous injection of 20% WGA-HRP solution into the lateral ventricle was performed after posttransplantation intervals of 6 weeks (one rat), 8 weeks (two rats), 9 weeks (two rats), 10 weeks (two rats), 11 weeks (two rats), and 12 weeks (one rat) in the same manner as the control animals. Light and electron microscopic analysis were also performed in the same manner for the control animals.

Results

Control Group

In the control rats ($n = 4$), all the experimental steps were successfully performed. On light microscopy, no pathological changes were observed in the spinal cord. By electron microscopy, the WGA-HRP reaction product was detected in the lateral ventricle but not in the spinal cord parenchyma, including the luminal space of the central canal.

Chronic Tonsillar Herniation Model

In six of ten rats receiving cancer transplantation, all the experimental steps were successfully performed. Tonsillar herniation was observed in two of these six rats at 8 and 9 weeks, respectively, after transplantation. The histological findings of the spinal cord and localization of the WGA-HRP reaction product in the two rats are described as follows.

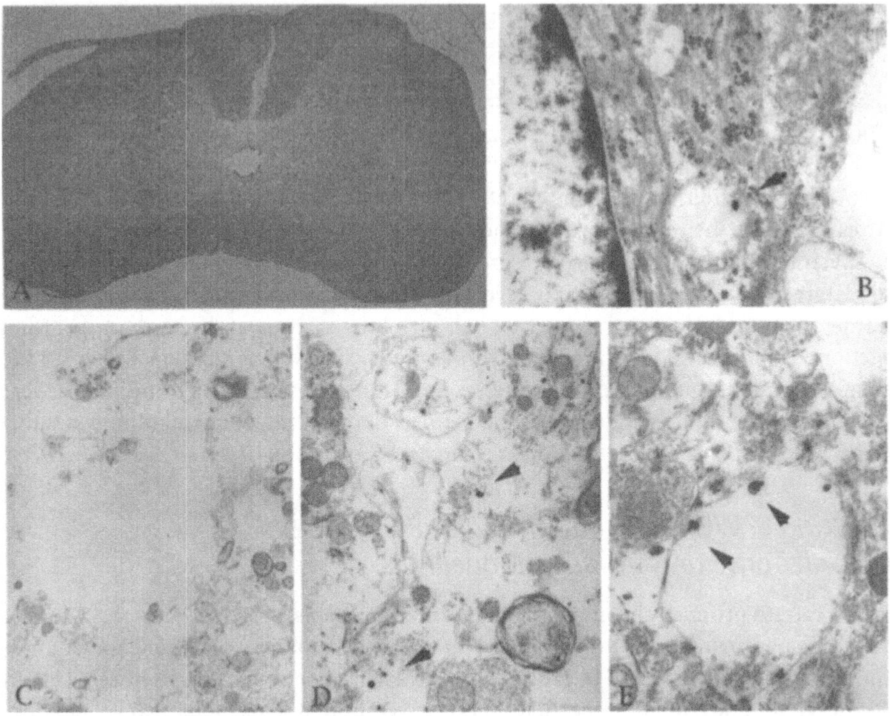

FIG. 1. **A** Photomicrograph of the cervical spinal cord (C5 segment). The central canal is dilated, and tissue loosening with a small syrinx cavity is apparent in the area extending from the dorsal side of the central canal to the ventral inner portion of the dorsal column. There is no evidence of arachnoiditis around the spinal cord. Hematoxylm and eosm (H&E). ×10. **B** Electron photomicrograph of an ependymal cell of the same specimen as **A.** A small vesicle including a wheat germ agglutinin-horse radish peroxidase (WGA-HRP) reaction product (*arrow*) and clear fluid is recognized in an ependymal cell. ×15 000. **C** Electron photomicrograph at site of a syrinx cavity shows no WGA-HRP reaction product in the cavity. ×3000. **D** Electron photomicrograph of peripheral portion of the syrinx cavity shows marked swelling and necrosis of the astrocytes. A few WGA-HRP reaction products (*arrows*) are visible. ×5000. **E** Electron photomicrograph of the subependymal gray matter. WGA-HRP reaction products (*arrows*) and clear fluid are recognized in the swollen astrocyte. ×16 000

Case 1: Killed 8 Weeks After Transplantation

In this rat, syrinx formation in the spinal cord was confirmed (Fig. 1A). Syrinx formation was prominent from the C5 to the T8 segments. On electron microscopy, some WGA-HRP reaction product was detected in the dilated central canal and in the ependymal cells, but not in the intercellular space between the adjacent ependymal cells (Fig. 1B). In the gray matter, WGA-HRP reaction product was seen in the swollen astrocytes around the central canal (Fig. 1E) and the peripheral portion of the syrinx cavity in the dorsal gray matter (Fig. 1D). No WGA-HRP reaction product was detected in the syrinx cavity itself (Fig. 1C) or in the extracellular space. At the level of the spinal cord, WGA-HRP reaction products were prominently observed from C5 to T8 segments.

Case 2: Killed 9 weeks After Transplantation

Tonsillar herniation had already occurred in this rat; however, histological changes of the spinal cord were still slight. The central canal was slightly dilated and mild swelling of astrocytes was observed in the dorsal gray matter. In contrast, a remarkable WGA-HRP reaction was observed. As shown in Fig. 2A, the reaction was recognized in the confined gray matter that was located around the central canal. On electron microscopy, much WGA-HRP reaction product was detected in the dilated central canal and in the ependymal cells (Fig. 2B). In the gray matter, copious WGA-HRP reaction products were detected in the swollen astrocytes around the central canal and in the dorsal gray matter reaching to the dorsal column (Fig. 2C). No WGA-HRP reaction product could be seen in the extracellular space in the gray matter. These findings were the same as in case 1; however, the amount WGA-HRP reaction product in the ependymal cells and the astrocytes was much greater than in case 1.

Transplanted Rats Without Tonsillar Herniation

In the transplanted rats without tonsillar herniation ($n = 4$), WGA-HRP reaction product was detected in the lateral ventricle but not in the spinal cord parenchyma, including the luminal space of the central canal, as in the control group.

Discussion

Chronic Tonsillar Herniation Model

Compared to the previously reported animal models of syringomyelia such as caused by kaolin hydrocephalus [3–6], our model is unique in achieving syrinx formation caused solely by chronic tonsillar herniation. Therefore, our model is more suitable than the kaolin-induced model for mimicry of syringomyelia in patients with posterior fossa abnormalities.

Dynamics of CSF: WGA-HRP Study

In the previous study, it was confirmed that the essential findings of the spinal cord following tonsillar herniation were that dilatation of the central canal, associated with histological changes of the ependymal cells and swelling of the astrocytic processes in the surrounding gray matter, preceded syrinx cavity formation. We therefore considered that the syrinx cavity was caused by an influx of CSF from the dilated central canal through the impaired ependymal cell layer and that astrocyte dysfunction might have been a contributing factor.

As shown in the results, WGA-HRP was detected in the spinal cord parenchyma, including the luminal space of the central canal, only in the rats with tonsillar herniation but not in rats without tonsillar herniation. In the spinal cord parenchyma, WGA-HRP was detected in the ependymal cells and astrocytes that were located

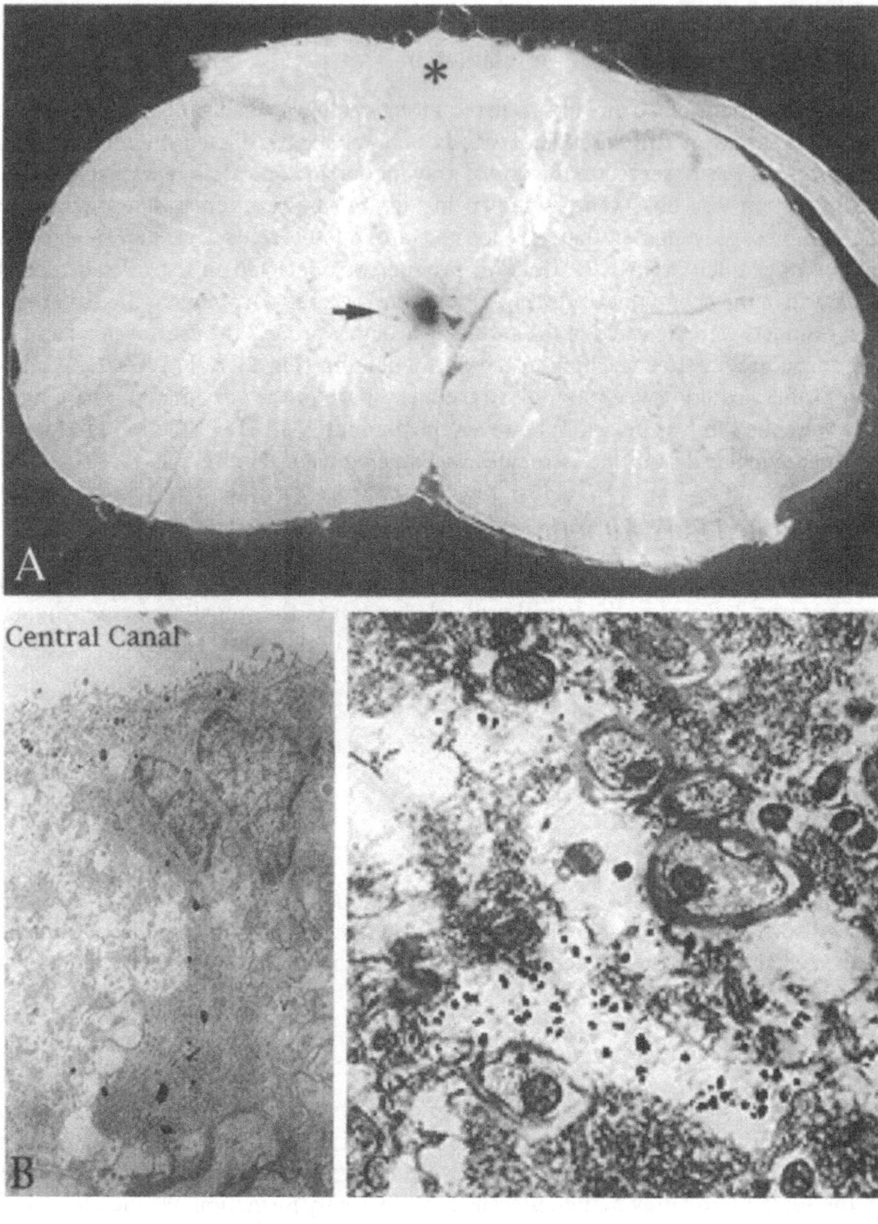

FIG. 2. **A** Stereoscopic photomicrograph of the cervical spinal cord (C5 segment). The WGA-HRP reaction is clearly observed in the gray matter located around the central canal (*arrow*), but no WGA-HRP reaction is recognized in the surface of the spinal cord. *Asterisk*, posterior column. ×10. **B** Electron photomicrograph of ependymal cells of the same specimen as **A**. Much WGA-HRP reaction product is recognized in the ependymal cells but not in the intercellular space. ×1500. **C** Electron photomicrograph of the subependymal gray matter. Copious WGA-HRP reaction products and clear fluid are recognized in the swollen astrocyte. ×6000

around the central canal reaching to the dorsal column, but not in the surface of the spinal cord. These results suggest that the CSF flowed into the central canal and then was transported into the spinal cord parenchyma. Furthermore, CSF transportation should have been accomplished by some biological function, not by mechanical pressure because WGA-HRP was present in the astrocytes and also in the ependymal cells but not in the intercellular space between the adjacent ependymal cells or in the extracellular space in the gray matter. This result suggests the existence of a system of active CSF evacuation by the ependymal cells and astrocytes. More WGA-HRP reaction products were observed in case 2 than in case 1. Degenerative changes of the spinal cord were mild in case 2 and remarkable in case 1. Based on these results, it can be said that biological functions of the ependymal cell and astrocyte might be still active in case 2, so that much WGA-HRP could be taken up by the spinal cord parenchyma.

Pathogenesis of Syringomyelia in Our Model

Based on the results of our current and previous study [1], the pathogenesis of syrinx formation in our chronic tonsillar herniation model is considered to be as follows. First of all, CSF flow at the foramen magnum is obstructed following tonsillar herniation. Then, CSF flows into the central canal and dilates it. To evacuate the surplus CSF in the central canal, an active CSF evacuation system may be initiated by the ependymal cells and the astrocytes. When the system reaches its limits, the overloaded astrocytes develop a swollen state and dysfunction, finally reaching necrosis. Syrinx formation is a result of these biological functions and their breakdown.

References

1. Yamazaki Y, Tachibana S, Ohta N, et al (1995) Experimental model of chronic tonsillar herniation associated with early stage syringomyelia. Acta Neuropathol (Berl) 90:425–431
2. Graham RC, Karnovsky MJ (1966) The early stages of injected horseradish peroxidase in the proximal tubule of mouse kidney: ultrastructual cytochemistry by a new technique. J Histochem 14:291–303
3. Becker DP, Wilson JA, Watson GW (1972) The spinal cord central canal: response to experimental hydrocephalus and canal occlusion. J Neurosurg 36:416–424
4. Dohrmann GJ (1972) Cervical spinal cord in experimental hydrocephalus. J Neurosurg 37:538–542
5. Mclaurin RL, Bailey OT, Schurr PH, et al (1954) Myelomalacia and multiple cavitations of spinal cord secondary to adhesive arachnoiditis. Arch Pathol 57:138–146
6. Rascher K, Booz KH, Donauer E, et al (1987) Structural alterations in the spinal cord during progressive communicating syringomyelia. An experimental study in the cat. Acta Neuropathol (Berl) 72:248–255

Biomechanical Changes of the Spinal Cord Caused by Chiari I Malformation

Tatsuya Nagashima[1], Kazuki Yamamoto[1], Ayumi Takahashi[1], Shogo Tamura[1], Mitsugu Nakamura[1], Norihiko Tamaki[1], Yukio Tada[2], and Shinichiro Asada[2]

Summary. Biomechanical and hydrodynamic analysis of the spinal cord was performed to understand the pathogenesis of syringomyelia associated with Chiari I malformation. A finite element analysis of intraspinal stress distribution was done by a newly developed two-dimensional elastic craniocervical model of Chiari I malformation. The finite element model was refined to simulate the effect of the generation of an intraspinal cavity on stress distribution. Three different models —normal, Chiari I malformation, and Chiari I malformation with syrinx—were constructed with triangular elastic elements. Different material properties such as brain, spinal cord, disk, bone, and cerebrospinal fluid (CSF) were added to each element. On neck extension and flexion, the calculated intraspinal stress was concentrated in the upper cervical spinal cord where the cerebellar tonsil had herniated. The presence of the intraspinal cavity generated stress around the cavity itself. Intraspinal stress concentration associated with the presence of Chiari I malformation may play a role in syrinx initiation, after which the formation of a small syrinx promotes further stress concentration around it and results in the progression of the syrinx.

Key words. Syringomyelia, Biomechanics, Chiari malformation, MRI, Computer simulation

Introduction

The questions we asked were "Where does the syrinx associated with Chiari I malformation start to grow in the spinal cord?" and "Is there any specific point from which the syrinx starts to grow?" We can consider two types of syrinx generation, one in which the syrinx start to grow from the cranial end and extends caudally, and the other where the syrinx starts to grow from elsewhere in the caudal spinal cord, extends cranially, and stops at the level of the tonsillar impaction. Since Gardner presented the

[1] Department of Neurosurgery, Kobe University, Graduate School of Medicine, 7-5-1 Kusunoki-cho, Chuo-ku, Kobe 650-0017, Japan
[2] Department of Computer and Systems Engineering, Faculty of Engineering, Kobe University, Kobe, Japan

"hydrodynamic theory," hydrodynamic factors have been extensively studied. However, biomechanical factors such as stress or tissue pressure change in the spinal cord have been much less studied. We therefore studied changes in stress distribution in the spinal cord caused by the presence of tonsilar impaction to answer the two questions asked earlier.

Materials and Methods

The finite element method (FEM), which is a method widely used in engineering fields from the design of airplanes to that of atomic plants, was applied to simulate intraspinal stress distribution in cases of Chiari I malformation. A craniocervical finite element model with elastic elements was constructed using triangular elements (Fig. 1, left). The cervical cord was constructed from fine elements to obtain details of stress distribution. This model represents mass, mass center, and moment of inertia of the head and neck, as well as anatomic dimensions and different material properties, such as those of bone, spinal cord, disks, ligaments, and cerebrospinal fluid (CSF). All materials were assumed to be elastic. Different

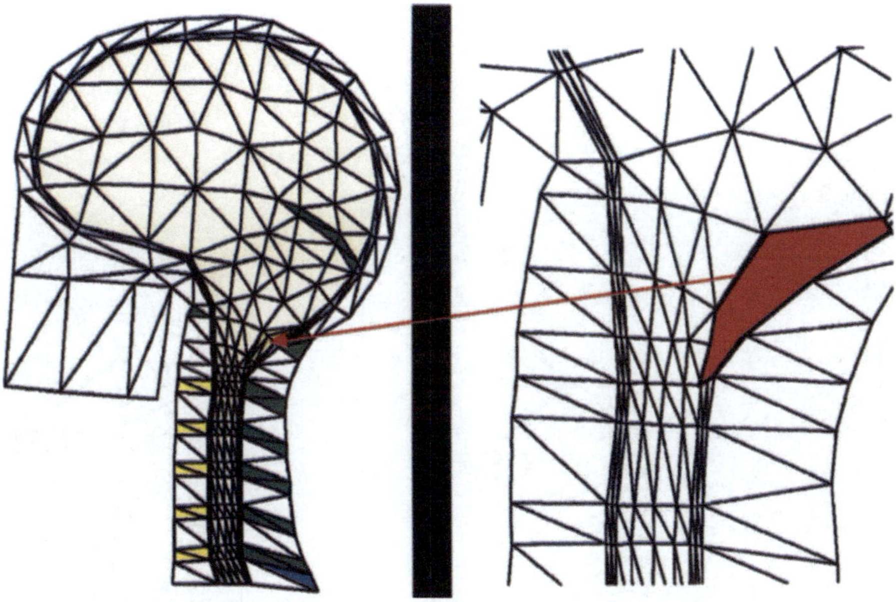

FIG. 1. *Left*: Finite element model of the normal brain and spinal cord. Fine triangular elements were employed to simulate details of the stress distribution in the spinal cord. Brain and spinal cord are shown in *light yellow*, disk in *yellow*, connective tissue in *green*, bone in *white*, and cerebrospinal fluid (CSF) in *light blue*. *Right*: In the Chiari I malformation model, the material properties of the elements at the cisterna magna (*red area*) were changed from those of CSF to those of the brain

material properties, Young's module, and Poisson ratio as reported in the literature were added to each element. In the Chiari I malformation model, CSF elements at the cisterna magna were changed to brain properties (Fig. 1, right) to mimic the descending tonsil. To simulate the presence of an early syrinx, material properties of several elements in the spinal cord corresponding to the area of stress concentration were changed to those of CSF. Changes in intraspinal distribution at neck flexion and extension were simulated, and the strength of effective stress was represented by the size of the circles.

Results

1. When neck flexion and extension were applied to the normal model, small and diffuse stress was exerted on the cervical spinal cord (Fig. 2). Neck flexion resulted in tensile stress on the dorsal side and compressive stress on the ventral side of the spinal cord. At extension, tensile stress appeared on the ventral side and compressive stress on the dorsal side of the spinal cord. There was no specific point from which the syrinx starts to grow in the spinal cord in the normal model.

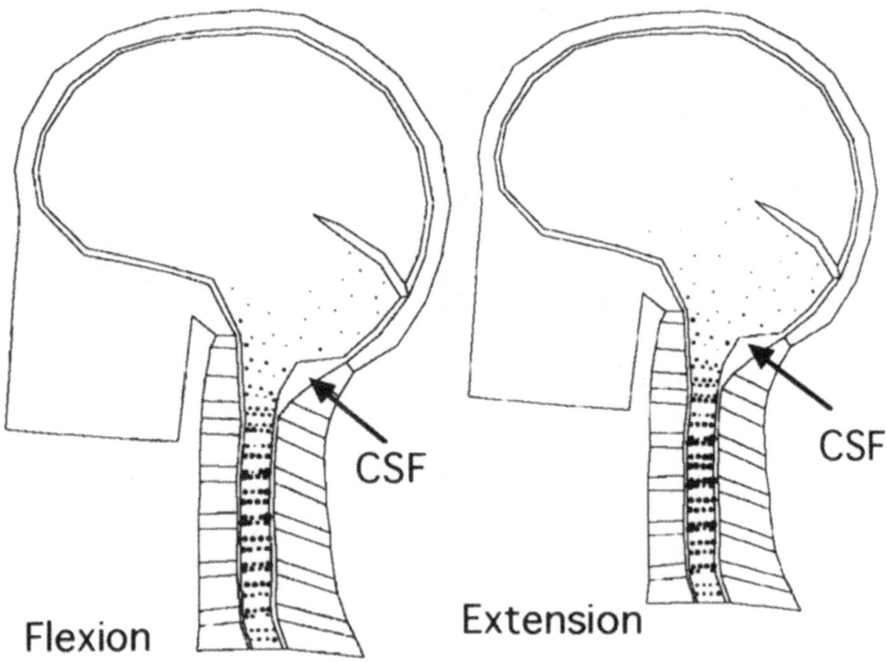

Fig. 2. Neck extension (*right*) and flexion (*left*) in the normal model. *Circles* represent intraspinal distribution of effective stress. Magnitude of stress is represented by the size of the circles. Midcervical stress seems to be relatively high, although there is no specific point from which the syrinx starts to grow. *CSF*, cerebrospinal fluid

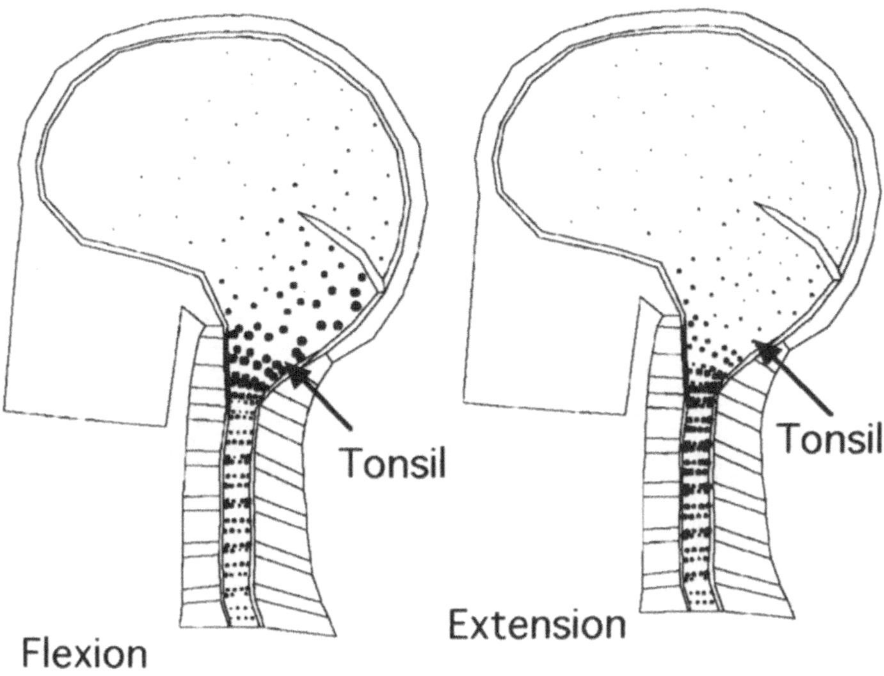

FIG. 3. Neck extension (*right*) and flexion (*left*) in the Chiari I malformation model. Stress concentration appears in the spinal cord adjacent to the descending tonsil. Stress in the upper and midcervical spinal cord does not change significantly

2. In the Chiari I model, on the other hand, marked stress concentration was generated at the craniocervical junction, especially in the spinal cord below the lower end of the descending tonsil (Fig. 3). From this specific point, the syrinx starts to grow. It is easy to see that this stress concentration also causes the neurological signs and symptoms of upper cervical cord compression in clinical cases.

3. When a small syrinx was generated at the point where the stress was concentrated, new stress concentration appeared around the syrinx (Fig. 4). This newly generated stress concentration may cause extension of the syrinx.

Discussion

There are many hypotheses concerning the mechanism of syrinx formation associated with Chiari I malformation [1–6]. Abnormality of CSF hydrodynamics at the foramen magnum is widely accepted as a mechanism of syrinx generation, but an hypothesis based on CSF hydrodynamics alone cannot explain the whole process of syrinx generation and evolution. Recent magnetic resonance imaging (MRI) findings have shown no communication between the syrinx and the fourth ventricle, so that current thinking favors some form of transparenchymal fluid migration as a mecha-

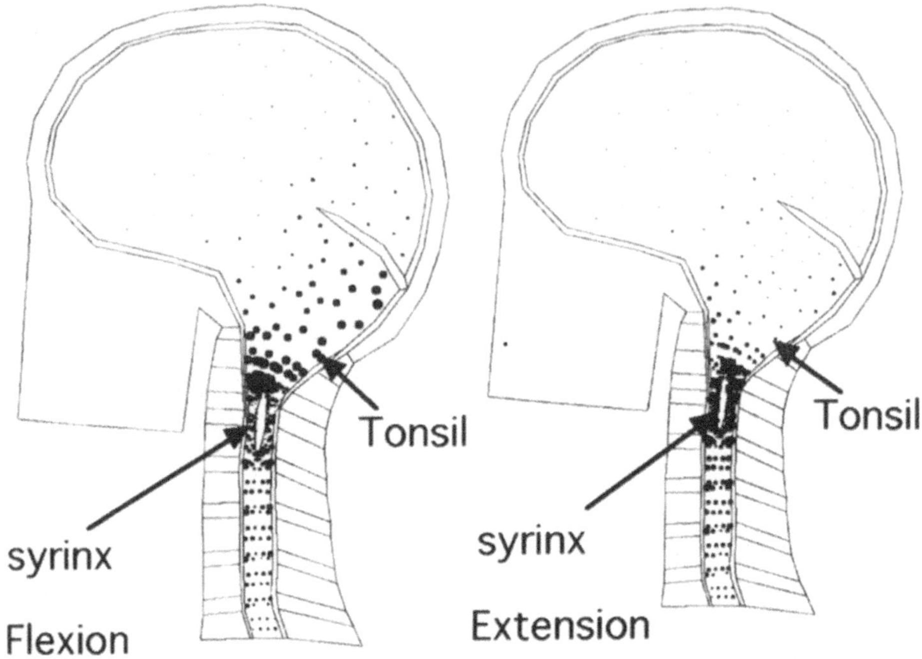

FIG. 4. Neck extension (*right*) and flexion (*left*) in the Chiari I malformation model with a small intraspinal syrinx. Stress concentration appeared around the small syrinx (*arrows*)

nism of syrinx formation. As for transparenchymal CSF migration, existence of a hydrostatic pressure gradient between the subarachnoid place and the syrinx must be assumed. However, in the very early stages of syrinx formation, i.e., when there is no syrinx in the spinal cord, it is impossible to assume a hydrostatic pressure difference between the two compartments.

Biomechanical factors are another important factor that needs to be discussed. Chiari I malformation can cause mechanical changes at the craniocervical junction such as intraspinal stress concentration. It is well known that the normal spinal cord can be elongated by neck flexion and shortened by neck extension [7]. This dynamic change generates changes in intraspinal stress distribution when smooth movement of the spinal cord is disturbed. Tachibana et al. reported that neck flexion causes narrowing of the ventral subarachnoid space at the foramen magnum and results in a positive Queckenstedt test in cases of Chiari I malformation [8]. They also demonstrated elevation of intraspinal cord pressure as a result of neck flexion and extension [9] in animal experiments. These findings indicate that biomechanical changes in the spinal cord caused by Chiari I malformation may play an important role in the development of syringomyelia.

The results of our study demonstrate that the stress is concentrated in the spinal cord adjacent to the descending cerebellar tonsil. This stress concentration can cause edema or microcystic changes in the spinal cord. When a small syrinx develops in the

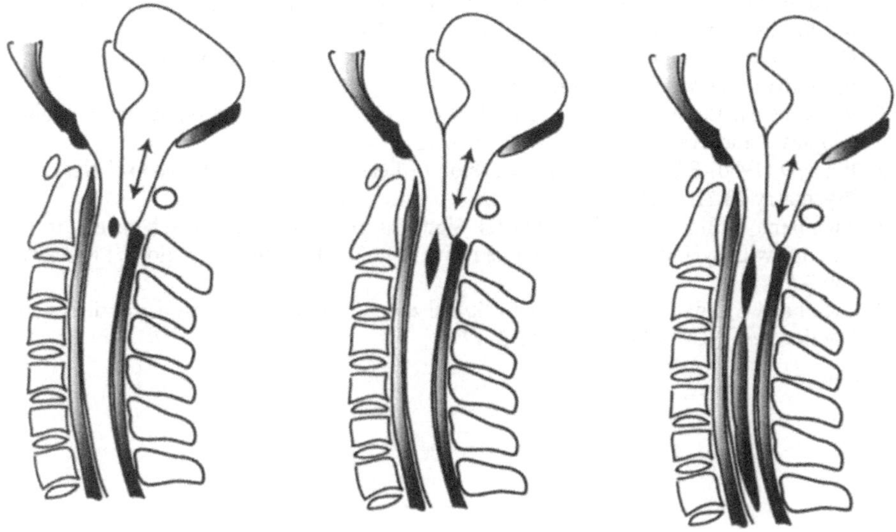

FIG. 5. Schematic representation of a hypothesis describing the process of generation and evolution of syringomyelia associated with Chiari I malformation

spinal cord, neck movement generates further stress concentration around the syrinx (Fig. 5). The stress concentration around the syrinx can then function as a driving force to extend the early syrinx. Oldfield used intraoperative ultrasonography to demonstrate piston-like movements of the descending tonsil, which are generated by pulsatile volume expansion of the brain by cardiac output. This type of tonsillar movement may cause a localized stress concentration in the adjacent spinal cord similar to that demonstrated in the simulation model.

Finally, a hypothesis for generation of a syrinx is presented in Fig. 5. Neck movements or piston-like movements of the descending tonsil generate stress concentration in the spinal cord. This stress concentration causes localized elevation of tissue pressure and microcystic change in the parenchyma. The tissue pressure elevation then becomes a driving force for the progression of the syrinx in a caudal direction.

In conclusion, biomechanical changes should be considered to reach an understanding of the mechanism of generation and extension of syringomyelia associated with Chiari I malformation.

References

1. Aboulker J (1979) La syringomyelia et les liquides intraarachdiens. Neurochirurgie 25(suppl 1):3–144
2. Ball MJ, Dyan AD (1972) Pathogenesis of syringomyelia. Lancet 2:799–801
3. du Boulay GH, O'Connell J, Currie J, et al (1972) Further investigations on pulsatile movements in the cerebrospinal fluid pathways. Acta Radiol 13:496–523

4. Gardner WJ (1965) Hydrodynamic mechanism of syringomyelia—its relationship to myelocele. J Neurol Neurosurg Psychiatry 28:247–259
5. Nagashima T, Hamano S, Tamaki N, Matsumoto S (1992) Intraspinal stress distribution in Chiari I malformation. Spinal Surg 6:91–96
6. Williams AL, Haughton VM, Pojunas KW, et al (1987) Differentiation of intramedullary neoplasm and cysts by MR. AJNR 8:527–532
7. Reid JD (1960) Effect of flexion-extension of head on spinal cord. J Neurol Neurosurg Psychiatry 23:214–221
8. Tachibana S, Iida H, Yada K (1992) Significance of positive Queckenstedt test in patients with syringomyelia associated with Arnold-Chiari malformations. J Neurosurg 76:67–71
9. Tachibana S, Iida H, Yada K (1995) Spinal cord intramedullary pressure: direct cord traction test. Neurol Med Chir 35:75–77

Physical Analysis of CSF Dynamics in the Spine

HAN SOO CHANG and HIROSHI NAKAGAWA

Summary. In various types of syringomyelia, the pathogenesis seems to be related to some derangement of cerebrospinal fluid (CSF) dynamics. In this report, we describe our mathematical model of CSF dynamics in the spine, and show how this model can effectively explain the pathogenesis of various types of syringomyelia. We constructed an electric circuit model of the CSF dynamics in the spine based on techniques of computational fluid mechanics. Using this model, we examined the behavior of this system to a step increase of pressure applied on the cranial side. We then simulated various conditions such as Chiari malformation, stenosis of the central canal, and adhesive arachnoiditis. The wall pressure across the central canal was sensitive to a decrease in capacitance at the cisterna magna. When the capacitance at the cisterna magna was decreased, as in Chiari I malformation, there was a marked increase of wall pressure, peaking at the low cervical segment of the spinal cord. If stenosis of the central canal was present, the wall pressure increased immediately proximal to the stenotic site. Blocking the subarachnoid CSF flow caused increased wall pressure of the central canal distal to the blocked site. Our mathematical model of CSF dynamics could explain the pathogenesis of various types of syringomyelia. It can serve as a useful working hypothesis in our future study of this disease.

Key words. Syringomyelia, Pathophysiology, Etiology, Cerebrospinal fluid, Computer simulation, Hypothesis

Introduction

Despite many hypotheses [1–6], we still do not have a clear understanding of the pathophysiology of syringomyelia. However, it seems that some derangement of cerebrospinal fluid (CSF) dynamics plays a major role in the pathogenesis of syringomyelia, whether it is related to Chiari malformation or to adhesive arachnoiditis. In this chapter, we aimed to provide a unifying theory that can explain various types of syringomyelia.

Department of Neurological Surgery, Aichi Medical University, 21 Yazako-Karimata, Nagakute-cho, Aichi-gun, Aichi 480-1195, Japan

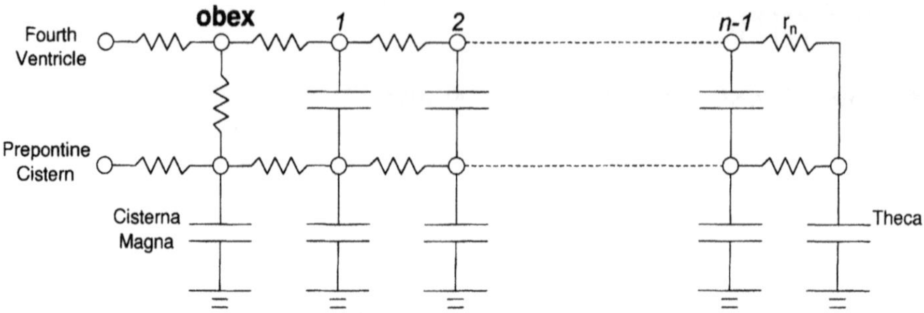

FIG. 1. The electrical circuit simulating cerebrospinal fluid (CSF) dynamics in the spine. Two rows of serially connected resistors represent two CSF pathways in the spine: the *upper row* represents the central canal, and the *lower row* represents the spinal subarachnoid space. The capacitors inserted between these rows represent the compliance of the central canal wall and the spinal cord; the capacitors inserted between the subarachnoid space and the ground represent that of the dural sac

Materials and Methods

We developed a model of CSF dynamics in the spine with an electric circuit that uses the following analogy: electrical resistance representing the resistance to flow, electrical capacitance representing the compliance of soft tissue and dural sac, and voltage accumulated in a capacitor representing pressure accumulated in soft tissue. Figure 1 shows the diagram of our circuit model. Two arrays of serially connected resistors represent two CSF pathways in the spine, namely, subarachnoid space and the central canal. Once we determine the values of these resistors and capacitors, albeit rather arbitrarily, we can calculate the response of this system to a step increase of voltage applied to the two cranial leads simultaneously. Mathematica version 3.0 (Wolfram Research, Champaign, IL, USA) running on a personal computer was used for this purpose.

Results

In this study, we were particularly interested in the distribution of voltage accumulated in the capacitors representing the compliance of the spinal cord. This pressure can be interpreted as the wall pressure across the central canal, namely, the pressure difference between outside and inside the central canal. For convenience, we just use the term central canal wall pressure, when we actually should use the term voltage accumulated in the capacitors representing the spinal cord soft tissue. We showed the spatial distribution of the central canal wall pressure along the long axis of the spinal cord, and its time course after a step increase of voltage was applied on the two cranial leads simultaneously.

When the capacitance of the cisterna magna was relatively large, there was almost no increase of wall pressure in response to the input. However, when the capacitance of the cisterna magna was decreased, there was a marked increase of the wall pressure peaking at the lower cervical segment (Fig. 2). On the other hand, if we increased the resistance at a certain point of the spinal subarachnoid CSF pathway, we observed an increased wall pressure of the central canal immediately caudal to the blocked point (Fig. 3).

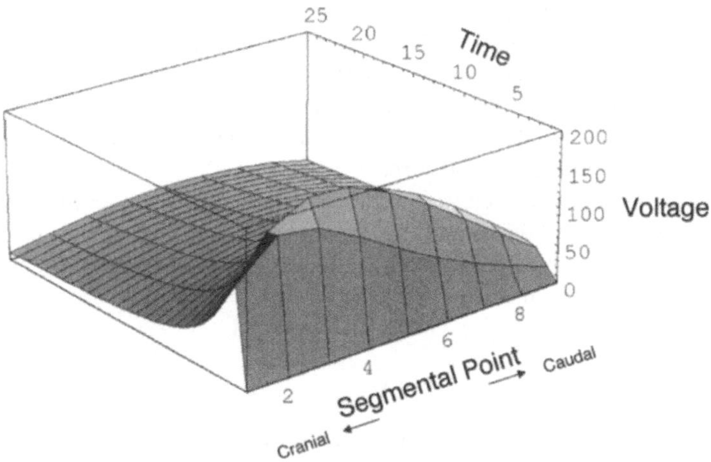

FIG. 2. Three-dimensional plot of the distribution and its time course of the voltage accumulated in the capacitors representing the wall of the central canal. A step increase of voltage is applied on the two cranial leads of the diagram in Fig. 1 at time zero

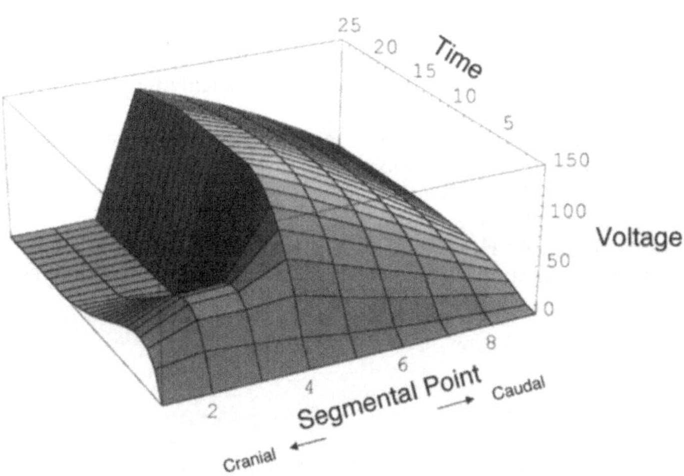

FIG. 3. The same plot as Fig. 2 except that the resistors of the subarachnoid space are increased between the segmental points *3* and *4*. A step increase of voltage is applied on the two cranial leads of the diagram in Fig. 1 at time zero

Discussion

Our mathematical model of CSF dynamics in the spine provides a good working space in which we can experiment with various settings simulating a number of pathological conditions. In this report, we showed the results of our computer simulation of Chiari malformation and adhesive arachnoiditis. Both results showed increased wall pressure across the central canal at locations where syringomyelia most often occurs. For syringomyelia associated with Chiari malformation, we can interpret the result as follows. In the normal situation, the cisterna magna functions as a shock absorber to pulsatile CSF waves coming from above. When the cistern is obliterated, as in Chiari malformation, the shock-absorbing function is lost, thereby causing increased central canal wall pressure in the cervical cord.

For syringomyelia associated with adhesive arachnoiditis, the result is interpreted as follows. Because the CSF pathway in the subarachnoid space is blocked, the CSF pressure outside the spinal cord distal to the blocked site is decreased, making the pressure inside the central canal relatively greater.

Conclusions

Our mathematical model of CSF dynamics can provide a working hypothesis explaining various types of syringomyelia. The validity of our hypothesis needs to be checked with future experiments and clinical experience.

References

1. Ball MJ, Dayan AD (1972) Pathogenesis of syringomyelia. Lancet 2:799–801
2. Gardner WJ (1965) Hydrodynamic mechanism of syringomyelia: its relationship to myelocele. J Neurol Neurosurg Psychiatry 28:247–259
3. Heiss JD, Patronas N, DeVroom HL, et al (1999) Elucidating the pathophysiology of syringomyelia. J Neurosurg 91:553–562
4. Oldfield EH, Murszko K, Shawker T, et al (1994) Pathophysiology of syringomyelia associated with Chiari I malformation of the cerebellar tonsils. J Neurosurg 80:3–15
5. Williams B (1969) The distending force in the production of "communicating syringomyelia." Lancet 26:189–193
6. Nishikawa M, Sakamoto H, Hakuba A, et al (1997) Pathogenesis of Chiari malformation: a morphometric study of the posterior cranial fossa. J Neurosurg 86:40–47

3. Pathophysiology of Syringomyelia

Hydrodynamics of Syringomyelia

Edward H. Oldfield, Hetty L. DeVroom, and John D. Heiss

Summary. Our studies demonstrate a mechanism of the pathogenesis of syringomyelia in which (1) the Chiari malformation partially obstructs the cerebrospinal fluid (CSF) pathways at the foramen magnum; (2) the normally rapid efflux and influx of CSF between the head and the spine, which normally compensates for brain expansion and contraction during the cardiac cycle, is blocked; (3) the cerebellar tonsils are displaced during the cardiac cycle, in lieu of CSF, creating a piston effect on the partially entrapped spinal subarachnoid space; (4) enlarged cervical subarachnoid pressure waves are created, which compress the spinal cord from without, direct CSF into the spinal cord, and cause pulsatile syrinx flow; which in turn (5) leads to syrinx progression. These findings are consistent with an origin of the syrinx fluid by pulsatile-facilitated transmission of CSF through the spinal cord. This mechanism of syrinx origin, progression, and resolution arises outside, not inside, the spinal cord. Thus, extraarachnoidal craniocervical decompression and duroplasty reverses the mechanism of syringomyelia progression without invading the central nervous system parenchyma or the CSF pathways and consistently provides a safe and effective treatment of patients with Chiari I and syringomyelia.

Key words. Syringomyelia, Chiari I malformation, Pathophysiology

Introduction

The Chiari I malformation, formation of the cerebellar tonsils below the foramen magnum, often is associated with syringomyelia. The mechanism of the origin of the Chiari I malformation, the mechanism of progression of syringomyelia, and the initial treatment of choice of syringomyelia associated with Chiari I malformation have been controversial issues for several decades. Disparate concepts of the origin, maintenance, and propagation of syringomyelia underly the development of a variety of surgical techniques used to treat patients with a Chiari I malformation and syringomyelia. Until recently, there have been two major theories on the origin and

Surgical Neurology Branch, National Institute of Neurological Disorders and Stroke, National Institutes of Health, Bethesda, MD 20892, USA

progression of syringomyelia, the Gardner "water hammer" theory [1,2] and the Williams theory [3–5].

Gardner was the first to convincingly demonstrate the frequent association of the Chiari I tonsillar malformation and syringomyelia. In his theory of the origin and progression of syringomyelia, he emphasized the embryological continuity of the central canal with the fourth ventricle [1,2]. He postulated that delayed opening of the outlet of the fourth ventricle leads to in utero hydrocephalus, which in turn was responsible for a retained communication of the central canal with the fourth ventricle, and he theorized that the etiology of syringomyelia associated with the Chiari I type of hindbrain malformation was a result of the transmission of the pulsatile transmission of fourth ventricular CSF into the central canal and the syrinx. Thus, with each arterial pulse, transmission of a "water hammer" effect of the pulse wave generated in the CSF by blood entering the choroid plexuses, as demonstrated by Bering [6], was stated to be the force responsible for the development and progression of cord cavitation. The continued partial obstruction of the outflow of CSF from the fourth ventricle directed the pulsations of CSF transmitted into the central canal. Based on these hypotheses, he advocated elimination of the obstruction to the normal route of CSF flow by surgical decompression of the tonsils, and occlusion of the route of CSF into the central canal, by plugging of the obex, to treat syringomyelia associated with a Chiari I malformation [2].

In support of Gardner's hypothesis are the dynamic movement of the CSF within the ventricular spaces, particularly the third and fourth ventricles, during systole, as shown on cine-radiography during ventriculography by du Boulay et al. [7,8], and the similarity of the syrinx fluid and the CSF. Arguments against his theory are that neither autopsy nor radiographic studies have demonstrated patency of a channel of sufficient size to transmit either a pulsatile flow of fluid or transmission of a sudden arterial pressure wave into the syrinx from the fourth ventricle. Further, obstructions to the normal CSF flow from the fourth ventricle have only occasionally been demonstrated in these patients, and no direct observations or measurements of pressure have been made that support the proposed mechanism.

Williams, who first emphasized the importance of the partial obstruction to the free flow of CSF by the tonsils at the foramen magnum, proposed that progression of syringomyelia is related to the pressure differences that arise within the cranial and spinal subarachnoid spaces shortly after a Valsalva maneuver because of one-way ball-valve obstruction to the downward flow of CSF shortly after straining, coughing, etc. [3–5]. His concept was that the increased thoracic and abdominal pressure associated with coughing, etc., compressed the spinal dural sac sending the spinal CSF upward into the cisterna magna. The tonsillar obstruction to the downward flow of CSF, the ball-valve obstruction, resulted in the diversion of the fourth ventricular CSF down a patent obex and central canal into the syrinx. Arguments against Williams' theory of the mechanism of progression of syringomyelia include that many patients with Chiari I malformations and syringomyelia do not have a block to transmission of CSF pressure at the foramen magnum, including Williams' own measurements [4,9] and the absence of a detectable communication between the fourth ventricle and the syrinx using high-resolution MRI and autopsy studies.

Hence, the principal difference in the premises offered by Gardner and Williams is that in the former the wave of pressure responsible for maintenance and progression of the syrinx is a pulsatile pressure from within the neural axis that acts centrifugally from the syrinx against the surrounding spinal cord, whereas in the latter a more prolonged wave of pressure associated with valsalva maneuvers acts on the cord from within.

Finally, Ball and Dayan [10] and Alboulker [11] hypothesized that the syrinx fluid is derived from CSF moving into the spinal cord and the syrinx cavity along the Virchow–Robin spaces as a result of sporadic elevations of increased CSF pressure associated with Valsalva and increased epidural venous pressure.

In the early 1990s, Oldfield et al. [12] studied the hydrodynamics of Chiari I-associated syringomyelia in six patients with intraoperative ultrasound at the cranio-cervical junction after removing the posterior lip of the foramen magnum and the posterior arch of C1. The goals were to compare the dynamics of the anatomy of the spinal cord, cerebellar tonsils, and the syrinx during the cardiac cycle and Valsalva maneuver (excess, sustained positive-pressure ventilation), before and after dural decompression. Phase-contrast and cine-MRI were also used to examine the rate and direction of fluid movement in the syrinx and spinal subarachnoid CSF during the cardiac cycle.

In that study, intraoperative ultrasound demonstrated dramatic pulsations of the wall of the syrinx cavity (the spinal cord surrounding the cavity) that were related to the cardiac cycle [12]. In addition, in several patients there was an obvious, occasionally striking, downward systolic excursion of the cerebellar tonsils associated with sudden compression of the upper portion of the spinal cord and syrinx. The pulsations of the walls of the syrinx cavity and of the tonsils that were linked to the cardiac cycle showed no correlation with the respiratory cycle. Similarly, they were not influenced by Valsalva maneuver, as forced inspiration did not produce cord expansion in any patient. After opening the dura, but with the arachnoid intact, the dramatic pulsations within the syrinx cavity and the abrupt, phasic downward movement of the cerebellar tonsils diminished and only then did expansion of the syrinx occur during forced inspiration. The patients had collapse of the syrinx on MRI and improvement or stabilization of their clinical syndrome after surgery. The results of the anatomic and cine-MRI studies demonstrated limited CSF movement across the subarachnoid space of the foramen magnum during the cardiac cycle, but downward systolic movement of the subarachnoid CSF and the syrinx fluid [12].

A New Theory

Based on these observations, one of us (E.H.O.) conceived a new theory of the basis of the origin and progression of syringomyelia (Fig. 1): (1) the Chiari malformation partially obstructs the CSF pathways at the foramen magnum; (2) the normally rapid efflux and influx of CSF between the head and the spine, which normally compensates for brain expansion and contraction during the cardiac cycle, is blocked; (3) the cerebellar tonsils are displaced during the cardiac cycle, in lieu of CSF, creating a piston effect on the partially entrapped spinal subarachnoid space; (4) enlarged cervical subarachnoid pressure waves are created that compress the spinal cord from without, direct CSF into the spinal cord, and cause pulsatile syrinx flow; which (5) leads to syrinx progression; (6) these anatomic and physiological abnormalities are reversed

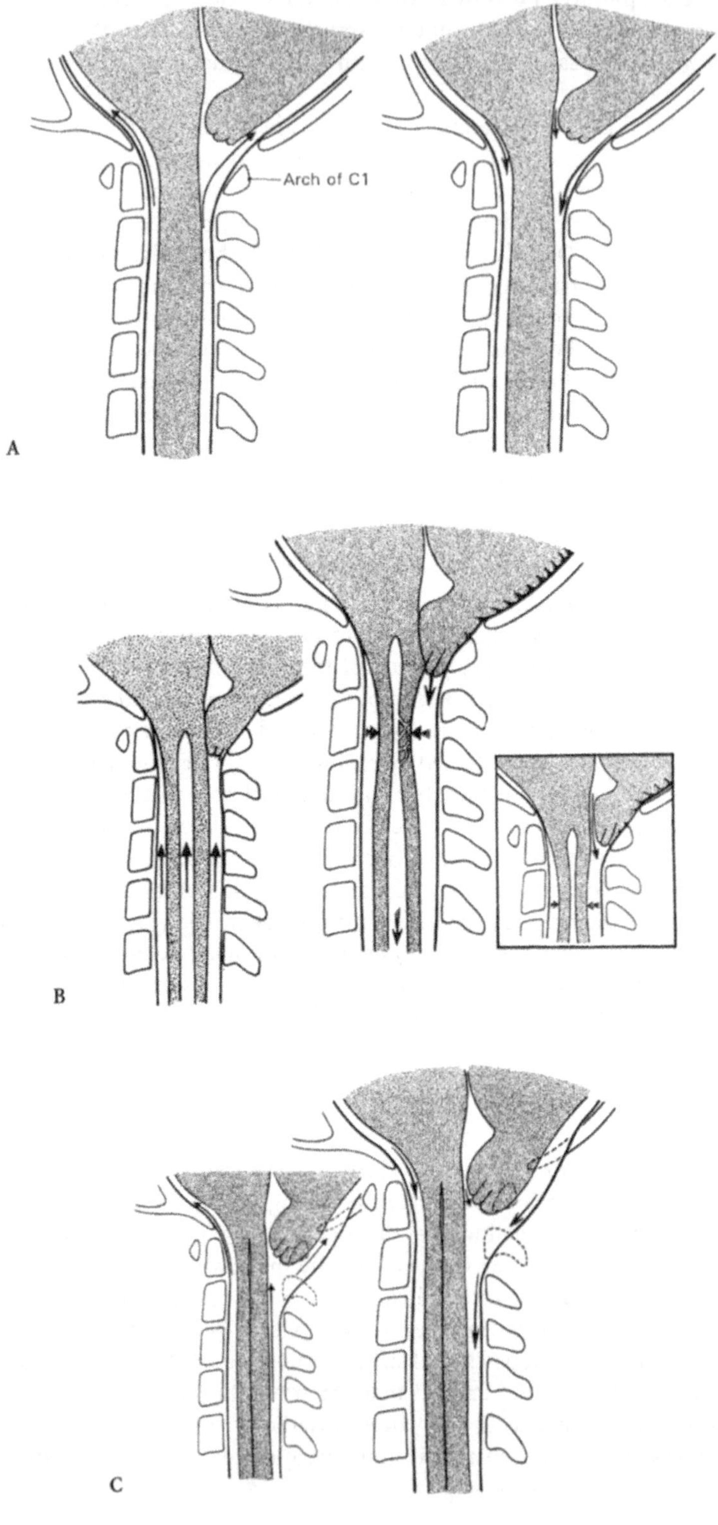
Arch of C1
A
B
C

by a simple surgical procedure to decompress the subarachnoid space at the foramen magnum [12]. It was further proposed that the origin of the syrinx fluid was by pulsatile-facilitated, not venous pressure-facilitated transmission of CSF through the spinal cord, as proposed by Ball and Dayan [10] and Alboulker [11].

To test this theory, a prospective study was designed and executed by Heiss et al. [13] to examine before and during surgery the anatomy and physiology of patients with Chiari I malformation and to compare the findings to measurements of the same features after surgery and to normal subjects. The following sections summarize the results of that study for each of the components of the proposed mechanism.

The Chiari Malformation Partially Obstructs the CSF Pathways at the Foramen Magnum, Blocking the Normally Rapid Efflux and Influx of CSF Between the Head and the Spine, Which Normally Compensates for Brain Expansion and Contraction During the Cardiac Cycle

The spinal cord was distended in all cases by syrinxes that ranged in diameter from 5 to 11 mm and extended longitudinally 2.4 to 40.0 cm. The studies demonstrated anatomic and physiological obstruction of the subarachnoid space at the foramen magnum by the cerebellar tonsils before and during surgery (before dural decompression), but which was relieved by simple decompressive surgery [13].

Anatomic Occlusion

The cerebellar tonsils consistently had a "pointed" shape with the tips lying below the foramen magnum (Fig. 2). The Chiari I malformation severely narrowed the anteroposterior (AP) diameter of the cerebrospinal fluid pathways at the foramen magnum on MRI, ventral to the medulla (Fig. 3A,B). Cine-MRI at the foramen magnum revealed

◀

FIG. 1A–C. Schematic drawings of the foramen magnum region, sagittal view, illustrating the proposed mechanism of origin and progression of syringomyelia associated with Chiari I malformation of the cerebellar tonsils. **A** In normal subjects during systole (*right*), as the brain expands with the reception of blood, cerebrospinal fluid (CSF) moves from the fourth ventricle into the cisterna magna; a larger volume of fluid passes from the basal cisterns to the subarachnoid space of the upper portion of the spinal canal. The magnitude of the systolic pressure wave that is conveyed to the CSF in the spinal canal dissipates with increasing distance inferiorly. During diastole (*left*), CSF flows rostrally across the foramen magnum. **B** With obstruction to the rapid to-and-fro movement of CSF in the subarachnoid space across the foramen magnum (ventrally by anterior displacement of the brain stem and posteriorly by the impacted cerebellar tonsils) during systole (*center*) and diastole (*left*), brain expansion during systole is accommodated by abrupt caudal movement of the tonsils. The piston-like effect of this movement on partially isolated spinal subarachnoid space imparts an accentuated systolic pressure wave to the spinal subarachnoid CSF. This pressure acts on the surface of the upper segments of the spinal cord, abruptly constricting the syrinx, propelling the fluid in it inferiorly and increasing bulk movement of CSF into the cord. In some patients, an inferior position of the foramen of Magendie may deposit CSF expelled from the fourth ventricle during systole into the spinal canal below the level of obstruction (*right*). **C** With surgical decompression of the foramen magnum and tonsils, occlusion of CSF flow across the foramen magnum is eliminated, normal physiology is restored, and syringomyelia disappears. (From [12], with permission)

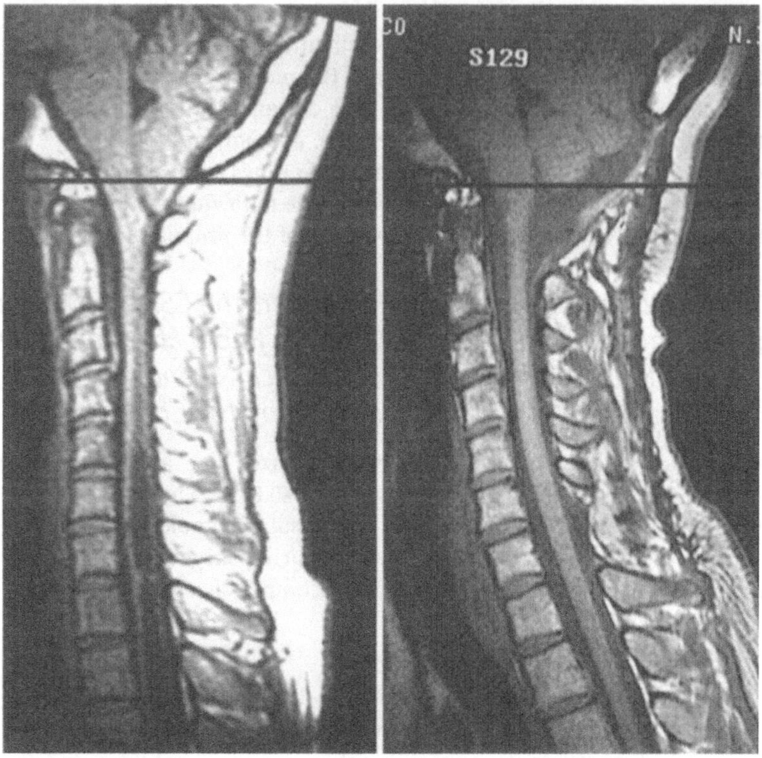

A B

FIG. 2. T_1-weighted MRI images of the posterior fossa and cervical spine in the midsagittal plane before surgery (**A**) and after craniocervical decompression and duroplasty (**B**). After decompressive surgery, the cerebellar tonsils become rounded and ascend into the posterior fossa and the subarachnoid space is enlarged ventrally and dorsally. *Horizontal black line* was added to align the images at the foramen magnum. (From [13], with permission)

that the cross-sectional area of the CSF flow pathway was reduced before surgery (Fig. 3C) compared to normal subjects [13].

Physiological Obstruction

Preoperatively, CSF pressure transmission across the foramen magnum was compromised, as shown by the slow rate of increase in the lumbar pressure during jugular venous occlusion, Queckenstedt's test (Fig. 4A,B). Cine-MRI demonstrated that the peak velocity of CSF at the foramen magnum during the cardiac cycle was increased in the inferior and superior directions (Fig. 5A).

After Surgery

Six months after surgery, T_1-weighted MRI images of the craniocervical area showed that ventral and dorsal CSF spaces at the foramen magnum had expanded and that the area of the CSF pathways at the foramen magnum had increased (see Fig. 3A–C).

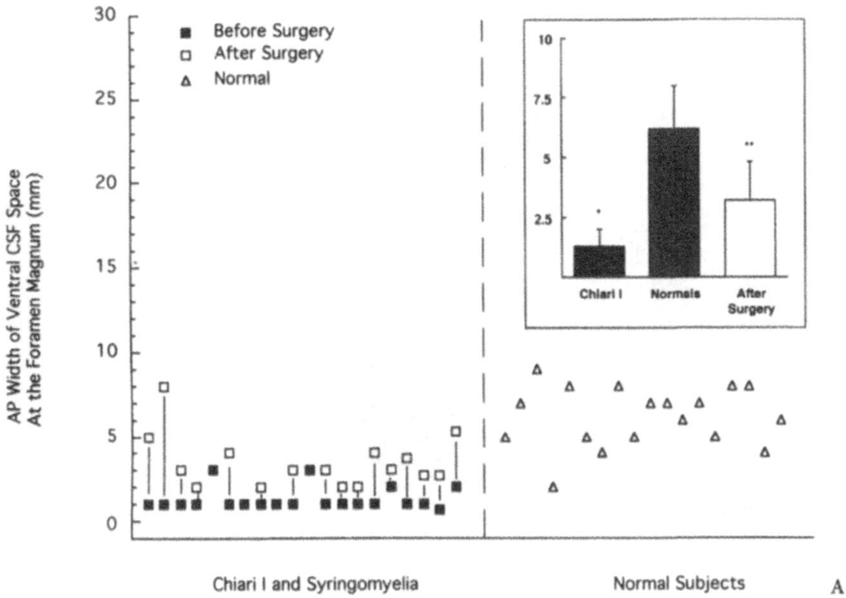

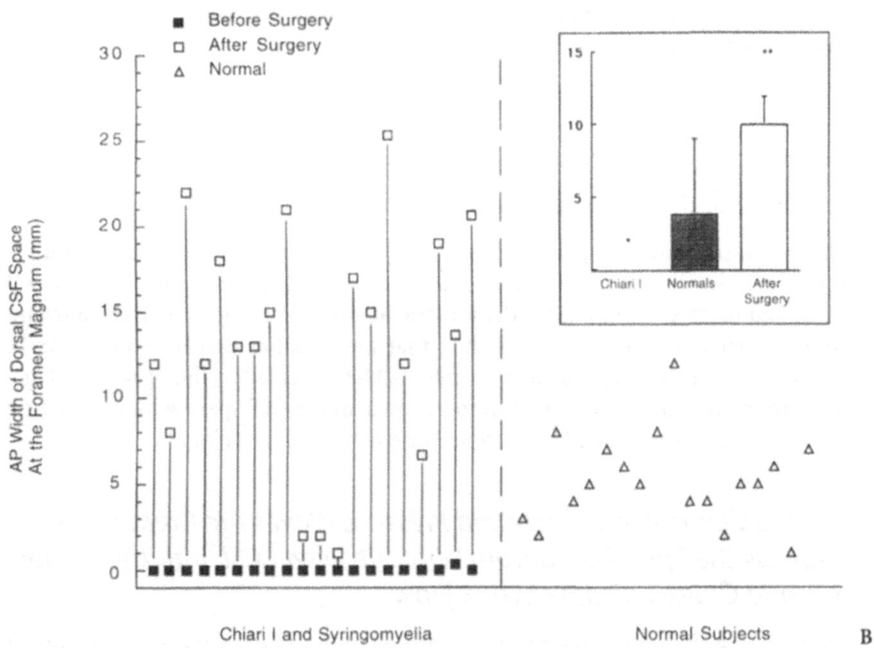

FIG. 3. Anteroposterior (AP) diameter of the subarachnoid space at the foramen magnum in normal subjects (*triangles*) and in patients with Chiari I and syringomyelia, before (*solid squares*) and after (*open squares*) surgery, ventral to the medulla (**A**) and dorsal to the cerebellar tonsils (**B**). **C** Cross-sectional area of the subarachnoid space at the foramen magnum. Measurements in **A** and **B** are from anatomic MRI and in **C** from cine-MRI studies. Six months after surgery, the ventral and dorsal CSF spaces at the foramen magnum and the cross-sectional area of the CSF pathways had expanded (**A–C**). *Column graphs* show mean ± 1 SD; *, $P < 0.0001$, patients before surgery versus normal subjects; **, $P < 0.0001$, before surgery versus after surgery. (From [13], with permission)

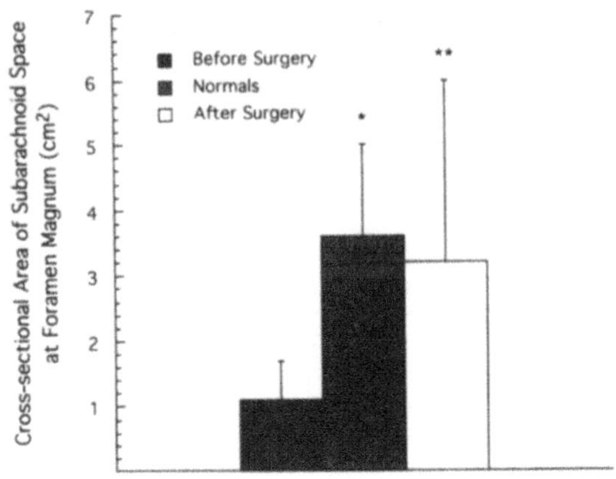

C

FIG. 3. *Continued*

The obstruction to the transmission of pressure across the foramen magnum was no longer present (Fig. 4).

The Cerebellar Tonsils Are Displaced During the Cardiac Cycle, in Lieu of CSF, Creating a Piston Effect on the Partially Entrapped Spinal Subarachnoid Space

At surgery, ultrasonography showed that the syrinx contracted in synchrony with tonsillar descent in all patients. Simultaneous ultrasonography and pressure testing that were linked in time with the EKG demonstrated abrupt systolic downward movement of the cerebellar tonsils and established that the tonsillar descent and syrinx contraction occurred during cardiac systole (200–600 ms after the R-wave) (Fig. 6). Furthermore, the tonsils were shown to act on a spinal CSF space with reduced compliance, which was reversed to a normal state after surgery (Fig. 7).

Enlarged Cervical Subarachnoid Pressure Waves Are Created That Compress the Spinal Cord from Without, Direct CSF into the Spinal Cord, and Cause Pulsatile Syrinx Flow

Before surgery, the mean cervical subarachnoid pressure was greater in patients than in the normal subjects, as was the cervical pulse pressure (Fig. 8A). At surgery, before the dura was opened syrinx pressure was identical to cervical subarachnoid pressure. Opening the dura while keeping the arachnoid intact reduced the amplitude of the pulsation of the cerebellar tonsils and eliminated the pulsatile compression of the upper pole of the syrinx. Cervical subarachnoid mean and pulse pressures and lumbar mean subarachnoid pressure decreased after surgery (Fig. 8B).

Preoperative cine-MRI revealed abrupt inferior movement of cervical subarachnoid CSF and syrinx fluid during systole and superior movement in diastole (see Fig. 5B).

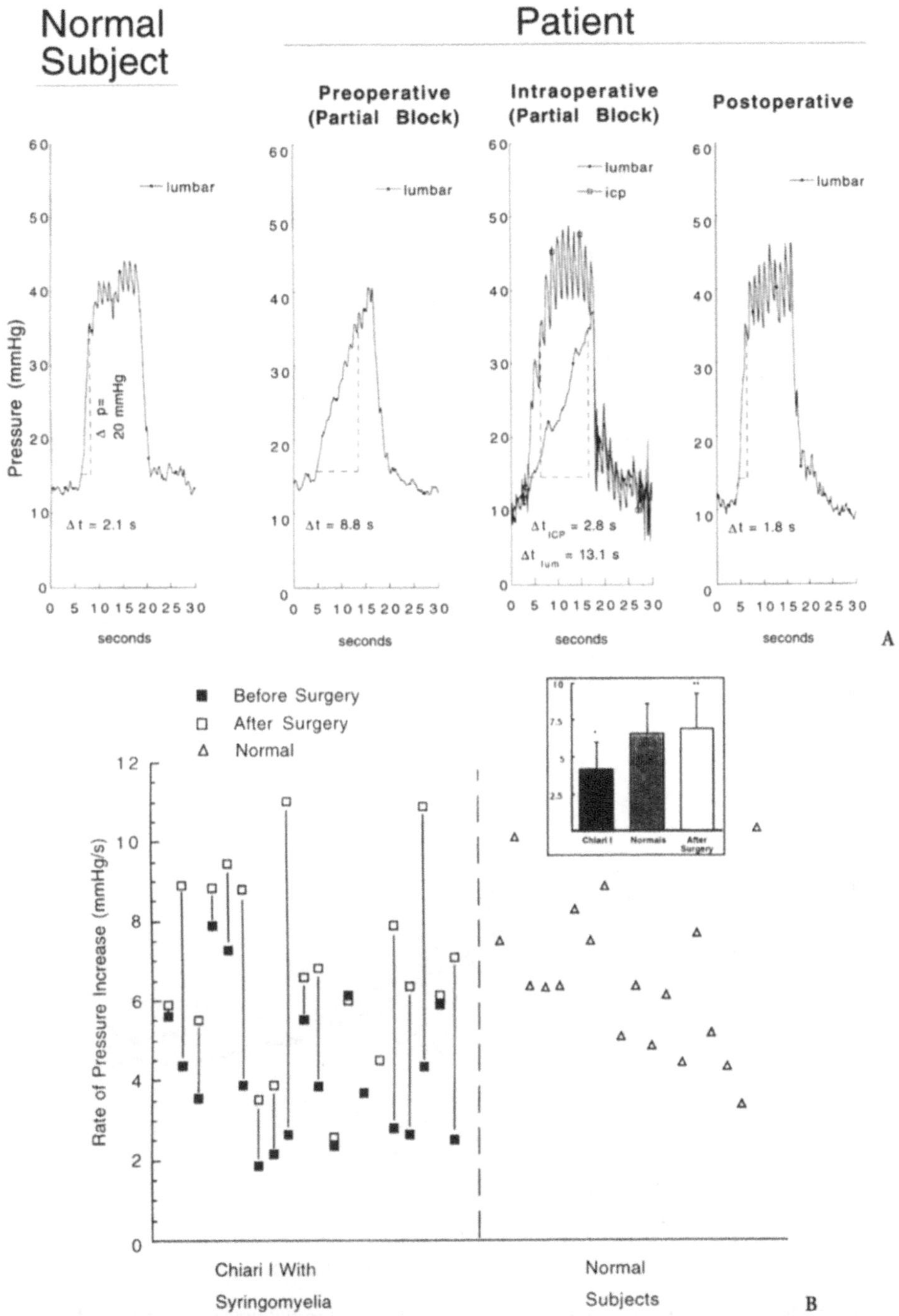

FIG. 4A,B. Partial occlusion of CSF flow at the foramen magnum. **A** Rate of rise in intrathecal pressure in a normal subject and in a patient with Chiari I and syringomyelia, before surgery and before the craniocervical junction is decompressed during surgery. After surgery, the rise in intrathecal pressure becomes normal. **B** Rate of rise in intrathecal pressure in patients with Chiari I and syringomyelia compared to normal subjects. After surgery, the rise in intrathecal pressure becomes normal. *Insert* shows mean ± 1 SD; *, $P < 0.0001$, patients before surgery versus normal subjects; **, $P < 0.0001$, before surgery versus after surgery. (From [13], with permission)

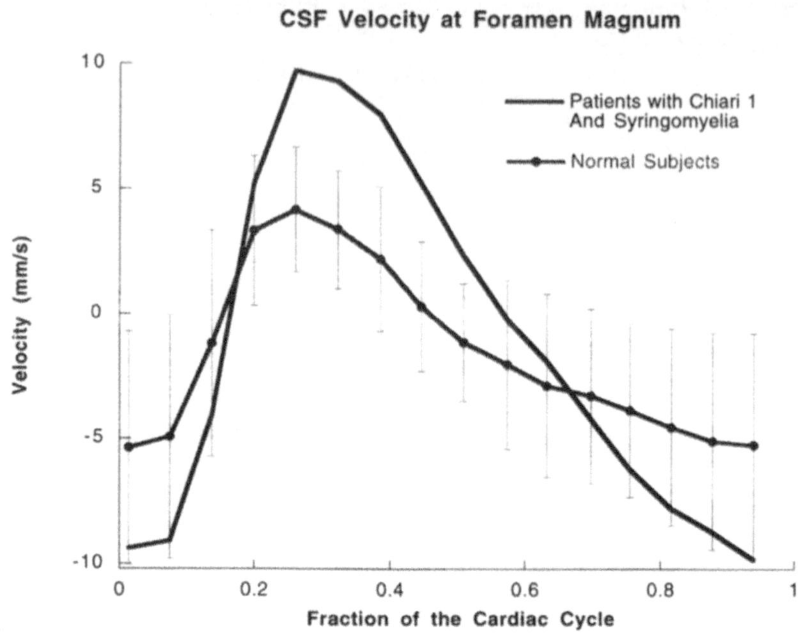

A

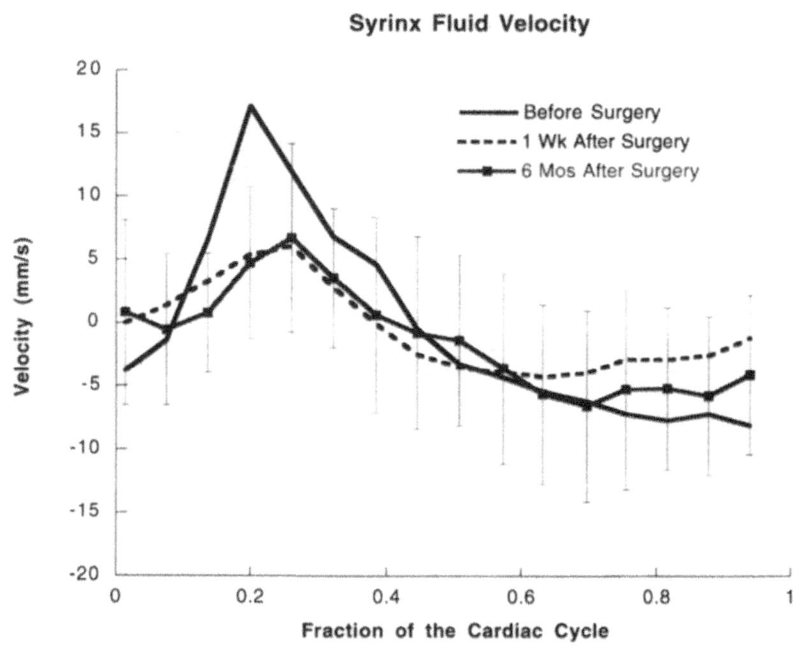

B

FIG. 5A,B. Phase-contrast cine-MRI studies were obtained in patients and normal subjects. In each patient, velocity was measured during 16 segments of the cardiac cycle. The mean velocity values for patients and normal subjects were plotted versus the fraction of the cardiac cycle after the R-wave of the ECG. *Positive values* indicate caudal flow and *negative values* indicate rostral flow; *error bars* indicate 1 SD from the mean. **A** The velocity of the CSF in the subarachnoid space at the foramen magnum and (**B**) the velocity of the syrinx fluid before and after surgery. The peak velocity of CSF during the cardiac cycle was increased in the inferior ($P = 0.0005$) and superior ($P = 0.008$) directions before surgery. (From [13], with permission)

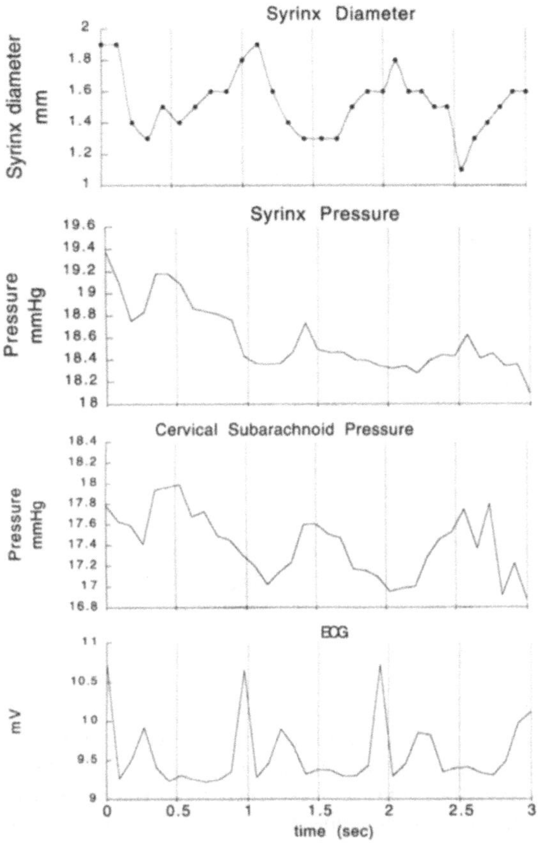

FIG. 6. Measurement of the diameter of the syrinx at C2 using cardiac-gated, intraoperative ultrasonography simultaneous with recording of the pressure within the syrinx and cervical subarachnoid space. The syrinx contracts during cardiac systole when the cervical subarachnoid pressure reaches its peak. (From [13], with permission)

After surgery the maximal velocity of the syrinx fluid in the inferior direction during systole decreased (see Fig. 5B).

These Anatomic and Physiological Abnormalities Are Reversed by a Simple Surgical Procedure to Decompress the Subarachnoid Space at the Foramen Magnum

The pathophysiological findings were consistently reversed by surgical decompression. In addition, by 6 months after surgery the longitudinal extent and diameter of the syrinx on MRI were much smaller (see Fig. 2). Before surgery, patients manifested the typical symptoms (headache, dysesthetic pain, weakness, clumsy gait, and loss of sensation) and signs (muscle weakness, atrophy, spasticity, sensory deficit, and ataxia) associated with syringomyelia and the Chiari I malformation. Symptoms improved more than signs on examination 6 months after surgery. Neurological examinations were repeated annually and remained stable in all patients.

Thus, the surgical procedure consistently corrected the pathophysiological consequences of the Chiari I malformation, induced remission of the syrinx, and stabilized

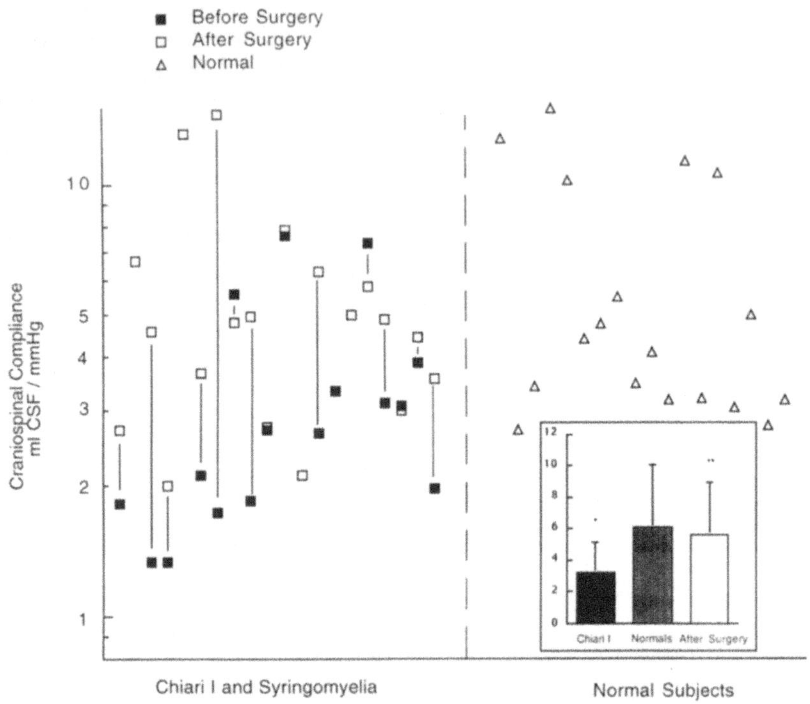

FIG. 7. Craniospinal compliance was compromised before surgery and returned to normal after surgery. Compliance (ml CSF/mmHg) was measured by dividing the amount of CSF removed (10 ml) by the reduction in intrathecal pressure (mmHg) that resulted. *Insert* shows mean ± 1 SD; *, $P < 0.0001$, patients before surgery versus normal subjects; **, $P < 0.0001$, before surgery versus after surgery. (From [13], with permission)

the patient's clinical picture, but was associated with limited improvement, presumably a result of preexisting irreversible injury to the spinal cord by the syrinx in most patients [13].

Is the Chiari I "Malformation" of the Cerebellar Tonsils Acquired by Relentless Tonsillar Impaction in the Foramen Magnum, Rather Than an Embryonic Dysgenesis?

Comparison of the pre-and postoperative T_1 MRI scans showed that surgical expansion of the posterior fossa results in a normal cerebellar morphology, with ascent of the cerebellar tonsils into the posterior fossa and the acquisition of a rounded, normal appearance, rather than the typical pointed, "beaked" shape before surgery (see Fig. 2). Because the Chiari I malformation results from the posterior fossa being smaller than normal in the majority of cases [14–16] and of insufficient size to contain the cerebellum and brainstem [17], rather than a primary abnormality of cerebellum, the surgical procedure directly addresses the underlying pathology.

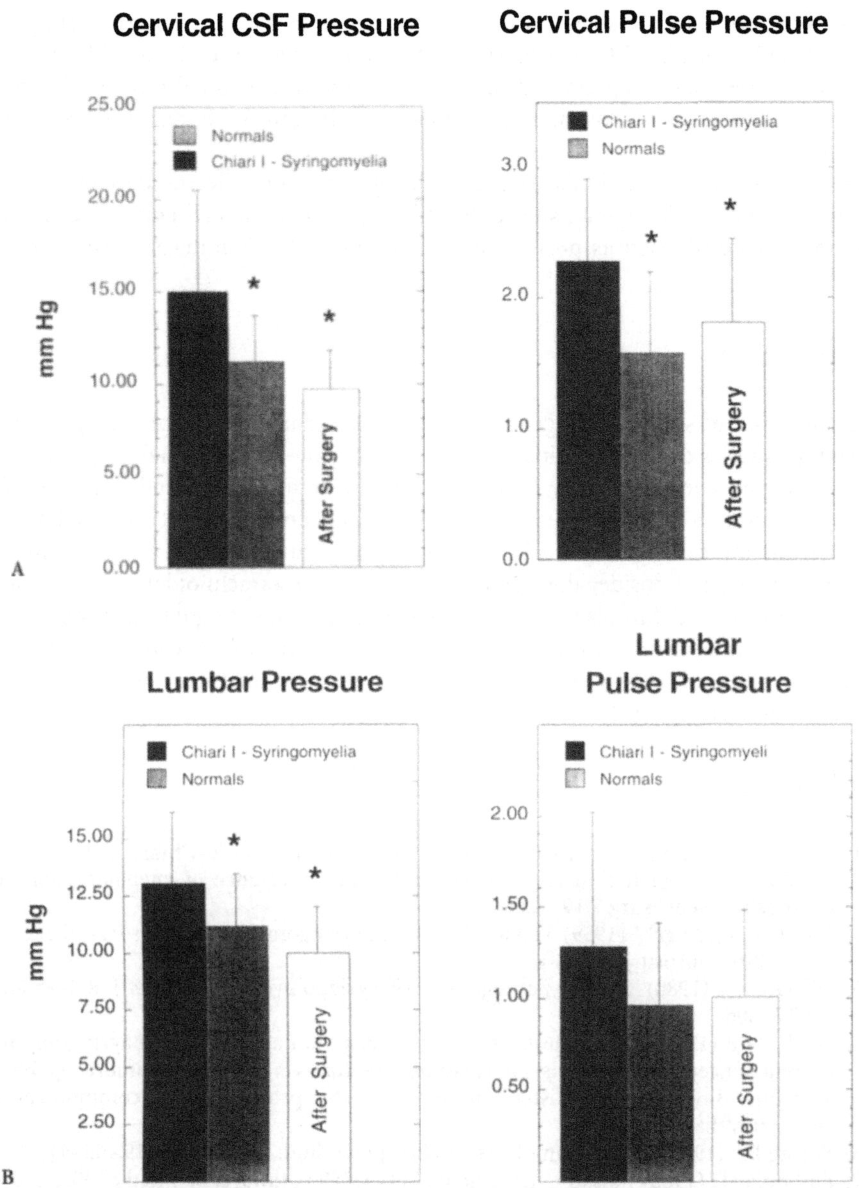

FIG. 8. **A** Before surgery, the mean cervical subarachnoid pressure was greater in the patients than in the normal subjects, as was the cervical pulse pressure. Cervical subarachnoid mean pressure decreased after surgery, as did lumbar mean subarachnoid pressure (**B**). Mean ± 1 SD; *, $P < 0.005$, before surgery versus after surgery and normal subjects. (From [13], with permission)

This return of tonsillar shape to normal also suggests that the abnormal shape of the cerebellar tonsils with the Chiari I malformation is acquired by tonsillar impaction in the foramen magnum and the upper portion of the spinal canal [13], rather than resulting from a congenital abnormality of the tonsils, as has been generally thought.

Finally, we note that similar pathophysiology may underlie the development of syringomyelia in other circumstances in which the spinal subarachnoid space is commonly obstructed, such as posttraumatic and arachnoiditis-induced syringomyelia [12,13].

Conclusions

Our proposal of syrinx pathogenesis has been confirmed by the physiological and anatomic studies during the initial study [12] and by the in-depth analysis performed before, during, and after craniocervical decompression for Chiari I and syringomyelia in our second, prospective study [13]. The findings are consistent from patient to patient and indicate that the mechanism of syrinx origin, progression, and resolution arises outside, not inside, the spinal cord. Thus, extraarachnoidal craniocervical decompression and duroplasty reverses the mechanism of syringomyelia progression without invading the central nervous system parenchyma or the cerebrospinal fluid pathways and consistently provides a safe and effective treatment of patients with Chiari I and syringomyelia.

References

1. Gardner W, Goodall R (1950) Surgical treatment of Arnold-Chiari malformation in adults. An explanation of its mechanism and importance of enephalography in diagnosis. J Neurosurg 7:199–206
2. Gardner WJ, Angel J (1959) The mechanism of syringomyelia and its surgical corrections. Clin Neurosurg 6:131–140
3. Williams B (1980) On the pathogenesis of syringomyelia: a review. J R Soc Med 73:798–806
4. Williams B (1991) Pathogenesis of syringomyelia. In: Batzdorf U (ed) Syringomyelia: current concepts in diagnosis and treatment. Williams & Wilkins, Baltimore, pp 59–90
5. Williams B (1992) The distending force in the production of communicating syringomyelia. Lancet 2:41
6. Bering EA (1962) Circulation of the cerebrospinal fluid. J Neurosurg 19:405–413
7. du Boulay G (1966) Pulsatile movements in the CSF pathways. Br J Radiol 39:255–262
8. du Boulay G, O'Connell J (1972) Further investigations on pulsatile movements in the cerebrospinal fluid pathway. Acta Radiol (Diagn) 13:496–523
9. Williams B (1986) Progress in syringomyelia. Neurol Res 8:130–145
10. Ball B, Dayan A (1972) Pathogenesis of syringomyelia. Lancet 1:799–801
11. Aboulker J (1979) La syringomyelie et les liquides intra-rachidiens. Neurochirurgie 25:1–144
12. Oldfield E, Muraszko K, Shawker T, et al (1994) Pathophysiology of syringomyelia associated with Chiari I malformation of the cerebellar tonsils: implications for diagnosis and treatment. J Neurosurg 80:3–15
13. Heiss J, Patronas N, DeVroom H, et al (1999) Elucidating the pathophysiology in syringomyelia. J Neurosurg 91:553–562

14. Nyland H, Krogness KG (1978) Size of posterior fossa in Chiari type I malformation in adults. Acta Neurochir 40:233–242
15. Stovner LJ, Bergan U, Nilsen G, et al (1993) Posterior cranial fossa dimensions in the Chiari I malformation: relation to pathogenesis and clinical presentation. Neuroradiology 35:113–118
16. Vega A, Quintana F, Berciano J (1990) Basichondrocranium anomalies in adult Chiari type I malformation: a morphometric study. J Neurol Sci 99:137–145
17. Nishikawa M, Sakamoto H, Hakuba A, et al (1997) Pathogenesis of Chiari malformation: a morphometric study of the posterior cranial fossa. J Neurosurg 86:40–47

Intraoperative Ultrasonography During Foramen Magnum Decompression for Syringomyelia Associated with Chiari I Malformation

Abesh Kumar Bhattacharjee, Norihiko Tamaki, Tatsuya Nagashima, and Kazumasa Ehara

Summary. Foramen magnum decompression (FMD) for syringomyelia associated with Chiari I malformation comprises a midline suboccipital expansive cranioplasty, C1 laminectomy, opening of the dura (with the arachnoid intact), and expansive duraplasty using Gore-Tex membrane. In this study we assess the utility of intraoperative ultrasound study for FMD. A Sonolayer α SSA-260A was used to perform an ultrasound study during FMD of 12 patients (7 women and 5 men), ranging in age from 13 to 60 years (average, 25.8 years). After craniotomy and laminectomy, the ultrasound scan was performed with the aid of a 7-MHz sector transducer both before and after the dura was opened. Before opening the dura, the ultrasound study demonstrated that the cerebellar tonsils abruptly descended during cardiac systole and ascended during diastole in all patients and that the syrinx contracted in synchrony with tonsillar descent. Opening of the dura reduced the amplitude of the pulsatile movement of the cerebellar tonsils and eliminated contraction of the syrinx. Postoperatively, all the patients were followed up (3 months–13 years; mean, 4.8 years) with neurological and radiological evaluations. MR imaging was used for all patients until the syrinx had disappeared. Increase in syrinx size was not observed in any patient. Ultrasound could detect craniocervical lesions very clearly in all cases. Pulsation of cerebrospinal fluid across the foramen magnum after surgery was confirmed intraoperatively. Ultrasound is quick, convenient, noninvasive, is performed in real time, and can be easily repeated to determine whether sufficient decompression has been achieved.

Key words. Foramen magnum decompression, Chiari I malformation, Syringomyelia, Intraoperative ultrasonography

Introduction

The objective of surgical treatment for syringomyelia associated with Chiari I malformation is elimination of the syrinx and prevention of progressive myelopathy. The optimal surgical treatment for Chiari I malformation with syringomyelia is still a

---

Department of Neurosurgery, Kobe University, Graduate School of Medicine, 7-5-1 Kusunoki-cho, Chuo-ku, Kobe 650-0017, Japan

matter of debate, but foramen magnum decompression (FMD) is often considered as the first choice of treament because it relieves impaction created by tonsillar herniation and may result in regression of the symptoms [1–3]. Foramen magnum decompression consisting of a suboccipital craniotomy, upper cervical laminectomy, and duraplasty has been shown to result in reliable reduction of the syrinx and clinical improvement [4,5].

The recent advent of magnetic resonance (MR) imaging has contributed to understanding of the pathophysiology of impaction at the foramen magnum and syrinx formation in the spinal cord. Furthermore, MR imaging is capable of detecting the flow dynamics of cerebrospinal fluid (CSF) preoperatively. Ultrasound has made it possible to intraoperatively examine pulsatility in nervous system structures as well as CSF dynamics before and after FMD. We review our experience with the treatment of syringomyelia associated with Chiari I malformation for patients who underwent FMD under ultrasonic guidance.

Clinical Materials and Methods

Patients and Clinical History

Twelve patients with syringomyelia associated with Chiari I malformation who underwent FMD were reviewed for this study. The patients comprised 7 women and 5 men with an age range from 13 to 60 years (average, 25.8 years). The FMD includes a midline suboccipital expansive cranioplasty combined with C1 laminectomy and expansive duraplasty using Gore-Tex membrane. All the patients had progressive myelopathy caused by syringomyelia; their clinical synopses are shown in Table 1. The diagnosis of syringomyelia and Chiari I malformation was made exclusively by means of MR imaging, which provides accurate identification of the rostral-caudal extent of the syrinx and anatomic delineation of the associated Chiari I malformation.

Ultrasound Study

Ultrasonic scanning was done with a Sonolayer α SSA 260 A (Toshiba, Odawara-shi, Japan), and a 7-MHz sector transducer was used to obtain images. By rotating the transducer head, both axial and sagittal scans could be obtained. The surgical field was filled with sterile warm saline solution to provide a fluid bath for the ultrasound. Such a bath reduces nearby field artifacts and allows the object of interest to be positioned within the focal zone. Most of the nervous system structure at the craniocervical junction was intersected by the sector scan. Conditions for satisfactory results were the complete absence of blood, fat drops, air bubbles, or alien bodies such as cotton or gelfoam in the sonographic window.

Results

Perioperative Findings for Ultrasound Study

The ultrasound study was used first to examine the anatomy and movement dynamics of the cerebellar tonsils, and next to assess the movement of the CSF and syrinx

TABLE 1. Clinical summary of the patients

Patient no.	Age/sex	Clinical presentation	Duration between onset of sign/symptoms and surgery	Level of syrinx	After foramen magnum decompression: Syrinx decreased/collapsed	After foramen magnum decompression: Symptoms improvement
1	45/F	Motor weakness in left and sensory disturbances in bilateral upper limb	2 years	C2–T4	Collapsed	No remarkable change
2	14/M	Scoliosis, no neurological deficit	9 years	C5–T2	Decreased	
3	17/F	Drop attack, no neurological deficit	3 months	C2–C5	Collapsed	
4	26/F	Disassociated sensory disturbance in right upper limb	4 years	C2–T3	Decreased	No remarkable change
5	14/M	Scoliosis, no neurological deficit	6 years	C6–T10	Collapsed	
6	60/F	Scoliosis, gait disturbances, motor weakness, and disassociated sensory disturbance	15 years	C2–T2	Decreased	Yes
7	48/F	Headache, no neurological deficit	4 months	C2–C4	Decreased	
8	17/F	Disassociated sensory disturbance	6 months	C2–L4	Collapsed	Yes
9	14/M	Scoliosis, no neurological deficit	3 years	C3–T9	Decreased	
10	24/M	Disassociated sensory disturbance	6 months	C2–T4	No remarkable change	Yes
11	17/M	Motor weakness and hypesthesia in left upper limb	3 months	C2–C3, and linear syrinx C3–T3	Decreased	Yes
12	13/F	Scoliosis and sensory disturbance in upper limb	4 years	C2–T12	Decreased	Yes

C, cervical; T, thoracic; L, lumbar; M, male; F, female.

at rest as well as during respiratory and cardiac cycles. In all patients the cerebellar tonsils were found to occlude the subarachnoid space at the foramen magnum. As the ultrasound study was performed during surgical exposure, the syringomyelia extending up to the craniocervical junction could be studied. None of the patients showed any patent communication between the fourth ventricle and the syrinx.

After the midline suboccipital craniotomy and first cervical laminectomy, the ultrasound study was performed first over the closed dura, then after opening of the dura (but with the arachnoid intact), and finally after the duraplasty. After bony decompression, the ultrasound studies over the closed dura demonstrated pulsatile downward movement of the cerebellar tonsils during cardiac systole and upward movement during diastole. The downward movement occurred synchronously with a sudden constriction of the spinal cord and syrinx. Dural scars or bands on the outside of the dura were identified in the form of overlapping, delineated high-density signals in addition to the signal produced by the dura itself. The subarachnoid space of all patients was obscured at the foramen magnum, and no CSF pulsation was observed across the foramen.

Dural scars or bands were eventually removed. Immediately after the dura was opened, ultrasound demonstrated that the pulsatile downward thrust of the cerebellar tonsils had diminished or disappeared. Surgical decompression was monitored with repeated ultrasonic scanning. After optimum decompression at the foramen magnum level had been achieved, a subtle gliding movement of the cerebellum on the medulla was observed in synchrony with the respiratory cycle, during which the spinal cord expanded with inspiration and contracted with expiration. Disappearance of pulsatile contraction of the syrinx and CSF movement across the foramen magnum were observed in all patients following surgery.

After a dural Gore-Tex graft (0.3 mm in thickness) was sutured into place, the reflection of ultrasound signals was partially diffused, although the signals from CSF pulsation remained obtainable.

Postoperative Magnetic Resonance (MR) Imaging

All the patients were followed up after surgery (3 months–13 years; mean, 4.8 years) on an outpatient basis and were evaluated by means of MR imaging, which was performed soon after surgery and then at regular intervals of 6 months until the syrinx had disappeared. In all patients anatomic MR imaging demonstrated that the size of the syrinx cavity had decreased within several days to weeks after surgery so that obstruction of the CSF flow at the foramen magnum was eliminated. Subsequent images showed a further reduction and eventual disappearance of the syrinx cavity (see Table 1). No clinically or radiographically detectable recurrence of syringomyelia occurred during the follow-up period. The tonsillar portion of the cerebellum first started to regain its normal shape and finally ascended into the posterior fossa in most of the patients.

An Illustrative Case

A 17-year-old female patient presented with right-hand numbness that had lasted for 6 months. Neurological examination revealed dissociated sensory disturbance (reduced pain and temperature sensation) at the C2–L4 spinal segments on the right side. There was no motor weakness. Preoperative MR imaging disclosed Chiari I mal-

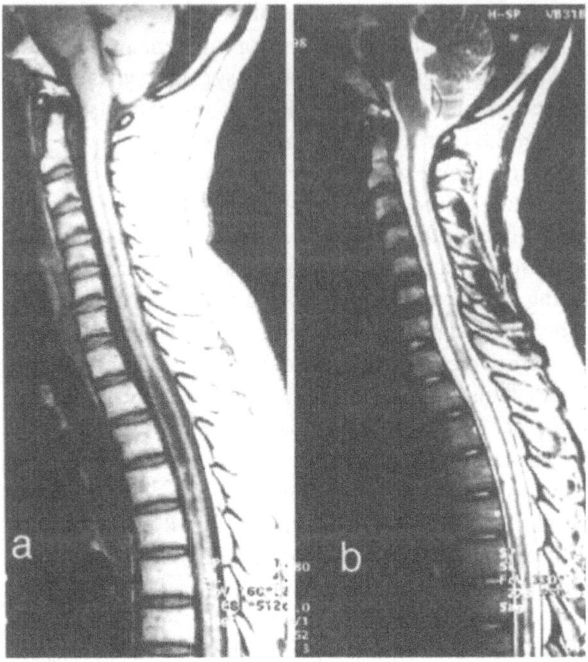

FIG. 1. **a** T_1-weighted image and **b** T_2-weighted image of 17-year-old female patient with syringomyelia associated with Chiari I malformation. Magnetic resonance (MR) imaging demonstrates herniation of the cerebellar tonsils and extension of the syrinx from the upper cervical to the lumbar segments of the spinal cord

formation with syrinx in the spinal cord extending over the C2–L2 segments of the vertebrae (Fig. 1a,b). The patient underwent FMD according to our protocol. Intraoperative ultrasound demonstrated impaction at the foramen magnum (Fig. 2a) and a piston-like downward thrust of the cerebellar tonsils in synchrony with cardiac systole. Immediately after opening of the dura, the pulsatile downward thrust of the tonsils disappeared and CSF movement across the foramen magnum was observed because decompression had created enough space for the CSF around the foramen magnum (Fig. 2b). Postoperatively, the first MR imaging was performed 2 weeks after surgery at discharge of the patient. The MR image showed reduced syrinx size and rounding of the previously herniated portion of the tonsil. The patient was followed up at regular intervals of 3 months on an outpatient basis, and MR imaging was performed twice in a year. One year and 6 months after surgery, MR imaging showed the syrinx had collapsed and that the tonsil had regained its normal shape and ascended into the posterior cranial fossa (Fig. 3a,b). The patient showed improvement in her dissociated sensory disturbance and had resumed a normal life.

Discussion

Ultrasonography has been used to localize brain tumors for more than 30 years [6], but its use during spinal operations is still limited. Recently, the development of a relatively small sector transducer with useful axial resolution allows for direct visualization of the spinal cord, even through a narrow window such as a hemilaminectomy, and thus makes intraoperative spinal sonography more practicable [7,8]. In addi-

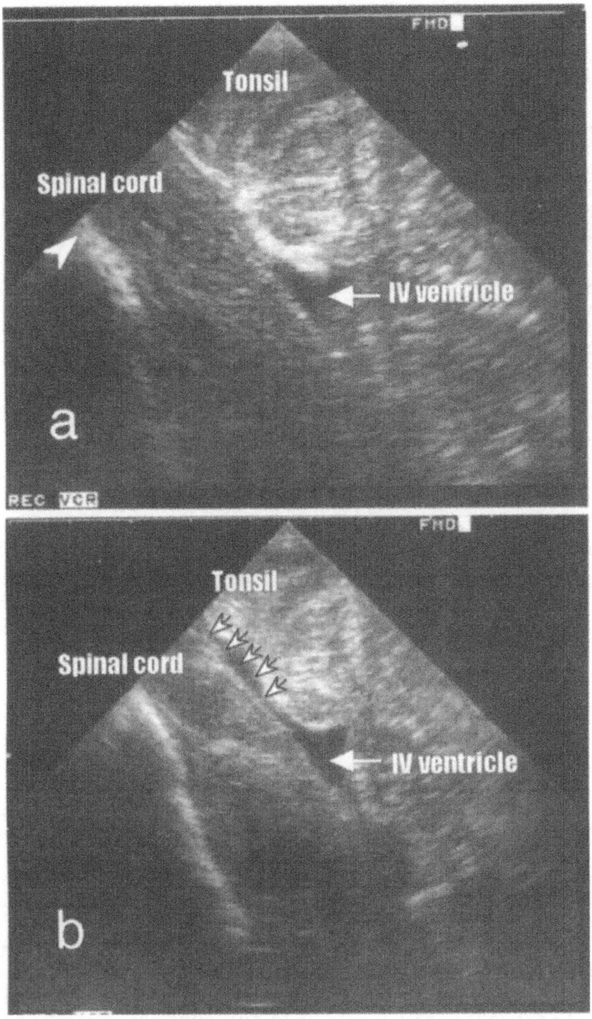

FIG. 2a,b. Intraoperative ultrasound scanning. **a** Before opening of the dura; *arrowhead* indicates impaction at the level of foramen magnum. **b** After opening of the dura, there is enough space for cerebrospinal fluid (CSF) movement (*arrows* indicate low-intensity signals in premedullary space), indicating that decompression has been achieved

tion, improved resolution of the real-time images obtainable with existing B-mode ultrasonography units makes possible detailed anatomic evaluation of spinal cord physiology (CSF pulsation, and the spinal cord) both before and after surgical manipulation. From a technical point of view, the fact that ultrasound scans can be performed in different planes (longitudinal and axial) and that dynamic movements can be observed on real-time images means more accurate assessment of the degree of foramen magnum impaction and decompression during surgery.

Intraoperative ultrasonography has proved to be as significant an advance in syrinx surgery as MR imaging has been in the diagnosis of spinal cord lesions. Ultrasound allows for a careful physiological assessment of the cord after suboccipital craniotomy and laminectomy and visualized pulsation of CSF and the cord. The surgeon can thus ascertain the degree of cord compression by Chiari I malformation in real time. Com-

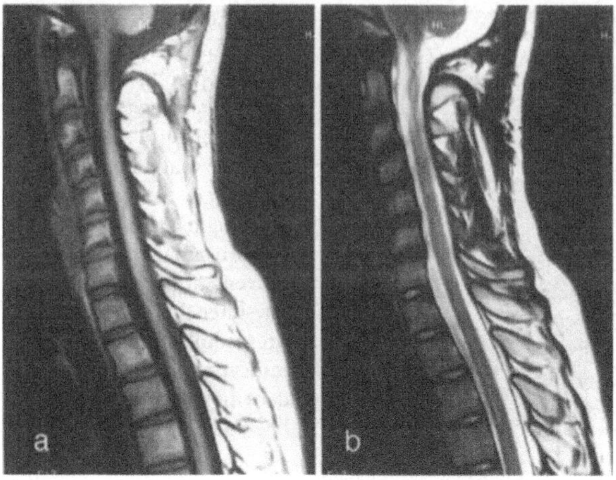

FIG. 3. **a** T_1-weighted image. **b** T_2-weighted image. These MR images were obtained 1 year and 6 months after foramen magnum decompression for syringomyelia associated with Chiari I malformation. The syrinx had collapsed and the tonsil had regained its round shape and ascended into the posterior cranial fossa

pared with recently introduced intraoperative computed tomography (CT) or MR imaging, ultrasonic monitoring is cost-effective, quick, convenient, and easy to repeat. In addition, ultrasound study does not necessitate any extension of total operating time.

This report summarizes the use of ultrasound in 12 cases requiring foramen magnum decompression. This technology proved to be both efficient and valuable for providing the neurosurgeon with direct and immediate information during and at the completion of the operation. Such information may modify the surgical approach. In addition, it allows the surgeon to assess the progress and final results of the operation before its completion.

References

1. Dubby MJ, Williams B (1991) Hindbrain migration after decompression for hindbrain hernia: a quantitative assessment using MRI. Br J Neurosurg 5:141–152
2. Isu T, Iwasaki Y, Akino M, Abe H (1990) Hydrosyringomyelia associated with a Chiari I malformation in children and adolescents. Neurosurgery 26:591–596
3. Dyste GN, Menezes AH, VanGilder JC (1989) Symptomatic Chiari malformation: an analysis of presentation, management, and long-term outcome. J Neurosurg 71:159–168
4. Heiss JD, Patronas N, Hetty L, et al (1999) Elucidating the pathophysiology of syringomyelia. J Neurosurg 91:553–562
5. Munshi I, Frim D, Stine-Reyes R, et al (2000) Effects of posterior fossa decompression with and without duraplasty on Chiari malformation-associated hydromyelia. Neurosurgery 46:1384–1390
6. Tanaka K, Ito K, Wagai T (1965) The localization of brain tumors by ultrasonic techniques. A clinical review of 111 cases. J Neurosurg 23:135–147
7. Montalvo BM, Quencer RM (1986) Intraoperative ultrasonography in spinal surgery: current state of the art. Neuroradiology 28:551–590
8. Rubin JM (1990) Ultrasonography in spinal cord surgery. In: Rubin JM, Chandler WF (eds) Ultrasound in neurosurgery. Raven Press, New York, pp 106–182

Intraoperative Subarachnoid Pressure to Predict the Result of Posterior Decompression in Syringomyelia Associated with Chiari Type I Malformation

Motoi Shoda, Shigehiko Kuno, Shinya Nagahisa, and Tetsuo Kanno

Summary. The surgical treatment for syringomyelia associated with Chiari type I malformation is reported. Surgical treatment is not yet established because the genesis of syringomyelia has not been clarified. We report here the subarachnoid cerebrospinal fluid flow findings during posterior decompression that correlate to the disappearance of syringomyelia.

During 1991 to 1999, among the patients with syringomyelia associated with Chiari type I malformation on whom we operated, we selected six cases with pos-terior decompression that avoided injuring the arachnoid. We describe here one male and five female patients from 17 to 54 years old (mean, 43.3 years old). Associated disorders were basilar impression, atlantoaxial dislocation, and assimilation of C1 to occipital bone in one patient, scoliosis in one patient, and Huntington's chorea in one patient. We incised the cervical dura linearly with extreme care, under a microscope, to not injure the arachnoid. The dura was incised in a Y-shape toward the cerebellar side. The subarachnoid usually bulged initially so we could avoid injuring the arachnoid. Subarachnoid pressure decreased when the incision was completed, to the cerebellar side, and pulsation was observed. We report how to evaluate subarachnoid CSF pressure during incision of the dura mater to predict the result of syringomyelia. There is good correlation between decompression and decreased syringomyelia size. This technique is not difficult and does not need any special equipment.

Key words. Syringomyelia, Chiari type I malformation, Intraoperative subarachnoid finding, Posterior fossa decompression

Introduction

The surgical treatment for syringomyelia associated with Chiari type I malformati on is not yet established because the genesis of syringomyelia has not been clarified [1].

Department of Neurosurgery, Fujita Health University, 1-98 Dengakugakubo, Kutsukake-cho, Toyoake, Aichi 470-1192, Japan

Since Gardner reported posterior decompression with muscle plugging to the obex, various surgeries have been reported for this pathology, such as posterior fossa decompression, expanding foramen magnum decompression, dural outer layer removal, tonsillectomy, and shunting operations [2–6]. As there are no clear criteria for selecting the surgical procedure for syringomyelia with Chiari type I malformation, surgeons select the manipulation according to their experience. We report here subarachnoid cerebrospinal fluid (CSF) flow findings during posterior decompression that correlate to the disappearance of syringomyelia.

Material and Methods

During 1991 to 1999, among the patients with syringomyelia associated with Chiari type I malformation on whom we operated, we selected six cases with posterior decompression that avoided injuring the arachnoid. We describe here one male and five female patients, from 17 to 54 years old (mean, 43.3 years old). Associated disorders were basilar impression, atlantoaxial dislocation, and assimilation of C1 to occipital bone in one patient, scoliosis in one patient, and Huntington's chorea in one patient (Table 1).

The standard surgical technique of posterior decompression was to remove the C1 or C2 lamina according to the position of tonsillar herniation. Posterior decompression was done with foramen magnum decompression. The removal range of the foramen magnum was 1.5–2.0 cm from the midline on each side. Then, we incised the cervical dura linearly with extreme care, under a microscope, to not injure the arachnoid. The dura was incised in a Y-shape toward the cerebellar side. The subarachnoid usually bulged initially so we could avoid injuring the arachnoid. Subarachnoid pressure will decrease when the incision is completed, to the cerebellar side, and pulsation will be observed. After the dural incision is completed, we use Gore-Tex to close the dura water tight.

Case Presentation

A 54-year-old woman was admitted because of right hand pain, loss of temperature sensation, and gait disturbance. She had shown marked myelopathy and numbness of the left side with pain and temperature sensation loss for several months before

TABLE 1. Syringomyelia with Chiari type I

Case	Age	Sex	Syrinx	Additional abnormality
1	46	F	+	—
2	17	F	+	Scoliosis
3	52	M	+	—
4	54	F	+	Huntington's chorea
5	37	F	+	—
6	54	F	+	Basilar impression, AAD, assimilation of C1

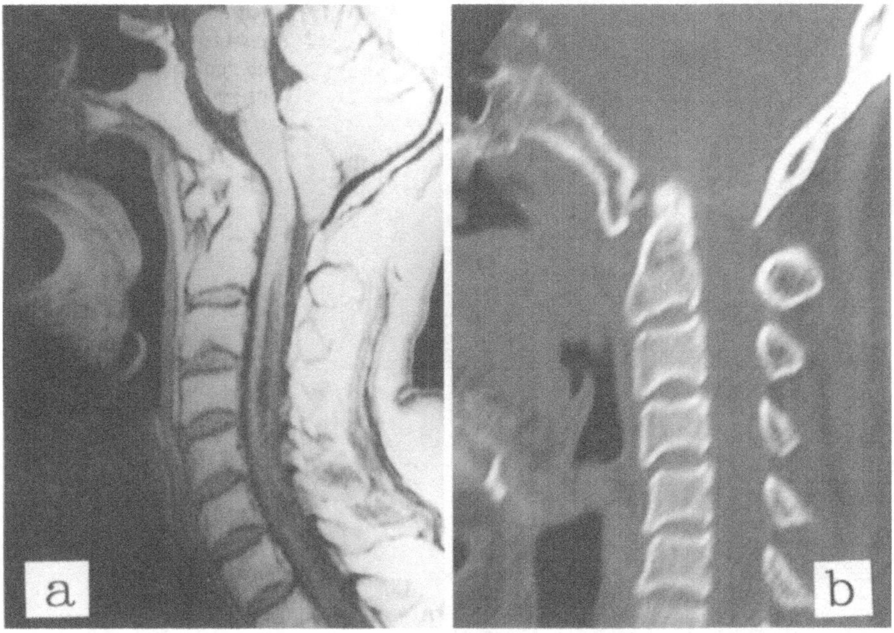

FIG. 1. **a** Preoperative magnetic resonance imaging (MRI) (T_1, WI) showed marked syringomyelia with tonsilar herniation and AAD. **b** CT reconstruction showed basilar impression assimilation of C1 and AAD.

presentation. Magnetic resonance imaging (MRI) and craniocervical X-ray examination revealed basilar impression, assimilation of C1, atlantoaxial dislocation, and Chiari type I malformation with syringomyelia.

We selected transoral odontoidectomy first and then posterior fossa decompression with dural plasty. The syringomyelia before surgery is shown in Fig. 1. Dural decompression without injury to the arachnoid was done and pulsation of the arachnoid observed (Fig. 2). Postoperative MRI showed marked improvement of syringomyelia (Fig. 3); the patient's neurological signs were also improved.

Discussion

Since Gardner reported muscle plugging to the obex [2], various surgical procedures have been reported for syringomyelia associated with Chiari type I malformation. The most common surgical procedures are classified as posterior fossa decompression and shunt operations. Posterior fossa decompression also has many variations, such as expanding foramen magnum decompression, outer layer removal, and tonsillectomy [2–6]. Because the origin of syringomyelia has not been investigated, standard procedures have not yet been established.

To select the surgical procedures, there are some important points that should be checked such as arachnoiditis, decompression range, occipital sinus, and subarach-

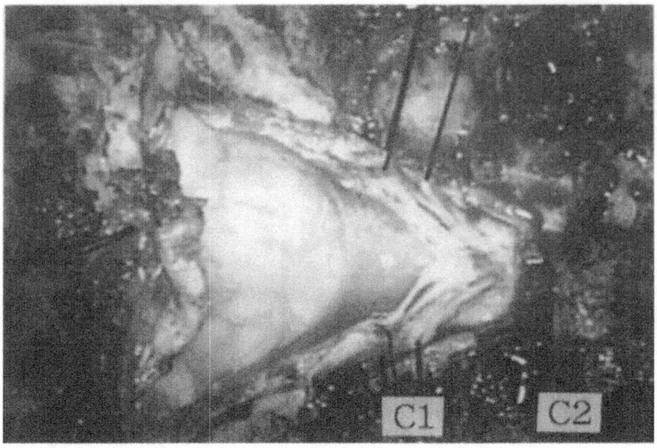

FIG. 2. After the dural incision, subarachnoid pressure was decompressed and good pulsation was observed

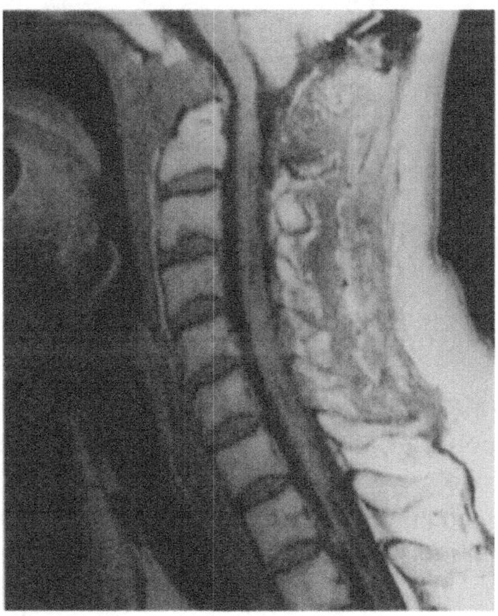

FIG. 3. Postoperative MRI showed marked improvement of syringomyelia

noid blood remaining. We selected posterior decompression with whole-layer dural plasty because we can clarity those points during surgery. Outer-layer removal surgery has the merit of arachnoid protection, but there is a risk of bleeding from the occipital sinus, and we could not determine the condition of arachnoiditis and subarachnoid space decompression.

Recent investigation provides more precise information about CSF flow around the craniovertebral area before surgery. The Q-test, % cardiac cycle, and cine-MRI are important examinations before surgery [7,8]. However, it is still difficult to assess the postoperative result of syringomyelia. It is very important that we evaluate decompression during surgery. We have observed the bulging of the arachnoid during incision of the cervical dura mater, and this subarachnoid bulging disappeared and showed pulsation after proper decompression of the cerebellar side of the dura mater.

Our technique is very useful to predict the postoperative results of treatment of syringomyelia. All cases, except one case of Huntington's chorea with arachnoiditis, showed a postoperative decrease in the size of the syringomyelia. This technique is important for evaluating the condition during surgery and does not need any special equipment.

Conclusions

Selection of surgical procedures for syringomyelia associated with Chiari type I malformation is controversial. The most common procedure is posterior fossa decompression, but we could not evaluate the surgical procedures to predict the postoperative outcome. We reported how to evaluate subarachnoid CSF pressure during incising the dura mater to predict the result of syringomyelia. There is a correlation between good decompression and decreased syringomyelia size. This technique is not so difficult and does not require any special equipment.

References

1. Moriwaka F, Tashiro K, Tachibana S, Yada K (1995) Epidemiology of syringomyelia in Japan: the nationwide survey. Rinsho Shinkeigaku 35(12):1395–1397 (in Japanese)
2. Gardner WJ, Angel J (1958) The mechanism of syringomyelia and its surgical correction. Clin Neurosurg 6:131–140
3. Goel A, Achawal S (1995) The surgical treatment of Chiari malformation association with atlantoaxial dislocation. Br J Neurosurg 9(1):67–72
4. Guyotat J, Bret P, Mottolese C, et al (1997) Chiari 1 malformation with syringomyelia treated by decompression of craniospinal junction and tonsillectomy. Apropos of 8 cases. Neurochirurgie 43(3):135–141
5. Hida K, Iwasaki Y, Koyanagi I, Abe H (1995) Surgical indication and results of foramen magnum decompression versus syringosubarachnoid shunting for syringomyelia associated with Chiari malformation. Neurosurgery 37(4):673–678
6. Isu T, Sasaki H, Tamura H, Kobayashi N (1993) Foramen magnum decompression with removal of the outer layer of the dura as treatment for syringomyelia occurring with Chiari 1 malformation. Neurosurgery 33(5):844–849
7. Tachibana S, Iida H, Yada K (1992) Significance of positive Queckenstedt test in patient with syringomyelia associated with Arnold-Chiari malformations. J Neurosurg 76(1):67–71
8. Tamaki N, Nagashima T (1995) Hydrodynamics of syringomyelia. Rinsho Shinkeigaku 35(12):1398–1399 (in Japanese)

Quantitative Analysis of Cerebrospinal Fluid Flow Dynamics in Syringomyelia Associated with Chiari I Malformation

Shogo Tamura[1], Norihiko Tamaki[1], Mitsugu Nakamura[1], Tatsuya Nagashima[1], and Junji Kitamura[2]

Summary. Two-dimensional phase-contrast (2D-PC) images can be used to evaluate cerebrospinal fluid (CSF) flow dynamics. The fast and active movement of CSF corresponds to cardiac pulsation. This report concerns the quantitative analysis of CSF flow dynamics using 2D-PC images. Since September 1996, we have obtained 35 2D-PC images each from 19 patients. We measured craniocaudal maximum CSF flow (peak velocity) and the position of peak velocity as a percentage of the R-R interval of the cardiac cycle (peak velocity position). In normal volunteers, peak velocity and peak velocity position were 4.67 cm/s and 19.3%, respectively, at the foramen magnum and 4.73 cm/s and 17.5% at the spinal subarachnoid space. In the 14 cases of syringomyelia, preoperative 2D-PC images showed delayed peak velocity position. Postoperative 2D-PC images showed shortened peak velocity position in improved patients. Preoperative CSF flow velocity in syringes was low and showed a phase contrary to that in the subarachnoid space. Postoperative CSF dynamics in syringes showed a normal pulsate pattern, although peak velocity was still low. 2D-PC images are useful for the evaluation of CSF flow dynamics and prediction of surgical results.

Key words. Syringomyelia, Phase-contrast MRI, Chiari, CSF

Introduction

Cerebrospinal fluid (CSF) hydrodynamics has been reported to be a major factor in the pathophysiology of syringomyelia [1–3]. Our purpose was to determine the clinical significance of pre- and postoperative spinal CSF flow dynamics for the management of syringomyelia. The fast and active movement of spinal CSF flow is synchronized with cardiac pulsation. For the analysis of CSF flow dynamics, we used two-dimensional phase-contrast (2D-PC) images obtained at the foramen magnum and the spinal subarachnoid space. We report the results of quantitative analysis of CSF flow dynamics using 2D-PC images in normal volunteers and syringomyelic patients.

[1] Department of Neurosurgery, Kobe University, Graduate School of Medicine, 7-5-1 Kusunoki-cho, Chuo-ku, Kobe 650-0017, Japan
[2] Kitamura Clinic, Ninomiya-cho, Chuo-ku, Kobe, Japan

Materials and Methods

Since September 1996, we have examined 27 patients with syringomyelia associated with Chiari I malformation and seven normal volunteers. Magnetic resonance (MR) measurements were performed on a 1.0-Tesla MRI system (Impact Expert; Siemens AG, Erlangen, Germany). All imaging was done with the following pulse sequence parameters: TR, 50–100 ms; TE, 11 ms; venc, 10–20; and ECG triggered.

We measured craniocaudal maximum CSF flow velocity (peak velocity) and the position of peak velocity as a percentage of the R-R interval of the cardiac cycle (peak velocity position). These values were measured before and after surgical treatment for syringomyelia. Statistical significance was calculated by means of Student's t test. We considered a P value of less than 0.05 mandatory for statistical significance.

Results

In normal volunteers, the dynamics of CSF flow velocity uniformly showed a biphasic waveform. The peak velocity and peak velocity position were 4.67 ± 0.9 cm/s and 19.3% ± 3.3% at the foramen magnum, and 4.73 ± 2.5 cm/s and 17.5% ± 1.9% at the spinal subarachnoid space. Figure 1 shows a normal CSF flow curve in the foramen magnum. At 0%–10% peak velocity position, the CSF flows in a cranial direction. The flow changed to a caudal direction and showed peak velocity at 15%–20% peak velocity position. The caudal CSF flow continued up to 45%–55% peak velocity position.

In cases of syringomyelia, preoperative 2D-PC images showed significantly delayed peak velocity positions (38.3% ± 8.0%, foramen magnum; 39.1% ± 10.1%, spinal

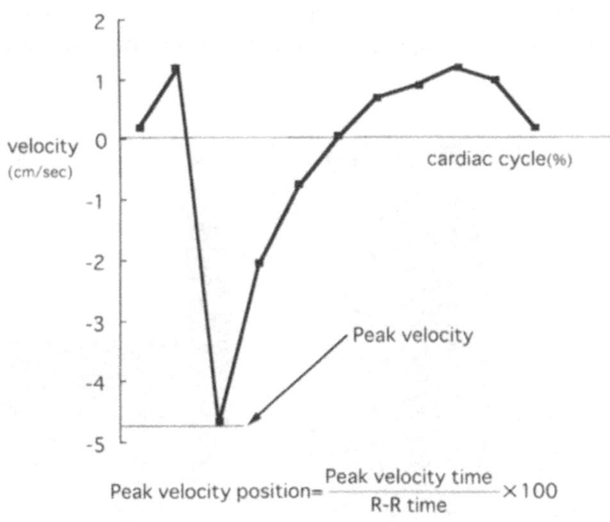

Fig. 1. Time-velocity curve in normal volunteers. The peak velocity is a craniocaudal maximal cerebrospinal fluid (CSF) flow velocity. The peak velocity position means the position of peak velocity as a percentage of the R-R interval of the cardiac cycle

subarachnoid space; $P < 0.05$). However, peak velocities (3.67 ± 1.8 cm/s, foramen magnum; 4.30 ± 1.4 cm/s, spinal subarachnoid space) were not very different from those of the normal control.

Twenty-five of the 27 patients with syringomyelia underwent foramen magnum decompression (FMD) and duraplasty. Postoperatively, the symptoms improved in 18 patients (group A) and remained unchanged in 7 patients (group B). In group A, peak velocity positions (26.7% ± 3.5%, foramen magnum; 23.9% ± 4.1%, spinal subarachnoid space) improved significantly ($P < 0.05$), although peak velocities (3.96 ± 1.8 cm/s, foramen magnum; 4.25 ± 1.3 cm/s, spinal subarachnoid space) did not change significantly. In group B, neither peak velocities (5.55 ± 3.1 cm/s, foramen magnum; 3.67 ± 2.2 cm/s, spinal subarachnoid space) nor peak velocity positions (38.3% ± 6.8%, foramen magnum; 42.5 ± 8.3%, spinal subarachnoid space) improved.

Case 1

A 17-year-old male experienced dysesthesia of the upper and lower extremities. Preoperative MRI showed Chiari I malformation and syringomyelia extended from the cervical to the upper thoracic segment of the spinal cord (Fig. 2). Preoperative 2D-PC images showed delayed peak velocity position (39.0%) and prolonged caudal CSF flow (Fig. 3). Dysesthesia improved after foramen magnum decompression and duraplasty. Postoperative MRI and 2D-PC images showed reduced syringes, improved peak velocity position (21.0%), and normalized CSF flow curve (Figs. 4, 5).

Discussion

With the aid of 2D-PC images, we could quantify the CSF flow dynamics in all patients and normal volunteers. In normal volunteers, the CSF flow showed a constant biphasic pattern that was compatible with that previously reported [4]. Du Boulay

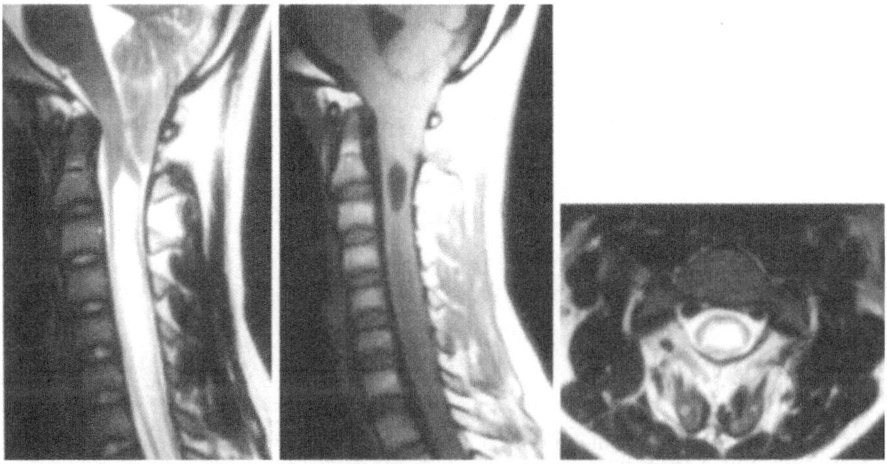

FIG. 2. Preoperative MRI shows that Chiari I malformation and syringomyelia extended from the cervical to the upper thoracic segment of the spinal cord

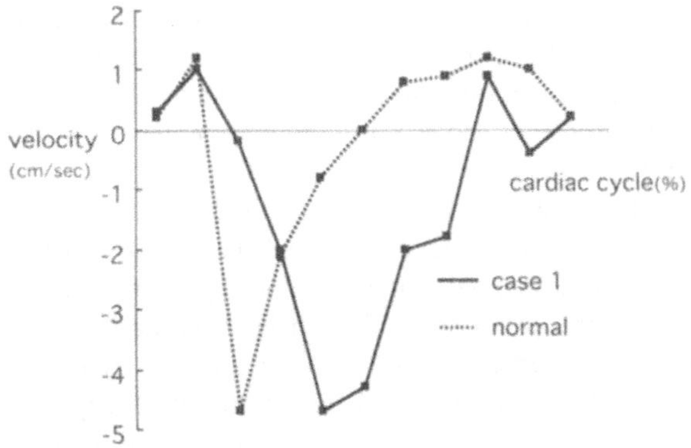

FIG. 3. Preoperative two-dimensional phase-contrast (2D-PC) image shows a delayed peak velocity position and prolonged caudal CSF flow

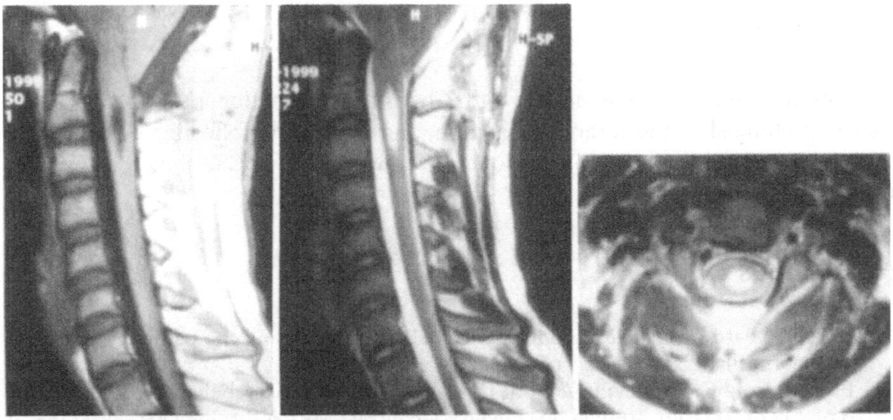

FIG. 4. Postoperative MRI shows well-reduced syringes

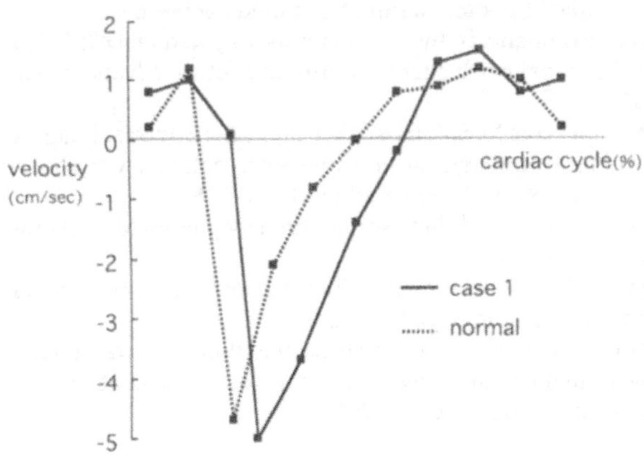

FIG. 5. Postoperative 2D-PC images show an improved peak velocity position (21.0%) and normalized CSF flow curve

used myelography to demonstrate that the CSF pulsation is synchronized with cardiac pulsation [5]. Recently, advanced MRI technology enabled us to see the pulsation of CSF without any invasiveness and to analyze it quantitatively [6–9]. We found that the craniocaudal CSF flow synchronized with the cardiac pulsation is generated by brain volume expansion induced by an increase in intravascular blood volume.

In cases of syringomyelia associated with Chiari I malformation, the subarachnoid space of the foramen magnum is restricted because the tonsil has fallen into the foramen magnum. Preoperative studies showed delayed peak velocity position in both the foramen magnum and spinal subarachnoid space. This delay was the result of blocking the normal CSF flow at the foramen magnum. Bhadelia et al. reported improvement in systolic CSF flow pulsations immediately below the foramen magnum after surgery [10]. In the patients who underwent foramen magnum decompression, peak velocity improved significantly ($P < 0.05$) and the CSF flow pattern became almost normalized. Postoperative reduction of peak velocity position thus corresponds to improvement of the patient's symptoms.

Conclusions

In cases of syringomyelia associated with Chiari I malformation, peak velocity position is prolonged at the foramen magnum, and it recovers following FMD. 2D-PC images are useful for pre- and postoperative evaluation of CSF flow dynamics in Chiari I malformation.

References

1. Heiss JD, Patronas N, De Vroom HL, et al (1999) Elucidating the pathophysiology of syringomyelia. J Neurosurg 91:553–562
2. Pujoa J, Roig C, Capdevilia A, et al (1995) Motion of the cerebellar tonsils in Chiari type I malformation studied by cine phase-contrast MRI. Neurology 45:1746–1753
3. Oldfield EH, Muraszko K, Shawker TH, Patronas NJ (1994) Pathophysiology of syringomyelia associated with Chiari I malformation of the cerebellar tonsils. Implications for diagnosis and treatment [see comments]. J Neurosurg 80:3–15
4. Kuroda S, Matsuzawa H, Iwasaki Y, et al (1994) CSF dynamics and pathophysiology in syringomyelia associated with Chiari I malformation. Noushinkei 46:59–64
5. du Boulay GH (1996) Pulsative movements in the CSF pathway. Br J Radiol 39:255–262
6. Sze G (1992) MR imaging of the spinal cord: current status and future advances. AJR Am J Roentgenol 159:149–159
7. Hofmann E, Warmuth Metz M, Bendszus M, Solymosi L (2000) Phase-contrast imaging of the cervical CSF and spinal cord: volumetric motion analysis in patients with Chiari I malformation [see comments]. AJNR Am J Neuroradiol 21:151–158
8. Enzmann DR, Pelc NJ (1993) Cerebrospinal fluid flow measured by phase-contrast cine MR. AJNR Am J Neuroradiol 14:1301–1307
9. Rubin JB, Wright A, Enzmann DR (1988) Lumbar spine: motion compensation for cerebrospnal fluid on MR imaging. Radiology 167:225–231
10. Bhadelia RA, Bogdan AR, Wolpart SM, et al (1995) Cerebrospinal fluid flow waveforms: analysis in patients with Chiari I malformation by means of gated phase-contrast MR imaging velocity measurements. Radiology 196:195–202

Deep Pain Loss in Syringomyelia and Other Spinal Cord Lesions

Shigekuni Tachibana and Sumito Sato

Summary. Deep pain is an important muscle nociception; however, testing for it has long been ignored in the clinical field. The authors studied the clinical significance of testing deep pain sensation in patients with spinal cord lesions. Deep pain sensations evoked by squeezing superficial muscles were examined in 19 patients with syringomyelia, 50 with cervical spondylosis, 2 with Hirayama disease, and 2 patients with spinal neurinoma. Deep pain sensitivity was graded as hyper-, normal, hypo-, and loss compared to that of the trapezius muscle in the intact side and was compared with other neurological findings. In those patients with syringomyelia, deep pain was diminished or lost in 14 (74%) patients. Only 24% of the patients with cervical spondylosis presented superficial sensory loss in the digits. In contrast, 70% presented deep pain diminution, especially in those muscles with diminished deep tendon reflex (except for Hirayama disease) or in those muscles innervated by the same segment with a dysesthetic dermatome. In the patients with spinal neurinoma, deep pain was lost in those muscles with diminished deep tendon reflex. Ten patients of 17 with syringomyelia underwent surgery and complained of residual pain postoperatively in spite of shrinkage of the syrinx. This residual pain was of two types, one being superficial dysesthetic pain and the other muscle aching pain. The latter presumably is related to the dysfunction of the system conveying muscle nociception. Deep pain loss is not uncommon in many spinal cord lesions. In addition, postoperative residual pain in syringomyelia should be recognized as superficial dysesthetic pain, deep muscle aching pain, or both. This approach will develop a successful measure of treatment of residual pain in the future.

Key words. Syringomyelia, Cervical spondylosis, Muscle nociception, Cutaneous nociception, Deep tendon reflex

Introduction

Several studies concerning muscle nociception and its pathway have been done [1–7]. However, most of these are basic research, and the subject has long been ignored in the clinical field. Dissociated sensory disturbance is a common clinical feature in

---

Department of Neurosurgery, Kitasato University School of Medicine, 1-15-1 Kitasato, Sagamihara, Kanagawa 228-8555, Japan

patients with syringomyelia. However, without exception, hypoalgesia or analgesia means superficial pain loss. In 1967, Magee and Schneider [8] reported a patient with syringomyelia who presented with deep pain loss but otherwise had normal cutaneous sensation; however, this topic has not received much attention. Our study aimed to evaluate the significance of neurological testing of muscle nociception (deep pain) in syringomyelia and other spinal cord lesions.

Materials and Methods

This study consisted of 19 patients with syringomyelia (3 men and 16 women; mean age, 47 years), 50 patients with cervical spondylosis (40 men and 10 women; mean age, 55 years), 2 patients with Hirayama disease (2 men, 20 and 25 years old), and 2 patients with spinal neurinoma (2 men, 28 and 57 years old). Most often the genesis of syringomyelia was Chiari malformation (Table 1).

Deep pain was elicited by simply squeezing superficial muscles and was graded as "hyper," "normal," "hypo," and "null" compared to that of trapezius muscle in the intact side. The results were compared with other clinical signs and symptoms.

Results

Patients with Syringomyelia

In 4 patients with syringomyelia, both deep and superficial sensation was normal. Each 2 patients presented diminished either superficial or deep pain sensation only; however, in 12, both deep and superficial pain sensation were diminished simultaneously (Table 2).

TABLE 1. Genesis of syringomyelia

Genesis	No. of patients
Chiari malformation	15
Arachnoiditis	2
Tumor	1
Unknown	1

TABLE 2. Relationship between deep and superficial pain loss in syringomyelia ($n = 19$)

	No. of patients	Percent
Normal	4	21.1
De	2	10.5
De + Su	12	63.2
Su	2	10.5

De, deep pain loss; Su, superficial pain loss.

TABLE 3. Relationship between levels of superficial and deep pain loss in syringomyelia ($n = 19 \times 2$)

Dermatome	No. of sides	Muscles	No. of muscles
C2	5		
C3	10		
C4	13	Trapezius	3
C5	15	Bicepa brachii	12
C6	15	Brachioradialis	15
C7	15	Triceps brachii	15
C8	15		
Th1	8		

TABLE 4. Relationship between deep tendon reflex (DTR) and deep pain in syringomyelia ($n = 19 \times 6$)

	Deep pain		
Reflex	Normal	Hypo-	Null
Areflexia	21	8	18
Hyporeflexia	12	2	1
Normal	25	8	6
Hyperreflexia	10	3	0

$\chi^2 = 14.4$; $P = 0.024$.

The spinal cord segments innervating those muscles with diminished deep pain and the dermatome with diminished superficial pain was distributed very similarly (Table 3). At the same time, diminished deep pain was observed at a significantly high rate in those muscles with diminished deep tendon reflex (DTR) (Table 4).

Among 19 patients with syringomyelia, 17 underwent surgery. A detailed interview revealed that 10 of them complained of residual pain postoperatively. This residual pain was of two types: one was superficial dysesthetic pain and the other muscle aching pain. Most of the patients rarely distinguished aching muscle accurately; however, they could distinguish deep pain from superficial dysesthetic pain. In 8 patients, pain was both superficial dysesthetic pain and deep muscle aching pain; in 2 of them, pain was only deep muscle aching.

Patients with Other Cord Lesions

In 50 patients with cervical spondylosis, the percentile of the patients who presented with dysesthesia (irrespective of initial symptom or on examination), deep pain loss, and superficial pain loss is shown in Table 5. Of the patients, 20% showed no sensory disturbance, 10% only superficial dysesthesia, 42% both dysesthesia and deep pain loss, 24% all the sensory modalities, and 4% only deep pain loss. In other words, subjective superficial dysesthesia is common in as many as 76% of patients with cervical spondylosis. At the same time, deep pain loss was also found at a high rate, 70%. In contrast, superficial pain was diminished only in 24% at the time of examination.

TABLE 5. Relationship between dysesthesia, deep pain loss, and superficial pain loss in cervical spondylosis ($n = 50$)

	No. of patients	Percent
Normal	10	20
Dy	5	10
Dy + De	21	42
Dy + De + Su	12	24
De	2	4

Dy, dysesthesia; De, deep pain loss; Su, superficial pain loss.

TABLE 6. Relationship between dysesthetic digits and deep pain loss in cervical spondylosis ($n = 50 \times 2$)

		No. of muscles			
Dysesthetic digits	No. of sides	Biceps brachii	Brachioradialis	Triceps brachii	None
None	46	2	8	8	40
All	5	3	8	7	2
First, second	16	3	12	6	2
Third	19	5	7	7	8
Fourth, fifth	14	1	1	10	3

TABLE 7. Relationship between DTR and deep pain loss in cervical spondylosis ($n = 50 \times 6$)

	Deep pain			
DTR	Hyper	Normal	Hypo	Null
Areflesia	0	21	12	31
Hyporeflexia	1	17	13	7
Normal	0	153	14	5
Hyperreflexia	0	19	6	1

$\chi^2 = 116.766$; $P < 0.0001$.

The relationship between initial dysesthetic digits obtained from the history and those muscles with deep pain loss at the time of examination is as follows. In those patients who started with dysesthesia in the first and second digits, in other words, at the dermatome of C6 segment, deep pain loss was common in the brachioradialis muscle, and in those who started at the fourth and fifth digits, deep pain was diminished in the triceps brachii muscle (Table 6).

The relationship between deep tendon reflexes (DTR) and deep pain sensitivities is shown in Table 7. In the muscle with diminished DTRs, deep pain loss was seen at a significantly high rate compared to that of either hypo- or normal reflex ($\chi^2 = 116.766$; $P < 0.0001$). In two patients with Hirayama disease (juvenile unilateral muscle atrophy), no deep pain loss was seen. In two patients with spinal neurinoma, one having extracanalicular plexiform neurinoma in the C6 root and the other a caudal single root neurinoma, no evidence of weakness of the muscle or diminution of superficial sensation was observed postoperatively. However, the DTR in the brachioradialis in the former and quadriceps femoris in the latter diminished postoperatively, and at the same time, deep pain was lost in these particular muscles.

Discussion

Vatine et al. [9] developed electric pressure algometry to elicit deep pain. By using this instrument, the result is more accurate; however, its use has not been popular. Squeezing a superficial muscle to provoke deep pain as used in this study is a rather rough method and the results can easily biased by the examiner; however, it is very convenient and easy for daily clinical examination without using any instrument.

In the patients with cervical spondylosis, dysesthesia in the digits is a common initial symptom; however, superficial sensory loss is not always proven on the neurological examination. In this study, 76% of patients presented with dysesthesia, although only 27% exhibited superficial sensory diminution in the digits on examination. This effect is well recognized as overlapping of the dermatome innervation of the superficial sensory system [10]. Irritation of a single root or segment radiates to the whole skin area innervated by this root; however, complete lesion in a single root hardly indicates superficial sensory loss. Deep pain loss was found in as many as 76% of the patients with cervical spondylosis, especially in those muscles with diminished deep tendon reflex, except for Hirayama disease, or those muscles innervated by the segment with initial dysesthetic dermatome. In addition, the result obtained in the patients with spinal neurinoma points out that a single root lesion can produce deep pain loss without superficial pain loss. These findings indicate that the deep pain system seems to have less complete overlapping.

On the other hand, superficial pain loss is a common feature in syringomyelia. This result presumably is caused by the syrinx being apt to extend longitudinally for several segments of the spinal cord; therefore, overlapping innervation of the superficial dermatome is insufficient and hypoalgesia or analgesia manifests. Furthermore, deep pain loss appeared to be very common in this disease. Most patients exhibited both superficial and deep pain loss. Only two patients presented dissociation of deep and superficial pain loss, as reported by Magee [8]. Magee attributed this dissociation of deep and superficial pain sensation to lamination of the spinothalamic tract. However, this would not be true, for several reasons. The syrinx is apt to extend not into the white matter but into the posterior lateral gray matter, destroying the posterior horn. In an animal experiment, fibers conducting superficial pain (C fiber) terminated to the first and second laminae of the posterior horn, although fibers conveying muscle nociception terminate at the first and fourth laminae [6,7]. Such difference of termination presumably causes dissociation in a few cases of this disease.

Postoperative residual pain is a great nuisance in syringomyelia [11,12]. Milhorat et al. [11] reported about 35% of patients suffered from residual dysesthetic pain. However, no one has paid attention to muscle aching pain or deep pain as a residual symptom of syringomyelia. In this study, a detailed interview revealed 71% of patients complained of deep muscular pain postoperatively in spite of shrinkage of the syrinx.

Electrical stimulation of the fibers, conveying deep pain by using a single-fiber technique, produced muscle clamping pain, therefore, this complaint is probably caused by dysfunction of the deep pain-conducting system, the same mechanism as that of residual dysesthetic pain [12,13]. The precise mechanism causing this type of pain is still unclear; however, for better understanding one should keep in mind the fact that these two types of pain exist.

Conclusions

Deep pain loss is not uncommon in many spinal cord lesions. It shows fewer false-negative results and indicates the affected sensory segment precisely. Therefore, testing deep pain is an important neurological examination for many spinal cord disorders. In addition, postoperative residual pain in syringomyelia should be recognized as superficial dysesthetic pain, deep muscle aching pain, or both. This understanding can develop a successful measure for treatment of residual pain in the future.

References

1. Hobbs SF, Chandler MJ, Bolser DC, Foreman RD (1992) Segmental organization of visceral and somatic input onto C3–T6 spinothalamic tract cells of the monkey. J Neurophysiol 68(5):1575–1588
2. Kniffki D, Mense S, Schmidt RF (1978) Responses of group IV afferent units from skeletal muscle to stretch, contraction and chemical stimulation. Exp Brain Res 31:511–522
3. Kniffki KD, Mense S, Schmidt RF (1977) The spinocervical tract as a possible pathway for muscular nociception. J Physiol (Paris) 73(3):359–366
4. Marchettini P, Simone DA, Caputi G, Ochoa JL (1996) Pain from excitation of identified muscle nociceptors in humans. Brain Res 740(1–2):109–116
5. Simone DA, Marchettini P, Caputi G, Ochoa JL (1994) Identification of muscle afferents subserving sensation of deep pain in humans. J Neurophysiol 72(2):883–889
6. Willis WD (1985) Nociceptive pathways: anatomy and physiology of nociceptive ascending pathways. Philos Trans R Soc Lond Ser B Biol Sci 308(1136):253–270
7. Willis WJ (1988) Dorsal horn neurophysiology of pain. Ann N Y Acad Sci 531(76):76–89
8. Magee KR, Schneider RC (2000) Syringomyelia. Loss of deep-pain sensation with otherwise normal sensory perception. JAMA 200(9):795–796
9. Vatine JJ, Shapira SC, Magora F, et al (1993) Electronic pressure algometry of deep pain in healthy volunteers. Arch Phys Med Rehabilitation 74(5):526–530
10. Haymaker W (1969) Bing's local diagnosis in neurological disease. Mosby, St. Louis
11. Milhorat TH, Kotzen RM, Mu HT, et al (1996) Dysesthetic pain in patients with syringomyelia. Neurosurgery 38(5):940–946
12. Milhorat TH, Mu HT, LaMotte CC, Milhorat AT (1996) Distribution of substance P in the spinal cord of patients with syringomyelia. J Neurosurg 84(6):992–998
13. Ovelmen LJ (1988) Abnormal physiology of the dorsal horn as related to the deafferentation syndrome. Appl Neurophysiol 51(2–5):104–116

Some Further Thoughts on the Etiopathology of Syringomyelia and Experience with Surgical Management

Pragnesh Bhatt[1], Venkatachalam Iyer[2], Windsor Gunawardena[3], and Charles Davis[2]

Summary. Syringomyelia has baffled neuroscientists throughout the world. The pathophysiological mechanism underlying this rather mystifying clinical condition remains controversial despite significant advances in all the fields related to this entity. We present here our views regarding the understanding of syringomyelia with reference to our observations in (1) the Cavalier King Charles Spaniel dog and (2) recently encountered clinical situation including monozygotic twin sisters who presented with Arnold–Chiari malformation type I, one of whom also had associated syringomyelia. At the end, we include our personal series of 25 patients treated (by one of the authors) for syringomyelia, majority of whom had hindbrain herniation (HBH). On the clinical front, we observed monozygotic twin sisters, the senior of whom presented initially with syringomyelia associated with Arnold–Chiari malformation type I. A few weeks later her younger sister was diagnosed to have Arnold–Chiari malformation type I, showing that syringomyelia is not a congenital condition and could be acquired during the birth process. We support the theory of John D. Heiss suggesting its origin outside the spinal cord.

Key words. Syringomyelia, Arnold–Chiari malformation, Syringopleural shunt, Etiopathology, Management

Introduction

Syringomyelia was first described by Ollivier in 1827, but resurgence of interest has largely followed the advent of MRI. Also, our understanding of this rather complex disease has been assisted by advances in all the related disciplines of neuroscience [1].

We (a senior author, CHGD) have been interested in this condition for more than 20 years. We have found interesting situations in humans as well as in animals and expand here on our observations with our experience in surgical management of this condition.

[1] The Gujarat Research and Medical Institute, Camp Road, Shahi Baug, Ahmedabad 380004, India
[2] Department of Neurosurgery, [3] Department of Neuroradiology, Royal Preston Hospital, Fulwood, Preston, UK

Materials and Methods

Twenty-five consecutive patients with syringomyelia were managed at the Gujarat Research & Medical Institute, Ahmedabad, India, from January 1992 to December 1998. Their age distribution is shown in Fig. 1. There were 15 males and 10 females. Their clinical presentation was typical of central cord disturbance (Table 1).

The duration of symptoms ranged from 3 months to 5 years with an average of 2.25 years. This range may be peculiar to our setting, where patients come late to medical attention, sometimes with quite advanced disease as two of our patients had Charcot's arthropathy (one had the shoulder and the other had his elbow affected). All patients had magnetic resonance imaging (MRI) of the craniovertebral junction; some underwent brain imaging as well to assess the size of ventricles (Table 2).

The extent of the syrinx cavity was classified according to the length of the spinal cord involved and an arbitrary classification, which had some bearing on the type of operation performed. They were further classified according to the underlying pathology, and the most striking feature was absence of posttraumatic syrinx due to the pattern of referral. The most common variety was related to hindbrain herniation [2],

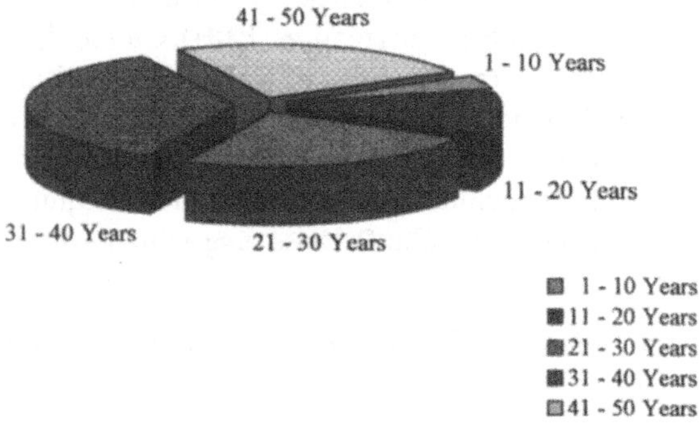

FIG. 1. Age distribution of patients

TABLE 1. Summary of clinical features

	No. of patients
Symptoms	
Neck pain	20
Upper limb paraesthesias	15
Numbness on the face	2
Upper limb weakness	22
Lower limb weakness	20
Signs	
Cranial nerve deficit	1
Cerebellar signs	10
UMN signs in lower limbs	15
LMN signs in upper limbs	21
Dissociate sensory loss	16

TABLE 2. Magnetic resonance imaging (MRI) findings

Finding	No. of patients
Arnold-Chiari type I	23
Intramedullary tumor	1
Hydrocephalus	2
Syrinx	1
Syringomyelia—extent of the syrinx cavity	23
Cervical	10
Cervicodorsal	8
Extensive	5

TABLE 3. Operations performed

Nature of operation	No. of patients
Foramen magnum decompression	23
Syringopleural shunt	5
Tumor excision	1
Ventriculoperitoneal shunt	2

and there was one case each due to postinflammatory arachnoiditis and intramedullary tumor. Their surgical management is listed in Table 3. Those who had hindbrain herniation (HBH) were subjected to foramen magnum decompression (FMD), in which the standard bony decompression was supplemented with duroplasty using a fascia graft.

After two patients developed hydrocephalus as a result of subarachnoid dissection, we restricted our dissection to extraarachnoid [1,3]. This primary procedure was supplemented by a syringopleural shunt, either at the same stage (three patients who had extensive syrinx) or as a secondary procedure when they continued to deteriorate following FMD (the remainder). For syringopleural shunt, a thecoperitoneal shunt (Chhabra) was used without a valve as suggested by Bernard Williams [2]. Similarly, for the ventriculoperitoneal shunt, Chhabra's medium pressure valved shunt was used in patients with hydrocephalus.

Results

These patients were followed up clinically for 1 to 7 years. MRI was repeated only when clinically indicated. Complications were encountered in eight patients (32%). The low rate of complication is probably because the main group comprised patients with HBH as seen by Batzdorf et al. [1]. Five required reoperation to treat the complication, which included a cerebrospinal fluid (CSF) leak in five, of which two patients required formal repair. Postoperative hydrocephalus occurred in two and was related to intraarachnoid dissection and blood spillage leading to adhesions. The shunt block in one patient, suspected to be a persistent syrinx on the repeat MRI, was confirmed at the revision.

The overall outcome was categorized, comparing neurology at follow-up, as (a) improved, (b) stable, or (c) deteriorated. Fifteen patients remained stable while the other two categories had 5 each.

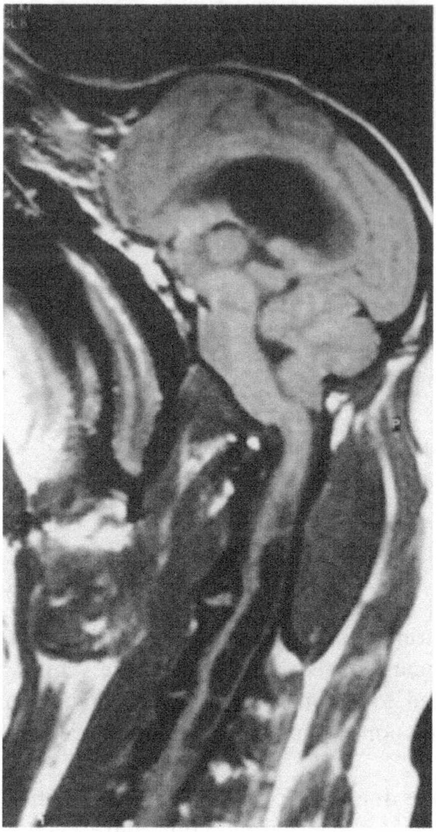

FIG. 2. Syringomyelia observed in a dog. Magnetic resonance imaging of the craniovertebral junction of a Cavalier King Charles Spaniel

Discussion

We present a peculiar group of patients in whom some of the factors relating to diagnosis as well as management are unique. First of all, the patients have presented late, often having symptoms for years and with quite advanced neurology, sometimes impossible to reverse. The group was mainly composed of the HBH-related cases with a striking absence of posttraumatic individuals due to the referral pattern. The follow-up is mainly clinical, reserving repeat MRI for those who showed progressive clinical deterioration. In three individuals, the syrinx was reduced in size and deterioration can only be explained on the basis of vascular mechanism [2]. One patient had an increased syrinx and required shunt revision; in the other, who had unchanged syrinx size, we thought the deterioration was due to a CSF leak-related infection.

We also observed syringomelia in a dog (see Fig. 2).

Conclusion

The origin of syringomyelia is multifactorial [4] and primarily acquired rather than congenital. The important issue is an anatomical as well as an physiological block to CSF circulation produced by hindbrain herniation [3]. It is also known that HBH results from a small posterior fossa rather than a primary abnormality of cerebellum [5–7].

Early diagnosis and treatment of syringomyelia are essential for good outcome and to prevent irreversible neurological deficits [3], as also evident in two patients with Charcot's arthropathy in our series.

The syringopleural shunt is preferred because it is technically easier [4], less likely to become infected or be blocked distally, as compared to a syringoperitoneal shunt [2], and, most important, is draining to a low-pressure cavity.

References

1. Batzdorf U, Klekamp J, Johnson JP (1998) A critical appraisal of syrinx cavity shunting procedures. J Neurosurg 89:382–388
2. Williams B, Page N (1987) Surgical treatment of syringomyelia with syringopleural shunting. Br J Neurosurg 1:63–80
3. Heiss JD, Patronas N, DeVroom HL, et al (1999) Elucidating the pathophysiology of syringomyelia. J Neurosurg 91:553–562
4. Davis CHG, Symon L (1989) Mechanisms and treatment in post-traumatic syringomyelia. Br J Neurosurg 3:669–674
5. Nyland H, Krogness KG (1978) Size of posterior fossa in Chiari type 1 malformation in adults. Acta Neurochirurgica 40:233–242
6. Stovner LJ, Bergan U, Nilsen G, et al (1993) Posterior cranial fossa dimensions in the Chiari 1 malformation: relation to pathogenesis and clinical presentation. Neuroradiology 35:113–118
7. Vega A, Quintana F, Berciano J (1990) Basichondrocranium anomalies in adult Chiari type 1 malformation: a morphometric study. J Neurol Sci 99:137–145

4. Syringomyelia Associated with Abnormalities of the Craniocervical Junction

Treatment of Syringomyelia Associated with Chiari I Malformation

Ulrich Batzdorf

Summary. Chiari malformation is a shorthand designation for a group of alterations in the posterior fossa architecture having the effect of reducing posterior fossa volume, causing descent of the cerebellar tonsils and often of the hindbrain; syringomyelia may be associated with these changes. Treatment today consists of suboccipital decompression, which should be planned in accordance with the particular variant of posterior fossa architecture. Establishment of optimal cerebrospinal fluid flow from the fourth ventricle and creation of a subtonsillar cistern is aided by reduction of the cerebellar tonsils and duraplasty. Repeat operations have been performed, when the original decompression was inadequate, for patients with cerebellar ptosis, pseudomeningocele, and scar formation.

Key words. Hindbrain descent, Chiari malformation, Syringomyelia, Cerebellar ptosis, Pseudomeningocele

Chiari Malformation: A Brief History and Definition

The entity we term the Chiari I malformation represents descent of the cerebellar tonsils through the foramen magnum. Although Hans von Chiari, a pathologist in Prague, provided the most detailed and systematized description of this condition in 1891 [1] and then more comprehensively in 1893 [2], it is clear that John Cleland's description of tonsillar descent in 1883 [3] preceded Chiari's. Chiari provided detailed drawings of the anatomy from autopsy specimens, and his descriptions of 23 cases were based on material from infants who died shortly after birth, all of whom also had hydrocephalus.

In translation, the four types of abnormality he described are as follows:

Type I: Elongation of the tonsils and the medial part of the inferior cerebellar lobes into conelike projections, which accompany the medulla into the spinal canal

Type II: Displacement of portions of the vermis and also of the pons and medulla into the spinal canal, and elongation of the fourth ventricle into the spinal canal

---

UCLA Medical Center, Division of Neurosurgery, Los Angeles, CA 90095-6901, USA

Type III: Displacement of virtually the entire hydrocephalic cerebellum into a cervical spina bifida

Type IV: Hypoplasia in the region of the cerebellum without displacement of portions thereof into the spinal canal

It is noteworthy that the focus of his descriptions was on the extent of hindbrain descent through the foramen magnum but, except for hydrocephalus, the descriptions did not address the other anomalies of the neuraxis, specifically the neural tube defects that we now associate with so-called Chiari II malformation, such as spina bifida.

Arnold's name was subsequently added, based on the analysis of an additional patient. It is reputed that two of Arnold's enthusiastic students were responsible for inserting Arnold's name ahead of Chiari's in designating the eponym the Arnold–Chiari Malformation. The trend in recent years, however, has been decidedly in the direction of simplifying the name to Chiari malformation and beyond that to eliminate the eponymic designation altogether, replacing it with the more anatomic term of hindbrain descent [4].

Surgeons who operate on patients with so-called Chiari I malformation, whether associated with syringomyelia or not, are aware that the strict definition as provided by Chiari does not, in fact, apply to all patients. In the author's experience the inferior portion of the fourth ventricle may be displaced to a level just below the foramen magnum, at least in some patients who otherwise meet the criteria of the "type I" malformation. There is also a wide range of descent of the tonsils and, recognizing that the tonsils may be immediately below the foramen magnum in otherwise normal individuals, attempts have been made to define an exact level of tonsillar descent that is to be considered pathological [5]. This attempt at further clarification of the definition became possible only because of the advent of magnetic resonance (MR) imaging, but has met with some criticism as MR scanning has brought some other aspects of hindbrain descent into focus, such as "fullness" of the posterior fossa with virtual absence of the cisterna magna, yet with levels of tonsillar descent that might previously have been considered within normal range [6] (Fig. 1).

Normal Posterior Fossa

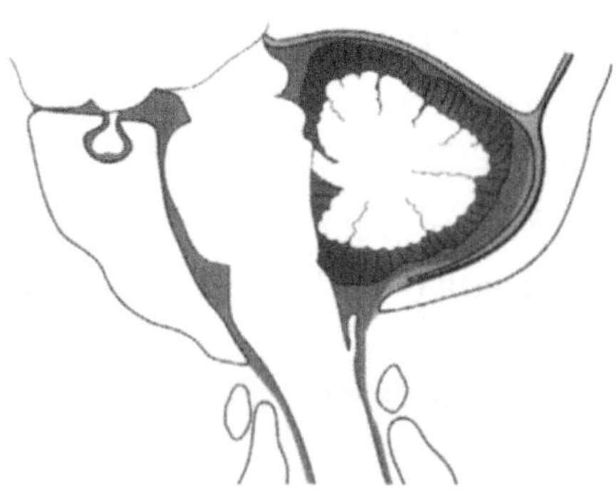

Fig. 1. Schematic diagram of usual posterior fossa relationships between cerebellum, tentorium cerebelli, occipital bone, and clivus and dens

As a result of the insights into this condition obtained from both MR scanning and surgical observation, it would appear that the designation Chiari I malformation today represents a range of abnormalities with varying extent of hindbrain descent, including partial descent of the fourth ventricle and tonsillar descent ranging from minimal to more than 1 cm. The term Chiari malformation thus has become a convenient "shorthand" in referring to this range of hindbrain abnormalities. It specifically does not include descent of the vermis through the foramen magnum, and should not include type II patients with neural tube defects such as meningomyelocele. Designations such as "congenital" or "developmental" are best avoided because there is still debate about the precise pathogenesis of this condition, which may, in fact, not be identical in all instances.

Syringomyelia, defined as a tubular, fluid-containing cavity within the spinal cord, is present in approximately 65% of patients with Chiari I malformation [7]. The syringomyelic cavity develops in the presence of partial obstruction of the subarachnoid space at the level of the craniocervical junction. Current thinking favors an explanation postulating that the descended cerebellar tonsils act as a piston on an essentially isolated spinal subarachnoid space [8]. The tonsils exhibit a to-and-fro motion caused by transmission of the normal cardiac and respiratory pulsations of cerebral spinal fluid (CSF) and drive spinal fluid into the parenchyma of the spinal cord along the Virchow–Robin spaces. It is not fully understood how this fluid coalesces to form a confluent cavity. Once the cavity is established, however, the same piston-like action of the tonsils and possibly intermittent distension of epidural veins may propel fluid within the cyst in an up-and-down direction, allowing the fluid to dissect the cord parenchyma and thereby enlarge the cyst [9]. Predicated on this theory, treatment of Chiari-related syringomyelia today aims to disable the piston action just described by enlarging the foramen magnum and expanding the subarachnoid space at the level of the craniocervical junction.

It is also recognized that there is a small group of patients in whom CSF flow restriction at the foramen magnum is not the result of wedging of the cerebellar tonsils into the foramen magnum but is caused by basilar arachnoiditis or tumors [10]. It has been postulated that arachnoiditis might result from hemorrhage at the time of traumatic birth [11,12]; inflammation may also result from meningeal infection.

Posterior Fossa Volume

The observation that the volume of the posterior fossa in patients with Chiari malformation is relatively small was first made by Marin-Padilla [13]. Traditional thinking has been that the skull enlarges in direct relationship to brain growth, so that the concept of disproportionate size of posterior fossa content and skull seems at first difficult to reconcile. It appears, however, that confinement within a relatively small posterior fossa allows the cerebellar tonsils and the hindbrain to escape through the foramen magnum to varying degrees, thereby setting into action the mechanism of restricted flow and its consequences. Studies attempting to quantitate the relative small size of the posterior fossa followed and confirmed the hypothesis [14–16].

Although such global assessments of disproportionate size of the posterior fossa to the rest of the calvarium are of value in focusing our thinking with respect to both underlying pathophysiology and treatment approaches, analysis of the variations of posterior fossa configuration has permitted a further breakdown, which has proved useful in planning surgical approaches. If one regards the walls of the posterior fossa separately, one may distinguish an *anterior wall*, normally formed largely by the clivus, a *roof*, formed by the tentorium cerebelli, and the *floor*, constituted by the occipital bone. Correspondingly, one may regard an abnormally small posterior fossa from four points of view:

A. Anterior type: encroachment of posterior fossa [17] (Fig. 2):
   Basilar invagination
   Platybasia
   Odontoid invagination into posterior fossa
B. Roof type: Low insertion of the tentorium cerebelli into the occipital bone, i.e., a low-lying torcula, resulting in what is sometimes referred to as an almost vertically oriented tentorium (Fig. 3).
C. Floor type (Fig. 4):
   1. Thickened occipital bone that may be a developmental variant, or is seen pathologically in hypophosphatemic (vitamin D-resistant) rickets [18].
   2. Shallow posterior fossa due to a horizontal orientation of the occipital bone, instead of the more usual slightly sloping orientation. At times, the anterior edge of the occipital bone even takes a slight upward turn, with the edge of the foramen thickened as well.
   3. Less commonly, one may see grossly thickened posterior fossa dura, and perhaps even thickened and hypervascular dura, as factors contributing to small posterior fossa size.
D. Mass type (Fig. 5): space-occupying lesions, most commonly represented by arachnoid cysts and extraaxial tumors [10,19], can effectively reduce the volume available to normal posterior fossa structures.

In the author's opinion it is essential that the MR scan window be large enough to distinguish these subcategories; this implies that the image must include the entire posterior fossa, not only the craniocervical junction. By obtaining a preoperative brain MRI to exclude the possibility of hydrocephalus, many patients will have undergone a complete posterior fossa study. These categories of reduced posterior fossa volume, along with illustrative MR scans, are shown in Figs. 1–5. All these subtypes of Chiari malformation allow for hindbrain descent and cerebellar tonsil descent through the foramen magnum; all may be accompanied by syringomyelia.

Treatment of Chiari Malformation Based on Subtypes

A. Anterior Type

Treatment of the anterior type of Chiari Malformation has been described extensively by Menezes [20–22]. Severe forms of anterior encroachment of the posterior fossa space, as seen in basilar invagination, often require transoral resection of the high-riding odontoid that indents the brainstem, followed by posterior fusion of the occiput to the cervical spine. Menezes' current recommendation is to perform a posterior

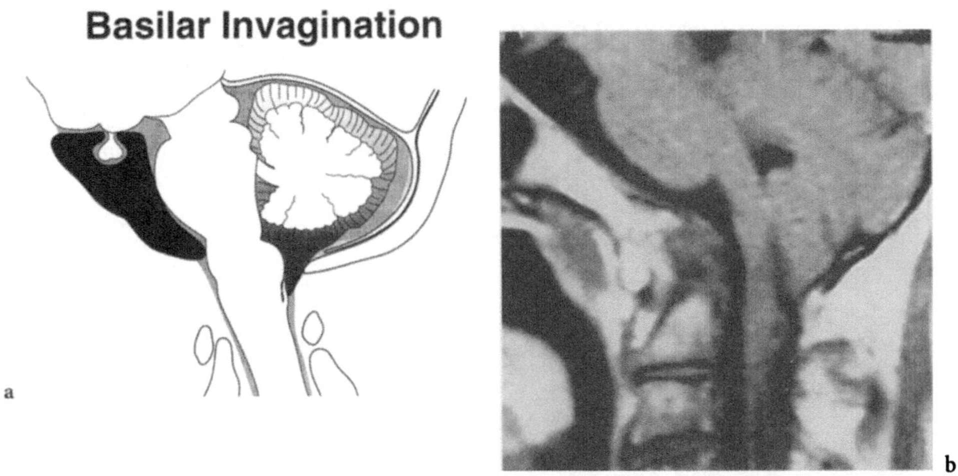

FIG. 2a,b. Anterior type of encroachment of posterior fossa. **a** Schematic diagram to represent the change in posterior fossa architecture with basilar invagination. **b** Magnetic resonance (MR) scan of adult man showing this type of deformity. Syrinx cavity extends into upper cervical spinal cord and was the cause of his symptoms

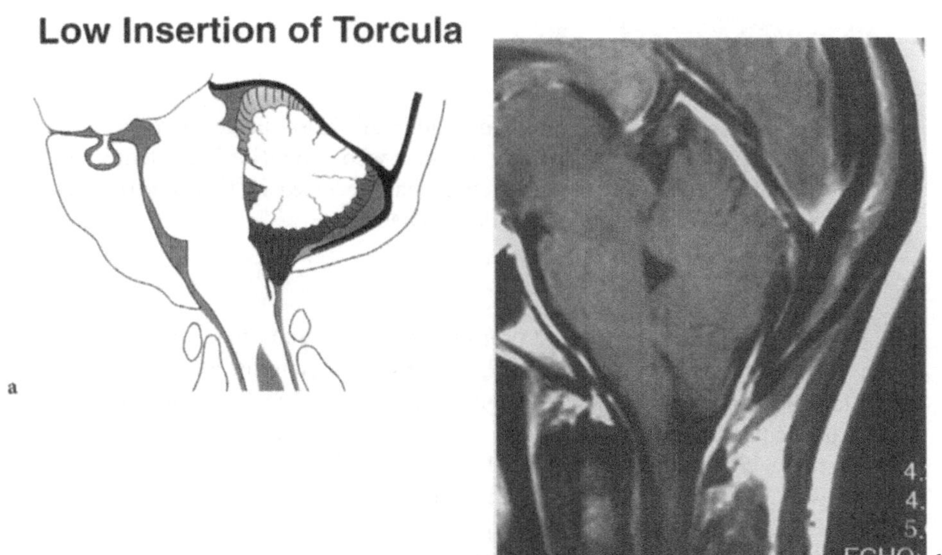

FIG. 3a,b. Roof type of encroachment of posterior fossa. **a** Schematic diagram of situation in which low insertion of the tentorium reduces the posterior fossa volume. **b** MR scan of 37-year-old woman who presented with this variant of Chiari malformation; this patient presented with headache but did not have a syringomyelic cavity

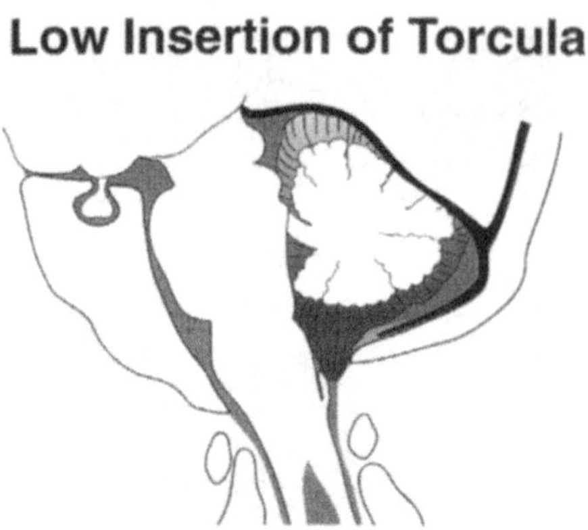

a

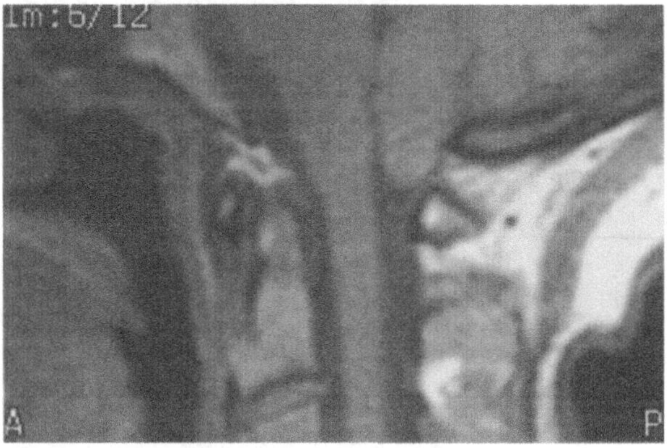

b

FIG. 4a,b. Floor type of encroachment of posterior fossa. **a** Schematic showing reduction of posterior fossa volume by thick, horizontally directed occipital bone. **b** MR scan of a 51-year-old woman who presented with headache and neck pain; she did not have a syrinx cavity

fusion in all patients who have undergone odontoid resection for anterior decompression of the posterior fossa. However, patients whose anterior brainstem indentation is reversible in extension and traction may be fused in this noncompressed position without undergoing transoral odontoidectomy.

B. Roof Type

Abnormally low insertion of the tentorium cerebelli results in a configuration in which extensive removal of bone, sometimes performed up to the torcula, may set the stage for postoperative downward descent of the entire cerebellar hemispheres. This seems particularly true when such extensive bone removal has been performed in conjunction with an expansile duraplasty, and especially when the duraplasty is performed with material capable of stretching. Fascia appears more capable of stretching than pericranium; certainly the addition of a nonstretching material such as polytetrafluoroethylene (ePTFE), or an external cranioplasty support, as advocated by some [14], reduces the likelihood of passive stretching of the posterior fossa dural closure.

Because the restriction of flow is the result of descent of the cerebellar tonsils, not the small posterior fossa volume per se, it is the author's opinion that it is particularly

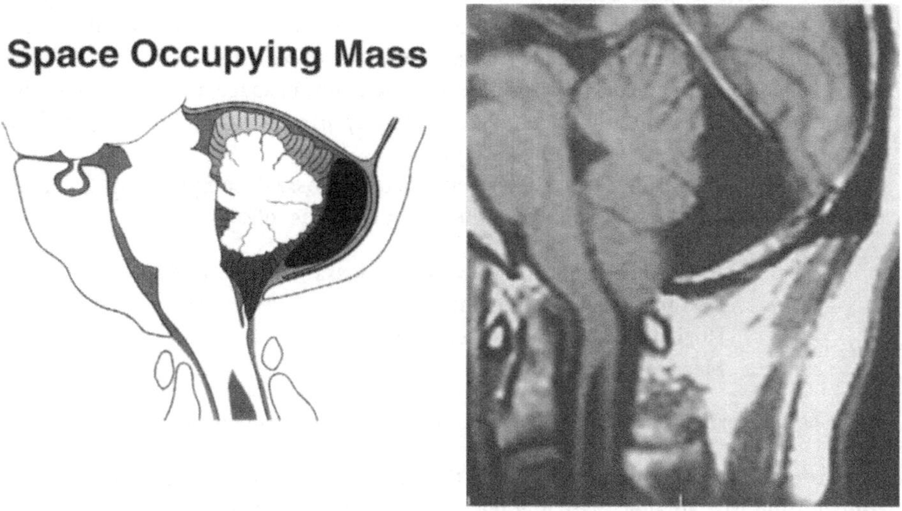

Fig. 5a,b. Mass type of encroachment of posterior fossa. **a** Schematic drawing illustrating crowding of posterior fossa contents by a mass. **b** MR scan of a 40-year-old man presenting with hand atrophy and sensory loss related to his extensive syringomyelia, which extended from C2 to T9. This patient has a large posterior fossa arachnoid cyst, in addition to having a horizontally oriented occipital bone

important to limit the bony decompression to a distance just above the cerebellar tonsils. This distance can be judged and measured from the sagittal scan image. The author's surgical technique includes reduction of the cerebellar tonsils (see following). Expansile duraplasty does not appear to add to the risk of cerebellar descent if the foregoing precautions are observed.

C. Floor Type

When the entire occipital bone is abnormally thick, horizontal in orientation, or particularly thick at the rim of the foramen magnum, one should remove sufficient bone from the margin of the foramen magnum that the remaining bone still permits support of the cerebellar hemispheres up to the point of their greatest diameter. This distance can also be measured from the MR scan, using the centimeter scale with which most scans are provided. Expansile duraplasty adds no additional risk of cerebellar descent under these circumstances (see Table 1).

D. Mass Type

Removal of a space-occupying tumor, insofar as possible, is the obvious solution to reduction of posterior fossa volume by a tumor mass. Klekamp et al. [10] have demonstrated resolution of the syrinx cavity following such tumor removal.

Treatment of a large posterior fossa arachnoid cyst in conjunction with a Chiari malformation and syringomyelia is perhaps more controversial. It has been the author's experience that treatment explicitly directly at the cyst is not necessary and that a standard decompression (see following) serves to restore normal CSF circulation at the level of the foramen magnum. In one of two patients so treated, this actually resulted in drainage of the cyst into the subarachnoid space; the cyst in the other patient remained essentially unchanged, but the syrinx cavity diminished greatly in size after bony decompression and duraplasty.

In a group of 82 patients who underwent posterior fossa decompression, the breakdown of these subtypes of Chiari I Malformation was as follows:

Anterior indentation of posterior fossa*	15/82
Low insertion of tentorium	35
Horizontally oriented occipital bone	34
Mass (arachnoid cyst)	2

*None of these patients had sufficient anterior indentation to require odontoid resection.

As is evident, in some patients more than one wall of the posterior fossa may be contributing to a smaller than adequate cavity, a factor that must also be taken into consideration in surgical planning.

Cerebellar Ptosis

Descent of the posterior fossa structures through a large craniectomy defect has been recognized by Duddy and Williams [23] and by Menezes [24], as well as in our series of reoperated patients [25]. In our experience there have been two conditions associated with cerebellar ptosis that have indicated a need for reoperation. Severe ptosis of the cerebellum may permit reformation of CSF flow restriction at the level of the foramen magnum, with reestablishment of a syrinx cavity. In such cases, one can hope that syrinx formation can be reversed when the cerebellum is supported with a limited cranioplasty.

Headache, presumably caused at least in part by stretching of the posterior fossa dura, is a more common problem leading to reoperation. It is of interest that asking patients to sleep in a position with the head lower than the body may occasionally temporarily relieve this type of headache. It is speculated that this position diminishes the gravitational force of cerebellar descent stretching the dura or dural graft. Attachment of the suboccipital musculature to a large area of exposed dura has also been cited as a source of postoperative headache (T.H. Milhorat, personal communication, 1999). Limited cranioplasty helps to deal with headache of dural stretch origin. The technique used by the author has been described [25].

Technique and Results

The surgical technique we currently employ, which has evolved over the course of the past 15 to 20 years, includes contributions of several surgeons who have treated patients with this problem and attempts to incorporate the principles already cited [26–31].

Diagnostic evaluation consists of MR scans of the craniocervical junction, to include the entire posterior fossa. Complete brain scans are advisable whenever there is a question of hydrocephalus, and for this reason are recommended at least in the initial evaluation. The initial scan should include the cervical spine to determine whether there is an associated syrinx cavity; if a cervical syrinx is present, a scan of the thoracic spine should also be obtained to assess the full extent of syrinx cavity formation.

Symptomatic patients who have marginal or very minimal descent of the tonsils, particularly in the absence of a syrinx cavity, are advised to undergo a cardiac-gated MR CSF flow study to rule out CSF flow impairment at the level of the foramen magnum. Patients who have a syrinx cavity in the absence of cerebellar tonsillar descent should be fully investigated to rule out a primary spinal cause of syrinx development, such as tumor, scar tissue, or arachnoiditis. Plain films of the head and upper cervical spine are often helpful in identifying associated skeletal abnormalities that might otherwise be missed, such as assimilation of the atlas, atlantoaxial problems, a midline posterior fossa keel, and even an anomalous vertebral artery ostium [28].

We perform suboccipital decompression procedures with the patient in the prone position, the head secured in a Mayfield clamp. The head and neck are maintained in neutral to slightly flexed position. Two incisions are marked out. The first is a midline incision from the external occipital protuberance to the palpable spinous process of the second cervical vertebra. A second incision to harvest pericranium is placed over the posterior parietooccipital area to one side or the other of the midline and away from the lambdoidal suture.

Soft tissue dissection is carried out to expose the foramen magnum and occipital bone just below the inion, the posterior arch of the atlas, and the rostral tip of the spinous process of the axis. Only in the unusual circumstance in which the tonsils descend well into the C2 region or below is it necessary to expose more of the cervical laminae. Based on measurements taken from the sagittal image of the preoperative scan, we measure the area of bone to be removed as the distance upward from the foramen magnum; this rarely exceeds 2 cm, but for reasons previously detailed, we have removed as little as 15 mm of bone from the edge of the foramen magnum. The side-to-side measurement of bone removal is approximately 25–30 mm. We do not encroach on the occipital condyles in our bone removal. The posterior arch of the atlas is resected in all patients to allow for the development of an artificial cisterna magna, which is an important goal of this operation [14]. The width of resection of the posterior arch of the atlas corresponds to the width of the suboccipital bone resection. Bone removal is accomplished with a combination of high-speed drill and thin-lipped rongeurs.

Ultrasonography may be employed over the intact dura and will confirm the position of the cerebellar tonsils. The dural opening is performed under the operating microscope as a midline dorsal incision over the spinal cord, extending laterally in the direction of each cerebellar hemisphere just above the craniocervical junction. Often the periosteal reflection from the outer table forms a distinct band at this level, which may enclose a small venous channel. Dissecting this band away from the midline for a distance of several millimeters assists in accomplishing a better dural closure at the end of the procedure. Extensive dural bands are sometimes encountered [32]. Microcoagulation forceps are used on the dural edge to control dural bleeders; large areas of dural coagulation may result in coagulation necrosis and pullout of dural closure sutures. On several occasions, we have encountered the unusual presence of very extensive venous vascular channels throughout the dural opening. This anomaly will require extensive and time-consuming hemostasis, and the resulting dural edge coagulation necrosis may then make it preferable to use the technique recommended by Williams [4,33], i.e., to stitch the remaining dura against the soft tissue wall of the wound cavity and follow this with a tight fascial closure, omitting a dural graft.

The arachnoid is then opened in the midline and connecting strands to underlying neural tissue are divided. The arachnoid is held against the dural edge with metallic clips that are removed during dural graft closure. They serve the purpose of allowing the closing suture to include the arachnoid, thereby preventing it from falling against the neural structures. At this point, the tonsils are assessed. Often one may see a concave indentation at the level of the foramen magnum; the position of the posterior inferior cerebellar arteries is noted. In most patients, the tonsils can be retracted laterally, away from each other; this often brings the lower fourth ventricle and sometimes a tuft of choroid plexus into view. Observations are also made on the appearance of pial vessels over the tonsils: long-standing compression often reduces the pial vasculature and the tonsils then may be gliotic.

Reduction of the Cerebellar Tonsils

Although surgical maneuvers to reduce the mass of the cerebellar tonsils have been carried out for many years [4,30,34], this remains a controversial step in the view of some surgeons [8,35]. Several reports suggest this step is not necessary. The rationale for reducing the size of the cerebellar tonsils is to establish unrestricted outflow of CSF from the fourth ventricle and to relieve direct pressure on the brainstem and upper spinal cord.

Fortunately, because of relatively early diagnosis of Chiari malformation today, as compared to the pre-MRI era, patients are relatively younger when the diagnosis is made. The tonsils are therefore less likely to be firm and gliotic, and lend themselves to shrinkage with the application of bipolar current on a low setting; this is applied to the dorsal, medial, and sometimes caudal aspect of the tonsils, staying away from major vessels and avoiding heat transference to nearby vessels by irrigating during coagulation. The pial surface remains intact. In most instances, this maneuver allows the tonsils to remain separated and will expose the fourth ventricle. Increased signal may be seen at the tonsillar tips on a postoperative MR scan, but this signal alteration gradually clears.

When the tonsils are firm and gliotic, subpial resection usually suffices. Ultrasonic aspiration has proved very helpful for this procedure; hemostasis is readily achieved with bipolar coagulation and temporary application of a hemostatic agent. The pial membrane is then reapproximated with one or two sutures of fine suture material, such as 6–0 polypropylene. Other steps are more rarely indicated [26,27].

Dural Closure

The exact technique employed for dural closure also varies considerably in current practice. The author currently prefers to use autologous pericranium, but in an attempt to reduce the likelihood of an adhesive reaction [36], places a layer of ePTFE beneath the pericranial graft. The ePTFE membrane is attached with small nonferromagnetic metallic clips; the pericranial graft is sutured in place with a continuous locked suture of 5-0 polypropylene or closely spaced, interrupted sutures of similar suture material. The suture line is checked for leaks with a Valsalva maneuver and is then covered with fibrin glue, prepared either from the patient's own blood or from a commercial source. To date this system of closure has been employed in approximately 40 patients without complications or long-term evidence of an adhesive reaction.

Shunting

Shunting of a syringomyelic cavity caused by Chiari malformation is reserved for those patients whose syrinx cavity failed to reduce in size following adequate posterior fossa decompression and whose studies do not reveal the presence of any of the factors cited earlier.

TABLE 1. Chiari malformation treatment results

Year	Procedure [reference]	*n*	Results
1983	Peerless and Durward (includes obex plug IVth) [37]	34	Improvement in 21/30
1988	Lapras et al. (arachnoid intact, no graft) [38]	20	"Good" in 13
1991	Batzdorf (dura, arachnoid open; duraplasty) [27]	24	Dural pain improved in 12/13 (92%) Dyesthesia pain improved in 7/14 (50%) Motor improved in 10/15 (67%) Sensory improved in 4/22 (18%)
1992	Menezes (anterior decompression) [22]	22	Improvement in 22/22
1992	Milhorat et al. (syringocisternostomy) [39]	6	Improvement in 6/6
1993	Williams (dura and arachnoid left open) [40]	100	Pain improved, 67% Motor improved, 29% Sensory improved, 34% Brainstem improved, 25%
1993	Isu et al. (outer layer of dura only) [35]	7	Improvement in 7/7
1994	Oldfield et al. (arachnoid intact, duraplasty) [8]	7	Improvement in 7/7
1994	Sahuquillo et al. (arachnoid intact, duraplasty) [14]	10	Improvement in 10/10
1998	Iskandar et al., Grabb and Oakes (no descent) [6]	5	Improvement in 5/5

Results

Surgical decompression of the posterior fossa and shrinkage of the syringomyelic cavity do not benefit all preoperative symptoms to the same degree. Overall improvement as noted in the literature is listed in Table 1.

Several authors have documented symptom-specific improvement. Table 2 compares the results of three series.

Imaging criteria for reoperation have been as follows:

Inadequate decompression of tonsils	4
Inadequate decompression of bone	2
Pseudomeningocele	5
Cerebellar ptosis	4
Intradural scar formation	4

TABLE 2. Symptom-specific improvement

Author	Symptoms	Return to normal (%)	Improved[a] (%)	Unchanged (%)	Worse (%)
Dyste et al. [41]	Pain	81	1	11	7
Batzdorf [27]	Headache and spinal pain		92	8	0
	Dyesthetic pain		50	44	7
Williams [40]			67	32	1
Dyste et al. [41]	Strength	21	70	3	6
Batzdorf [27]			67	33	0
Williams [40][b]			29	67	4
Dyste et al. [41]	Sensation	29	6	61	4
Batzdorf [27]			18	72	0
Williams [40]			34	63	3
Dyste et al. [41]	Cranial nerve function	36	18	43	3
Williams [40]			25	74	1
Batzdorf [27]	Spasticity		64	36	

[a] The series by Batzdorf [27] did not separate patients who reported complete normalization of their symptoms from those reporting improvement, but did distinguish between dural stretching and dysesthetic pain.
[b] Motor.

TABLE 3. Results of late repeat posterior fossa reoperation

	Better	No change
Inadequate decompression		
Tonsils	3/4	1/4
Bone	2/2	
Pseudomeningocele	3/5	2/5
Ptosis	3/4	1/4
Scar	2/4	2/4
Graft reduction	1/1	

In addition, one patient has undergone reoperation for a probable reaction to graft material. Secondary anterior decompression, although not performed by the author to date, should also be considered when indicated. Improvement in this group of patients is not always seen, although no patients were made worse by reoperation (Table 3).

The techniques employed for reoperation procedures for inadequate decompression are in accord with those described by us. When tonsils have not been reduced, that step is undertaken; when inadequate bone has been removed, we proceed with bone removal as described. Pseudomeningocele repair often requires replacement of the dural graft [42]; the technique for dealing with cerebellar ptosis is described in detail elsewhere [25]. Scar resection is, of course, self-explanatory. In the one patient with presumed graft reaction, a bovine pericardial graft was replaced with autologous pericranium.

References

1. Chiari H (1891) Ueber Veränderungen des Kleinhirns infolge von Hydrocephalie des Grosshirns. Dtsch Med Wochenschr 42:1172–1175
2. Chiari H (1896) Ueber Veränderungen des Kleinhirns, des Pons und der medulla oblongata in Folge von genitaler Hydrocephalie des Grosshirns. Denkschr Akad Wiss Wien 63:71–116
3. Cleland J (1883) Contribution to the study of spina bifida, encephalocele and anencephalus. J Anat Physiol 17:257–291
4. Williams B (1986) Progress in syringomyelia. Neurol Res 8:130–145
5. Barkovich AJ, Wippold JF, Sherman JL, et al (1986) Significant cerebellar tonsillar position on MR. Am J Neuroradiol 7:795–799
6. Iskandar BJ, Hedlund GL, Grabb PA, et al (1998) The resolution of syringohydromyelia without hindbrain herniation after posterior fossa decompression. J Neurosurg 89(2):212–216
7. Milhorat TH, Chou MW, Trinidad EM, et al (1999) Chiari I malformation redefined: clinical and radiographic findings for 364 symptomatic patients. Neurosurgery 44(5):1005–1017
8. Oldfield EH, Muraszko K, Shawker TH, et al (1994) Pathophysiology of syringomyelia associated with Chiari I malformation of the cerebellar tonsils. Implications for diagnosis and treatment. J Neurosurg 80:3–15
9. Williams B, Terry AF, Jones HWF, et al (1981) Syringomyelia as a sequel to traumatic paraplegia. Paraplegia 19:67–80
10. Klekamp J, Samii M, Tatagiba M, et al (1995) Syringomyelia in association with tumours of the posterior fossa. Pathophysiological considerations, based on observation on three related cases. Acta Neurochir 137:38–43
11. Williams B (1977) Difficult labour as a cause of communicating syringomyelia. Lancet II:51–53
12. Newman PL, Terenty TR, Foster JB (1981) Some observations on the pathogenesis of syringomyelia. J Neurol Neurosurg Psychiatry 44:964–969
13. Marin-Padilla M, Marin-Padilla T (1981) Morphogenesis of experimentally induced Arnold-Chiari malformation. J Neurol Sci 50:29–55
14. Sahuquillo J, Rubio E, Poca M, et al (1994) Posterior fossa reconstruction: a surgical technique for the treatment of Chiari I malformation and Chiari-I/syringomyelia complex: preliminary results and magnetic resonance imaging quantitative assessment of hindbrain migration. Neurosurgery 35(5):874–884

15. Badie B, Mendoza D, Batzdorf U (1995) Posterior fossa volume and response to suboccipital decompression in patients with Chiari I malformation. Neurosurgery 37:214–218
16. Nishikawa M, Sakamoto H, Hakuba A, et al (1997) Pathogenesis of Chiari malformation: a morphometric study of the posterior cranial fossa. J Neurosurg 86:40–47
17. Menezes AH (1995) Primary craniovertebral anomalies and the hindbrain herniation syndrome (Chiari I): data base analysis. Pediatr Neurosurg 23:260–269
18. Kuether TA, Piatt JH (1998) Chiari malformation associated with vitamin D-resistant rickets: case report. Neurosurgery 42:1168–1171
19. Williams B (1979) Subarachnoid pouches of the posterior fossa with syringomyelia. Acta Neurochir 47:187–217
20. Menezes AH, VanGilder JC, Graf CJ, et al (1980) Craniocervical abnormalities: a comprehensive surgical approach. J Neurosurg 53:444–455
21. Menezes AH (1991) Chiari I malformations and hydromyelia. Pediatr Neurosurg 92:146–154
22. Menezes AH (1992) The anterior midline approach to the craniocervical region in children. Pediatr Neurosurg 18:272–281
23. Duddy MJ, Williams B (1991) Hindbrain migration after decompression for hindbrain hernia: a quantitative assessment using MRI. Br J Neurosurg 5:141–152
24. Menezes AH (1991–1992) Complications of surgery at the craniovertebral junction: avoidance and management. Pediatr Neurosurg 17:254–256
25. Holly LT, Batzdorf U (2001) Management of cerebellar ptosis following craniovertebral decompression for Chiari I malformation. J Neurosurg 94:21–26
26. Batzdorf U (1988) Chiari I malformation with syringomyelia: evaluation of surgical therapy by magnetic resonance imaging. J Neurosurg 68(5):726–730
27. Batzdorf U (1991) Syringomyelia related to abnormalities at the level of the craniovertebral junction. In: Batzdorf U (ed) Syringomyelia: current concepts in diagnosis and treatment. Williams & Wilkins, Baltimore, pp 163–182
28. Batzdorf U (1993) Infratentorial procedures. Part 13, Congenital malformations: Chiari malformation and syringomyelia. In: Apuzzo LJ (ed) Brain surgery, complication and avoidance and management, vol 2. Churchill Livingston, New York, pp 1985–2002
29. Batzdorf U (1996) Syringomyelia, Chiari malformation and hydromyelia. In: Youmans JR (ed) Neurological Surgery, 4th edn, vol 2. Saunders, Philadelphia, pp 1090–1109
30. Halamandaris CG, Batzdorf U (1989) Adult Chiari malformation. Contemp Neurosurg 11(26):1–6
31. Klekamp J, Batzdorf U, Samii M, et al (1996) The surgical treatment of Chiari I malformation. Acta Neurochir 138:788–801
32. Nakamura N, Iwasaki Y, Hida K, et al (2000) Dural band pathology with Chiari type I malformation. Neuropathology 1:38–43
33. Williams B (1978) A critical appraisal of posterior fossa surgery for communicating syringomyelia. Brain (Part II) 101:223–250
34. Bertrand G (1973) Dynamic fac6tors in the evolution of syringomyelia and syringobulbia. In: Clinical Neurosurgery, vol 20. Waverly Press, Baltimore, pp 322–333
35. Isu T, Sasaki H, Takamura H, et al (1993) Foramen magnum decompression with removal of the outer layer of the dura as treatment for syringomyelia occurring with Chiari I malformation. Neurosurgery 33(5):845–850
36. Inoue HK, Kobayashi S, Ohbayashi K, et al (1994) Treatment and prevention of tethered and retethered spinal cord using Gore-Tex surgical membrane. J Neurosurg 80:689–693
37. Peerless SJ, Durward QJ (1983) Management of syringomyelia: a pathophysiological approach. Clin Neurosurg 30:531–576
38. Lapras C, Guilburd JN, Patet JD (1988) La malformation de Chiari type II. Neurochirurgie 34(suppl 1):53–58

39. Milhorat TH, Johnson WD, Miller JI (1992) Syrinx shunt to posterior fossa cisterns (syringocisternostomy) for bypassing obstructions of upper cervical theca. J Neurosurg 77:871–874
40. Williams B (1993) Surgery for hindbrain related syringomyelia. Adv Tech Stand Neurosurg 20:107–164
41. Dyste GN, Menezes AH, Van Gilder JC (1989) Symptomatic Chiari malformations. An analysis of presentation, management, and long-term outcome. J Neurosurg 71:159–168
42. Paré LS, Batzdorf U (1998) Syringomyelia persistence after Chiari decompression as a result of pseudomeningocele formation: implications for syrinx pathogenesis: report of three cases. Neurosurgery 43(4):945–948

Craniovertebral Junction Abnormalities with Hindbrain Herniation and Syringomyelia: Regression of Syringomyelia After Excision of Ventral Craniovertebral Compression

Arnold H. Menezes

Summary. The hindbrain herniation syndrome occurs frequently with craniovertebral junction (CVJ) abnormalities that reduce posterior fossa volume. Syringohydromyelia (SHM) is often present. Posterior fossa dorsal decompression (PFD) is customary, but has an adverse outcome when ventral bony abnormality exists in these circumstances. The results of a prospective study on CVJ abnormalities with Chiari malformation I (CM1) and SHM are presented. Between 1984 and 1999 (MRI era), 428 patients aged 6–68 years underwent operation for CM1; 154 had ventral CV abnormalities; 44 had associated SHM. Twelve had bone softening states with secondary basilar impression (6 previous PFD and 6 fusions); 26 had primary basilar invagination (10 had PFD, 9 previous syrinx–subarachnoid shunts and syrinx to peritoneal shunts). Symptoms reflected brainstem and high cervical myelopathy and cranial nerve deficits. Neurodiagnostic imaging included CT and MRI in dynamic modes and cine flow studies. All 44 patients had irreducible ventral CVJ bony invagination and underwent transpalatopharyngeal decompression of the cervicomedullary junction and dorsal occipitocervical fusion. Cervicothoracic SHM was present in 30, thoracic in 6, and holocord in 6. Brainstem symptoms regressed in 36 of the 44 patients; myelopathy regressed in 38 of 44 patients; and SHM showed MRI resolution in 34 of 44. Neurological improvement and SHM resolution can occur with ventral cervicomedullary junction decompression in patients with basilar invagination and basilar impression, likely because of relief of the neural encroachment and reestablishment of CSF pathways.

Key words. Chiari I, Syringomyelia, Craniovertebral abnormalities, Spinal fusion, Posterior fossa decompression

Introduction

Hans Chiari described four cerebellar anomalies, later termed the Chiari malformation [1,2]. A type I Chiari malformation is associated with caudal descent of the cerebellar tonsils and at times a kink of the lower medulla at the level of the foramen

Department of Neurosurgery, University of Iowa Hospitals and Clinics, 200 Hawkins Drive, Iowa City, IA 52242, USA

magnum. Adhesions are usually present between the cerebellar tonsils, and scar tissue may involve the arachnoid and tonsils and the dorsal surface of the medulla. Hydromyelia is present in 50% to 75% of patients. Posterior fossa bony abnormalities are recognized in 20% to 45% of individuals [3–6]. The type II Chiari malformation is best described from autopsy data of patients with myelomeningocele, with which it is most often associated. This type reveals a more extensive abnormality of the cervicomedullary junction as well as the cerebellum and the brain. The type III Chiari malformation, although rarely seen, occurs as herniation of posterior fossa tissue into the cervical canal through an upper cervical spina bifida. The Chiari IV malformation anomaly consists of hypoplasia of the cerebellum. One of the most common abnormalities associated with the Chiari I malformation is the presence of syringohydromyelia.

In the course of a review of radiographic findings in syringomyelia and syringobulbia at the Montreal Neurological Institutes, McRae found that 38% of patients had bony anomalies in the region of foramen magnum [7]. He identified atlantoaxial instability, basilar invagination, and the Chiari I malformation. De Barros et al. [8] expressed a long interest in basilar impression and the Chiari malformation in the 1950s and 1960s. They compiled a total of 66 patients in the pre-computed tomography (pre-CT) era with "basilar impression and the Arnold-Chiari malformation." Thirty-two were verified at operation. Twenty-two of these individuals had basilar invagination associated with the Chiari malformation.

In a detailed prospective database analysis of 2100 symptomatic patients referred to this author (Menezes) for primary craniovertebral junction abnormalities between 1977 and 1994, there were 100 patients with hindbrain herniation syndrome and irreducible median or paramedian invagination reflecting fourth occipital sclerotome abnormalities [9]. This association had been pointed out by Marin-Padilla in 1979 [10]. An abnormality of the occipital bone due to the occipital somite (originating from the paraaxial mesoderm) reflected overcrowding in the posterior fossa, which contained a normally developed hindbrain. Studies on basilar invagination showed an associated severe downward herniation of the hindbrain due to severe underdeveloped occipital enchondrium, which further exacerbated the overcrowding of the posterior cranial fossa [4,11,12]. Volumetric calculations for the posterior fossa by Milhorat and colleagues [6] revealed a significant reduction of the total volume and a 40% reduction of the cerebrospinal fluid (CSF) volume with normal brain content. The finding of a decreased volume of the posterior cranial fossa was substantiated by numerous publications [11–14]. The hindbrain herniation syndrome has been recognized to occur over a period of time in patients with secondary basilar invagination such as the bone softening syndromes of osteogenesis imperfecta, Paget's disease, and the Hajdu–Cheney syndrome. The developmental features of basilar invagination have been presented by this author with the progressive features of tonsillar ectopia into the cervical canal and subsequent development of syringohydromyelia [9].

Posterior fossa decompression, as treatment for the symptomatic Chiari I malformation with syringohydromyelia, has shown relatively satisfactory results except in the presence of ventral bony abnormalities. In this latter circumstance, adverse outcomes have been noted either immediately or several months to years after operation. This sequela occurs because of the peg effect of the ventral bony abnormality into the ventral cervicomedullary junction during the operative procedure for posterior fossa decompression, and also because of the persistence of CSF blockage at the foramen magnum and possible cerebellar tonsil reimpaction, which thus increases the dissociation between the cranium and the spinal CSF pressures. This latter in itself may lead to the formation of the syringohydromyelic cavity and its propagation. Various theories have been set forth for this by Gardner, Williams, Aboulker, Ball and Dayan, and Oldfield [15–19]. Thus, the question that has been unanswered for quite some time, despite the advent of magnetic resonance imaging (MRI), has been the ideal management of syringohydromyelia with a hindbrain herniation syndrome in the presence of ventral craniovertebral junction abnormalities.

A prospective study of Chiari I malformations in the MRI era, between 1984 and 1999, was undertaken at the University of Iowa Hospitals and Clinics. There were 428 patients who underwent operation; 154 of these 428 patients had a ventral craniovertebral junction irreducible bony abnormality. Of these, 44 patients fulfilled the criteria of having the ventral craniovertebral junction bony abnormality with the Chiari I malformation and syringohydromyelia. These 44 patients form the basis of this chapter.

Clinical Materials and Methods

The craniovertebral junction (CVJ) database is a prospective study of patients with abnormalities of the CVJ and has been recorded since 1977 by the author at the University of Iowa Hospitals and Clinics. A similar database is present for patients with the Chiari I malformation; 428 patients underwent operation for hindbrain herniation syndrome without myelodysplasia (Chiari I malformation), and 154 of these patients had ventral CVJ abnormalities. There were 44 patients who had a syringohydromyelia associated with the Chiari I malformation and a ventral bony abnormality indenting into the cervicomedullary or pontomedullary junction (Fig. 1).

This chapter focuses on these 44 patients. Twelve individuals had bone softening syndrome with secondary basilar impression. Six of these had undergone previous

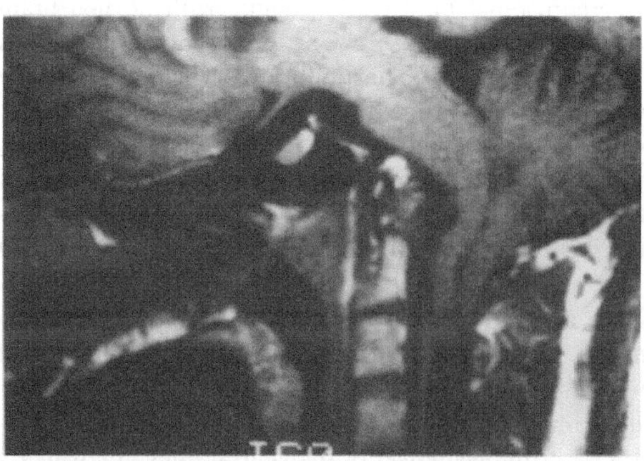

Fig. 1. Midsagittal T_1-weighted magnetic resonance imaging (MRI) of craniovertebral junction (CVJ) in a 20-year-old man with headaches, difficulty swallowing, and weakness of the hand. Note the short clivus, cerebellar tonsillar herniation into the cervical canal, ventral pontomedullary bony compression, and the cervical syringohydromelia (SHM)

posterior fossa decompression, and 6 had posterior fossa-occipitocervical fusions made before our evaluation. Twenty-six individuals had atlas assimilation with basilar invagination. Ten of these individuals had previously undergone a posterior fossa decompression with worsening of their existing neurological deficits. In 6 other individuals, proatlas segmentation abnormalities were noted. Nine patients had a primary syrinx to subarachnoid shunt with marked worsening of their neurological state.

All patients underwent MRI for their craniospinal investigation. This procedure identified hydrocephalus, syringohydromyelia, and the hindbrain herniation syndrome as well as bony abnormalities of the craniovertebral junction. Studies include dynamic flexion and extension views in the sagittal and parasagittal planes in both the T_1 and T_2 modes to identify the presence of instability as well as the best position for relief of the CSF blockage (Fig. 2). CSF flow studies were made in half the individuals using quantitative cine-mode magnetic imaging with analysis of CSF dynamics [20,21]. The MRI was repeated at 1 week as well as 6 months after surgery. Computed tomography in both two-dimensional (2-D) as well as 3-D imaging in the last 6 years was used to better define the bony abnormalities.

The age at presentation for neurological symptoms was 6 years to 68 years. The syringohydromyelia was located in the cervicothoracic cord in 30 of 44 individuals; it was thoracic in location in 6 and in the holospinal cord in 6. The symptoms and signs at presentation reflected brainstem dysfunction, high cervical myelopathy, and lower cranial nerve deficits.

The treatment algorithm for patients with a Chiari I malformation and syringohydromyelia with ventral craniovertebral junction abnormalities consisted of identification of hydrocephalus as a prime feature. If hydrocephalus was present, a supratentorial ventriculoperitoneal shunt was installed [4,22]. Patients who did not have hydrocephalus underwent flexion and extension dynamic studies to identify the reducibility of the bony abnormality. A reducible lesion was one in which the bony

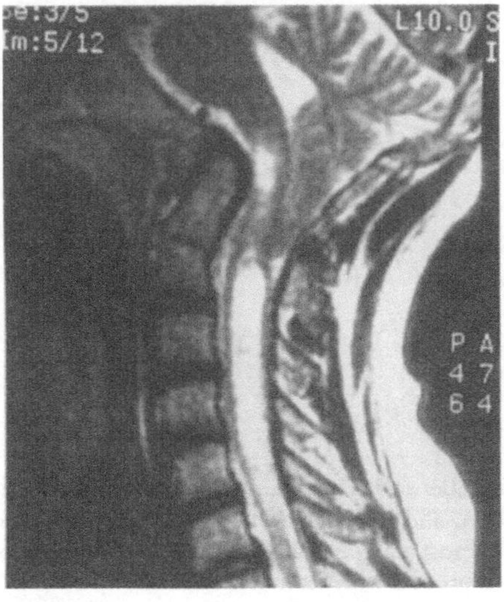

Fig. 2. Midsagittal T_2-weighted MRI of posterior fossa and cervical canal in a 16-year-old quadriparetic boy with trigeminal pain and swallowing difficulty. There is an abnormal clivus-canal-odontoid angle with atlas assimilation, basilar invagination, and syringomyelia with syringobulbia. The cerebellar tonsils extend below the posterior axis arch. Note the lack of cerebrospinal fluid (CSF) at the foramen magnum

compression was relieved with neck position or with cervical traction. Anatomic realignment then meant that posterior fossa decompression and a fusion were mandated. The 44 patients described here had an irreducible craniovertebral junction abnormality. Thus, a primary ventral decompression was made. Before 1991, 16 individuals were identified who had a ventral decompression via the transoral route. The MRI was done between the ventral decompression and the posterior fossa decompression–fusion, which were approximately 1 week apart. After 1991, 28 individuals underwent both the ventral and the dorsal procedures on the same day. Their MRIs were then carried out after the operative procedures.

The ventral procedure consisted of a transoral-transpalatine resection of the offending bony pathology with the patient in cervical traction. Resection of the anterior arch of the atlas, clivus, and the odontoid axis body was made (dictated by preoperative MRI) with preservation of the tectorial membrane (Fig. 3A,B). This procedure was followed by dorsal foramen magnum bony decompression with lateral resection of any paramesial invagination. Intraoperative ultrasonography was accomplished without opening the dura to identify the position of the tonsils and document the extent of the ventral bony decompression. CSF flow was recorded on ultrasonography as well as pulsations of the tonsils and the cervicomedullary junction. A C1 laminectomy was made, if needed. A dorsal occipital–C2 fusion was carried out with rib grafts and, more recently, the addition of internal instrumentation with a titanium loop and titanium cables. Postoperative immobilization was accomplished in a halo vest or a Minerva brace in an older individual. A duraplasty was only made if the CSF flow was found to be impeded on ultrasonography.

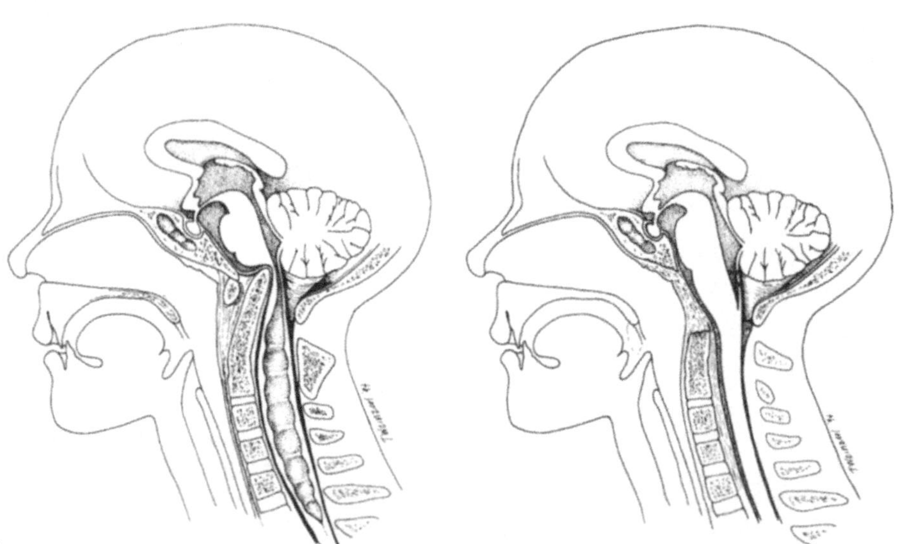
A B

Fig. 3. **A** Line drawing of midsagittal section of patient with atlas assimilation, basilar invagination with ventral cervicomedullary indentation, and tonsillar herniation. The easiest and shortest route for removal of the odontoid is the transpalatopharyngeal one. **B** Line drawing of patient in **A** after transoral resection of odontoid process with resection of SHM

All patients underwent follow-up MRI at 1 week and 6 months if the syringomyelia had not resolved. A yearly follow-up was made with both MRI and neurological evaluation. If patients had primary syrinx shunts that had been installed before our evaluation, these were removed at the time of the dorsal operative procedure.

Results

The brainstem dysfunction and cranial nerve findings were markedly improved in 36 of 44 individuals. Cervical myelopathy resolved in 38 of 44 individuals. Syringohydromyelia as documented by MRI (before 1991) resolved within the first week after ventral transoral decompression in 9 of 16 patients without posterior fossa decompression or fusion (Fig. 4A,B). In the remaining 7 individuals, the syrinx was markedly reduced in 3 by the 6-month MRI; in the other 4, the patient had clinical improvement without much change in the size of the syrinx. In the 28

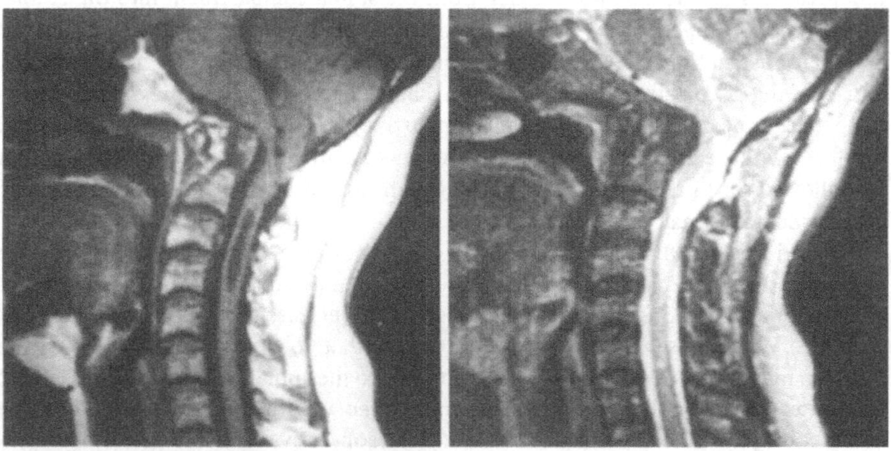

A

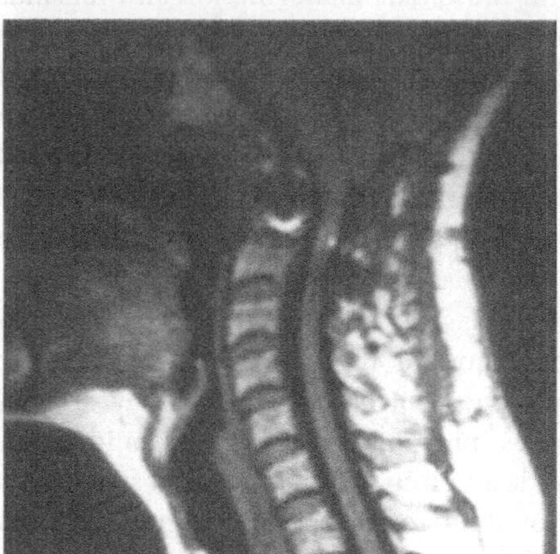

B

FIG. 4. **A** Composite of midsagittal T_1 (*left*) and T_2 (*right*) MRI of CVJ in 42-year-old woman with facial numbness, nasal regurgitation, poor hand coordination, and headaches. Note fixed atlantoaxial dislocation, odontoid invagination into the ventral medulla, Chiari I malformation, and cervical SHM. **B** Midsagittal T_1-weighted MRI of CVJ made 1 week after transoral resection of the odontoid process. Note the medullary compression, ascension of the cerebellar tonsils, and resolution of the SHM

individuals who underwent both the ventral and the dorsal operative procedures on the same day (between 1991 and 1999), the MRI showed resolution of the syrinx in 20 of the 28 within the first 6 months. In 4 others, this condition had improved by the 6-month MRI.

Discussion

Several pathogenetic theories have been put forward to explain the development of syringohydromyelia in the presence of Chiari malformations. Williams modified Gardner's theory of a "water hammer" effect wherein an arterially generated pulse wave deflected CSF into the central canal through an opening near the obex in patients in whom the normal outlet foramina of the fourth ventricle were not patent [16]. This, according to Milhorat [23] and Oldfield [19], is anatomically present in only a small percentage of individuals with the Chiari malformation and syringohydromyelia. Williams' modified theory suggested that normally occurring Valsalva maneuvers resulted in epidural venous congestion and caused intracranial as well as intraspinal CSF pressures to rise. The flow of CSF from the spinal compartment into the cranial aspect was not impeded by CVJ abnormalities whereas the caudal flow was delayed by outlet obstructions as well as hindbrain adhesions and hindbrain malformation, thus creating a "cork in a bottle effect." This blockage resulted in a pressure differential between the cranial and the spinal compartments. The pressure differential could last for several seconds to minutes, causing a worsening of the hindbrain impaction that allows CSF to enter via the abnormal pathways in front of the fourth ventricle into the central canal.

Ball and Dayan [18] as well as Aboulker [17] hypothesized that CSF under pressure may enter the spinal cord through Virchow–Robin spaces and gave direct evidence of their theory by demonstrating dilated vessels and perivascular spaces in spinal cord autopsies. When these anomalies are combined with an obstruction at the level of the foramen magnum, CSF accumulates and enters into the spinal cord, leading to a syrinx formation [24]. Aboulker proposed a similar theory with fluid entering along the dorsal roots [17]. Oldfield et al. used MRI and intraoperative ultrasonography to determine systolic pressure waves in patients with the Chiari malformation and tonsillar impaction [19]. Oldfield believed that this prevented pressure from diffusing from the spinal subarachnoid space to the cranial subarachnoid space. The pressure buildup in the relatively isolated spinal space forced fluid through the perivascular spaces into the spinal cord parenchyma with the tonsils acting as a piston. This theory differed from that of Williams in that it proposes that a CSF movement into the spinal cord is propelled by the systolic pressure wave rather than by the increased venous pressure from a Valsalva maneuver.

Stoodley and Jones, using horseradish peroxidase as a tracer in sheep, supported the hypothesis that there is a unidirectional flow of fluid from the perivascular spaces across the interstitial space and into the central canal, driven by arterial pulsations [25]. Under normal circumstances, presumably the fluid would travel through the central canal to the fourth ventricle and into the subarachnoid space. This model helps to explain the accumulation of fluid in noncommunicating syrinxes where there are isolated spinal segments. Milhorat et al. suggested that there is a normal flow of CSF from the spinal cord parenchyma to the central canal that may serve a lymphatic function, cleansing the interstitial space of metabolites and neurotransmitters [26].

These aforementioned theories describe the accumulation of fluid in syrinxes. The common denominator is a CSF block that occurs at the level of foramen magnum or above it; this is well seen in patients with a posterior fossa reduced in size as a result of basilar invagination or secondary basilar impression and is more common in patients with atlas assimilation. In the author's series of 400 patients with atlas assimilation and basilar invagination, the hindbrain herniation syndrome was present in 38% [27]. The acquired hindbrain herniation syndrome akin to the Chiari I malformation in bone softening states is well recognized [28–32]. The current literature certainly supports the proposition that the hindbrain herniation syndrome is a disorder of mesodermal origin. This idea is supported by the fact that several large series have recognized the presence of bony abnormalities in patients with the Chiari I–hindbrain herniation syndrome [3–6,33]. In addition, the neural abnormalities present, such as syringomyelia and hydrocephalus, are attributable to the secondary effects of chronic tonsillar herniation. The incidence of reduced height of the posterior fossa and the osseous abnormalities at the craniovertebral junction are consistent with a defect of paraaxial mesoderm.

Several important points are raised by the occurrence of syringohydromyelia in the setting of hindbrain herniation syndrome with CVJ abnormalities. The first is the pathogenesis of the syrinx under these conditions. It is more than likely that this is caused by the progressive reduction in posterior fossa volume, the tonsillar impaction, and its effect on subarachnoid blockage and the systolic pulse pressure wave. The bony abnormality in conjunction with the hindbrain herniation syndrome then causes a craniospinal CSF dissociation. The proof of this is in patients with osteogenesis imperfecta who develop a progressive reduction in the size of the posterior fossa leading to the secondary invagination and hindbrain abnormalities with later development of the syringohydromyelia (Fig. 5A,B). The next important question to be answered is the deterioration of patients with ventral CVJ abnormalities who undergo posterior fossa decompression as a primary procedure. It is likely that this deterioration is caused by the angulation that takes place at the cervicomedullary junction by the offending ventral pathology during the operation in a prone position, the presence of craniovertebral instability that may not be detected, and the effect of adhesions. The progressive worsening may be delayed by the gradual appearance of instability and cranial settling; this latter is caused by the cantilever effect of the cranium leading to further instability over a period of time. The possibility of cerebellar reimpaction despite the posterior fossa decompression (due to a large decompression and "slump") further aggravates the ventral angulation that may have occurred.

The issue that is paramount to this presentation is the significance of the syrinx disappearing after ventral CVJ decompression in the face of hindbrain herniation. It is more than likely that this results from the removal of the CSP block at the level of the foramen magnum and also from restoration of the posterior fossa volume. Postoperative cine studies of the CSF flow have failed to convincingly prove the reversal of craniospinal dissociation after removal of the CSF block. However, a combination of events must take place to provide for significant clinical as well as radiographic improvement [22,34,35].

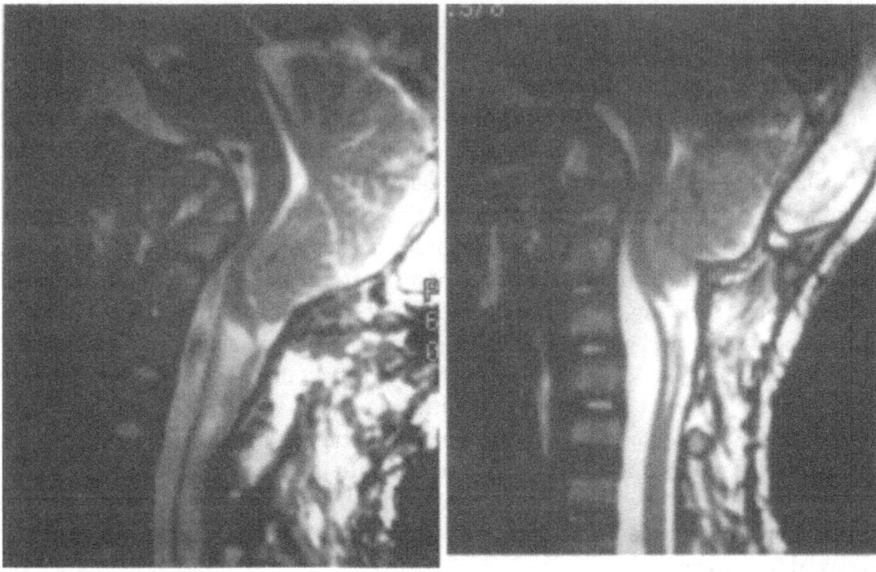

A B

Fig. 5. **A** Midsagittal T_2 MRI of CVJ in a 12-year-old boy with acroosteolysis. He had previously undergone ventriculoperitoneal shunting and posterior fossa dorsal decompression for basilar impression. The tonsils are now impacted below the C2–C3 interspace with a large SHM present. **B** Postoperative midsagittal MRI (T_2) made after high transpalatopharyngeal approach to resect the clivus and odontoid mass. The SHM is much reduced

References

1. Chiari H (1891) Ueber Veränderungen des Kleinhirns infolge von Hydrocephalie des Grosshirns. Dtsch Med Wochenschr 17:1172–1175
2. Chiari H (1896) Ueber Veränderungen des Kleinhirns, des Pons und der Medulla Oblongata infolge von congenitaler Hydrocephalie des Grosshirns. Denschr Akad Wiss Wien 63:71–116
3. Dyste GN, Menezes AH, VanGilder JC (1989) Symptomatic Chiari malformations. An analysis of presentation, management and long-term outcome. J Neurosurg 71:159–168
4. Menezes AH, Smoker WRK, Dyste GN (1990) Syringomyelia, Chiari malformation and hydromyelia. In: Youmans JR (ed) Neurological surgery. Saunders, Philadelphia, pp 1421–1459
5. Nohria V, Oakes WJ (1990–1991) Chiari I malformation: a review of 43 patients. Pediatr Neurosurg 16:222–227
6. Milhorat TH, Chou MW, Trinidad EM, et al (1999) Chiari I malformation redefined: clinical and radiographic findings for 364 symptomatic patients. Neurosurgery 44:1005–1017
7. McRae DL (1960) The significance of abnormalities of the cervical spine. Caldwell lecture 1959. AJR 84:3–25
8. De Barros MC, Farias W, Ataíde L, et al (1968) Basilar impression and Arnold-Chiari malformation. A study of 66 cases. J Neurol Neurosurg Psychiatry 31:596–605
9. Menezes AH (1995) Primary craniovertebral anomalies and the hindbrain herniation syndrome (Chiari I): data base analysis. Pediatr Neurosurg 23:260–269

10. Marin-Padilla M (1979) Notochordal-basichondrocranium relationships: abnormalities in experimental axial skeletal (dysraphic) disorders. J Embryol Exp Morphol 53:15–38
11. Nishikawa M, Sakamoto H, Hakuba A, et al (1997) Pathogenesis of Chiari malformation: a morphometric study of the posterior cranial fossa. J Neurosurg 86:40–47
12. Greenlee J, Garell PC, Stence N, et al (1999) Comprehensive approach to Chiari malformation in pediatric patients. Neurosurg Focus 6(6):article 4
13. Badie B, Mendoza D, Batzdorf U (1995) Posterior fossa volume and response to suboccipital decompression with Chiari I malformation. Neurosurgery 37:214–218
14. Stovner LJ, Bergan U, Nilsen G, et al (1993) Posterior cranial fossa dimensions in the Chiari I malformation: relation to pathogenesis and clinical presentation. Neuroradiology 35:113–118
15. Gardner WJ, Angel J (1959) The mechanism of syringomyelia and its surgical correction. Clin Neurosurg 6:131–140
16. Williams B (1980) On the pathogenesis of syringomyelia: a review. J R Soc Med 73:798–806
17. Aboulker J (1979) La syringomyelie et les liquides intra-rachidiens. Neurochirurgie 25(suppl 1):1–44
18. Ball MJ, Dayan AD (1972) Pathogenesis of syringomyelia. Lancet 2:799–801
19. Oldfield EH, Muraszko K, Shawker TH, et al (1994) Pathophysiology of syringomyelia associated with Chiari I malformation of the cerebellar tonsils: implications for diagnosis and treatment. J Neurosurg 80:3–15
20. Armonda RA, Citrin CM, Foley KT, et al (1994) Quantitative cine-mode magnetic resonance imaging of Chiari I malformations: an analysis of cerebrospinal fluid dynamics. Neurosurgery 35:214–224
21. Wolpert SM, Bhadelia RA, Bogdan AR, et al (1994) Chiari I malformations: assessment with phase-contrast velocity MR. AJNR 15:1299–1308
22. Dyste GN, Menezes AH (1988) Presentation and management of pediatric Chiari malformations without myelodysplasia. Neurosurgery 23:589–597
23. Milhorat TH, Nobandegani F, Miller JI, et al (1993) Noncommunicating syringomyelia following occlusion of the central canal in rats: experimental model and histological findings. J Neurosurg 78:274–279
24. Citow JS, Dohrmann GJ, Batzdorf U (2000) Syringomyelia. Neurosurg Q 10(3):159–168
25. Stoodley MA, Jones NR (1997) Syringomyelia. In: Clark C (ed) The cervical spine. Lippincott, Philadelphia, pp 110–140
26. Milhorat TH, Johnson RW, Johnson WD (1992) Evidence of CSF flow in rostral direction through central canal of spinal cord in rats. In: Matsumoto N, Tamski N (eds) Hydrocephalus: pathogenesis and treatment. Springer, Tokyo, pp 202–217
27. Menezes AH, Ryken TC, Brockmeyer DL (2000) Abnormalities of the craniocervical junction. In: McLone DG (ed) Pediatric neurosurgery: surgery of the developing nervous system, 4th edn. Saunders, Orlando, pp 400–422
28. Elisevich K, Fontaine S, Bertrand G (1987) Syringomyelia as a complication of Paget's disease. J Neurosurg 67:611–613
29. Harkey HL, Crockard HA, Stevens JM, et al (1990) The operative management of basilar impression in osteogenesis imperfecta. Neurosurgery 27:782–786
30. Nyland H, Krogness KG (1978) Size of posterior fossa in Chiari type I malformation in adults. Acta Neurochir 40:233–242
31. Sawin PD, Menezes AH (1997) Basilar invagination in osteogenesis imperfecta and related osteochondrodysplasias: medical and surgical management. J Neurosurg 86:950–960
32. Kurimoto M, Ohara S, Takaku A (1991) Basilar impression in osteogenesis imperfecta tarda. Case report. J Neurosurg 74:136–138

33. Menezes AH (1991–1992) Chiari I malformations and hydromyelia—complications. Pediatr Neurosurg 17:146–154
34. Ghanem IB, Londono C, Delalande O, et al (1997) Chiari I malformation associated with syringomyelia and scoliosis. Spine 22(12):1313–1318
35. Muhonen MG, Menezes AH, Sawin PD, et al (1992) Scoliosis in pediatric Chiari malformations without myelodysplasia. J Neurosurg 77:69–77

T-Tube Syringoperitoneal Shunts for the Treatment of Syringomyelia Associated with Chiari I Malformation

Shu-Yuan Yang and Yong-Zhong Gao

Summary. To assess the outcome of surgical management of syringomyelia associated with Chiari I malformation, we report 22 cases in which a T-tube syringoperitoneal shunt was used. After a mean follow-up of 26.6 months, the outcome in all patients was classed as excellent or good, and in this period there was no recurrence of the syrinx. We believe that the T-tube syringoperitoneal shunt is a reasonable treatment of first choice for syringomyelia associated with a Chiari I malformation.

Key words. Syringomyelia, Chiari I malformation, T-tube shunting, Outcome

Introduction

With a reported prevalence of 8.4 cases per 100000 population, the effective management of syringomyelia is an important problem [1]. Because the pathological findings and pathogenesis of syringomyelia remain controversial [1–9], various surgical procedures have been used for the treatment of syringomyelia associated with Chiari I malformation. These treatments have included foramen magnum decompression (FMD), with or without obex plugging, syringostomy, syringosubarachnoid shunt (SS), syringoperitoneal shunt (SP), and shunting to the pleura or cisterna magna [2,10–25]. Since January 1992, we have used a T-tube syringoperitoneal shunt, and report here the results in 22 cases of syringomyelia associated with Chiari I malformation.

Materials and Methods

We have reviewed the records of 22 patients with syringomyelia associated with Chiari I malformation who underwent a T-tube syringoperitoneal shunt from January 1992 in the Department of Neurosurgery, General Hospital, Tianjin Medical University. There were 16 men and 6 women, aged 14 to 55 years with a mean of 33.9 and median of 31.2 years. The duration of the illness was from 1.5 to 20 years, with a

Department of Neurosurgery, General Hospital, Tianjin Medical University, 154 AnShan Road, Tianjin 300052, People's Republic of China

mean of 7.5 and a median of 7.1 years. Of the 22 patients, 20 suffered from a variety of dysesthesias and pain, and 20 from wasting of the muscles of the hands, arms, and shoulders. In 10 there was autonomic trunk pain, which became more marked year by year, in 6 lower cranial nerve paresis, and in 6 nystagmus. Scoliosis was present in 8 patients. In all 22 cases, the diagnosis was made by magnetic resonance imaging (MRI), demonstrating both the syringomyelia and the Chiari I malformation. The shortest syrinx was between C2 and T2 vertebral levels, and the longest from the medulla to T12.

Operative Procedure

Under general anesthesia with the patient in the left lateral position, a laminectomy is performed over one or two levels where the syrinx is largest. Under the microscope, a 2-mm myelotomy is made in the midline of the dorsum of the spinal cord. A T-tube CSF-Lumboperitoneal shunt is inserted (P.S. Medical, Goleta, CA, USA). This shunt is fabricated from barium-impregnated silicone elastomer tubing, 1.5 mm in outer and 0.7 mm in inner diameter. The T-section is 8 cm in length, open-ended, and perforated with 28 pairs of flow holes approximately 2.5 mm apart (Fig. 1). It is threaded into the syrinx through the myelotomy, trimmed if the tube is longer than the cavity, and when in place sutured to the pia mater of the cord. The stem of the T is 87 cm in length and is provided with slit valves and a radiopaque marker at the distal end. It is tunneled subcutaneously and inserted into the peritoneal cavity (Fig. 2).

Results

In this group there was no operative mortality and no postoperative infection. One case developed saddle anesthesia. Follow-up is available for all patients for 24 to 50 months after surgery (mean, 26.6 months). At 12 months, the clinical condition was related to the preoperative state, using the simple criteria described by Tator et al. [22]. An excellent result is defined as a reduction of the neurological deficit. In a good result, the neurological deficit has not progressed, and in a poor result there is further deterioration of neurological function. By these criteria there was an excellent result in 8 cases, a good result in 9 cases, and a poor result in 5. Reassessment at 2 years showed an excellent result in 15 cases and a good result in 7. In each case MR imaging was repeated annually during follow-up. This method showed that after operation the syrinx became slitlike or could not be identified; there was no recurrence (Fig. 3).

Discussion

It is becoming increasingly clear that syringomyelia cannot be regarded as a condition with a uniform pathology. Differing views of the etiology and natural history of the condition have generated much controversy regarding its management [1–9].

The two major types of syringomyelia are the communicating and the noncommunicating. In the former, there is a direct communication of the syrinx with the fourth ventricle. MR imaging, however, has shown that this connection is present in only a minority of cases. In noncommunicating syringomyelia, there is a focal dilata-

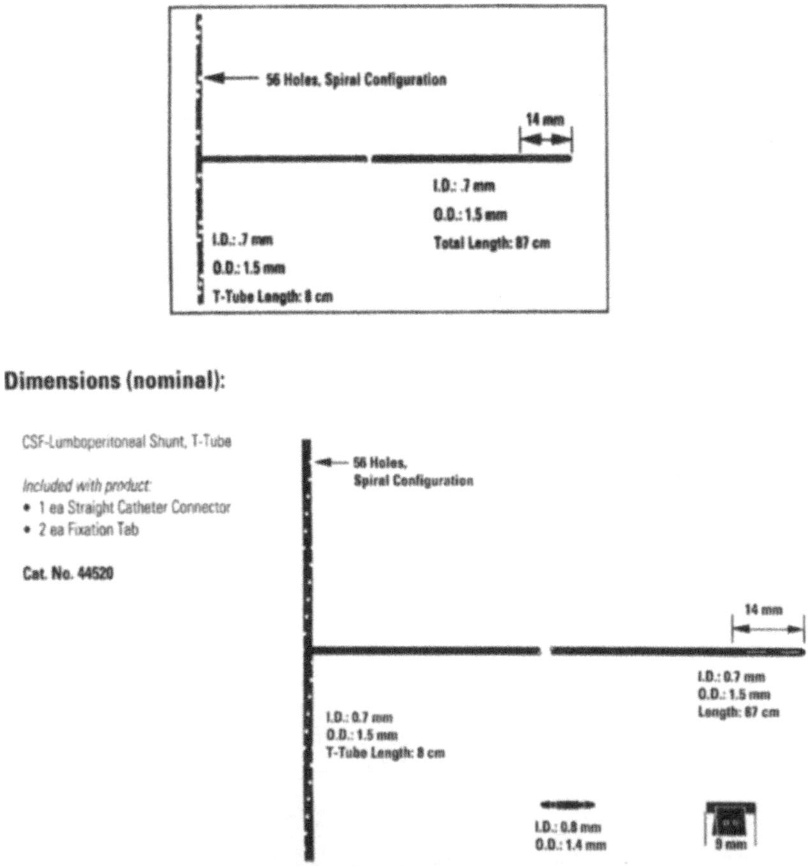

Fig. 1. T-tube for syringoperitoneal shunt is fabricated of barium-impregnated silicone elastomer. The long section of the T-tube is designed for peritoneal placement; it is 87 cm long, with four slit valves located approximately 14 mm from the end. The tip is filled with radiopaque tantalum-impregnated silicone elastomer so that its position can be checked

tion of the central canal that is separated from the fourth ventricle by a syrinx-free segment of spinal cord. This is the lesion that is encountered predominantly in adults and is associated with the Chiari I malformation [4]. The patients in the present series were all in this group.

The several theories of pathogenesis of syringomyelia have generated a variety of surgical procedures for its management. Current methods in clinical use are posterior fossa decompression (PFD), Gardner's operation (PFD with plugging of the obex), and shunting the syrinx, either to the subarachnoid space or the peritoneum [2,14,15,17,20–22,24,26].

Which is the best option has given rise to considerable controversy. The majority of neurosurgeons favor posterior fossa and C1 decompression (PFD), with or without duraplasty and with or without closure of the obex. Plugging of the obex was originated by Gardner and advocated by Williams [2,11,21,27]. According to Gardner's theory, the obstruction by the Chiari I malformation at the craniocervical junction

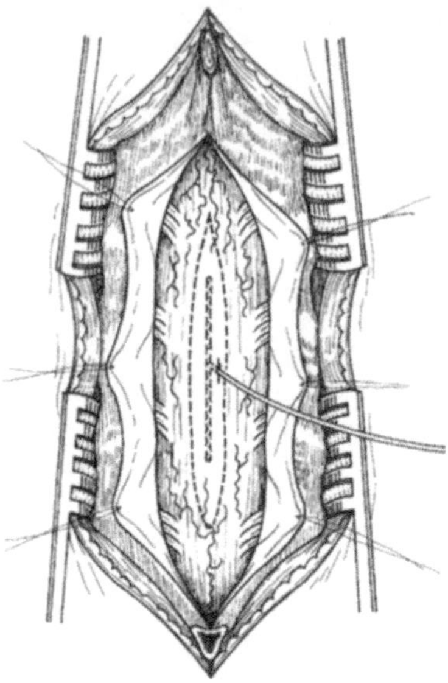

FIG. 2. The T-tube in place in the syrinx

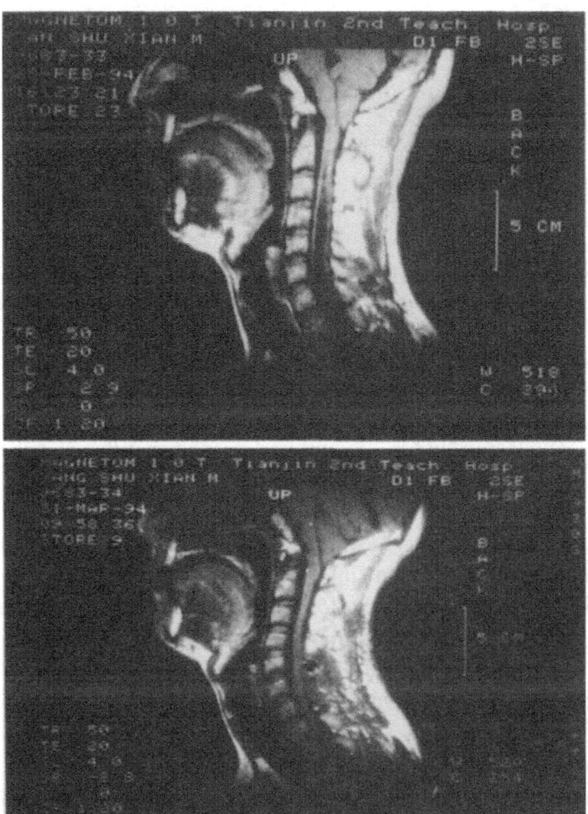

a

b

FIG. 3. **a** Syringomyelia with Chiari I malformation. **b** After T-tube shunting, the syrinx could not be identified

causes cerebrospinal fluid (CSF) to enter the central canal of the cervical cord. However, in the majority of patients the connection with the central canal does not exist, so that this theory cannot explain the formation of the syrinx. In practice the Gardner operation is technically not easy and risks injury to the hypoglossal and vagal nuclei in the medulla. Matsumoto and Symon [2] reported the use of Gardner's operation in 22 cases; 6 patients deteriorated and 2 died. The improvement that does occur with the Gardner operation is probably due to the decompression of the hindbrain hernia rather than blockage of a presumed communication between the fourth ventricle and the central canal.

Heiss et al. [1] studied 20 cases of syringomyelia associated with the Chiari I malformation. They thought that the syringomyelia progressed because the cerebellar tonsils partially occluded the subarachnoid space at the foramen magnum and, with the cardiac pulsation, then acted on the spinal CSF as a piston, resulting in increased cervical subarachnoid pressure waves. These waves were transmitted through the wall of the syrinx, propagating the fluid caudally and leading to its enlargement. This view was supported by cine MR imaging, which showed that the velocity of CSF flow at the foramen magnum was increased in either direction, and that there was a downward flow of subarachnoid and syrinx fluid with systole which was reversed in diastole. Intraoperative measurements confirmed that the syrinx contracted during cardiac systole in synchrony with the tonsillar descent. These observations were repeated after PFD. The CSF passages at the foramen magnum had enlarged, the maximum flow rate of CSF with cardiac systole had increased, and transmission of pressure across the foramen with jugular compression was normal. The mean and pulse cervical CSF pressure had decreased to normal. MR imaging showed reduced velocity and flow of the syrinx fluid. The cerebellar tonsils assumed a normal form and size. Clinical symptoms and signs improved or remained stable in all patients. All these findings were inconsistent with the view that dilatation of the central canal is caused by CSF pressure waves from the fourth ventricle, and therefore there was no justification for blockage at the obex.

Other reports in the recent literature confirm favorable results from FMD, with improvement of clinical symptoms or signs or stability with no progression in 30% to 82% of cases [2,11,14,16,19,21]. An example is that of Hida et al. [14], who reported a series of 70 patients, 33 of whom were treated by FMD and 37 by syringosubarachnoid shunting. In the 33 patients treated by FMD, postoperative MRI showed that the syrinx had collapsed or decreased in size in 94%.

Shunting the syrinx fluid to either the subarachnoid space or the peritoneum is the most direct method of reducing the pressure within the syrinx. There have been many reports of improvement or stabilization in 50% to 100% of cases [14,15,17,22–24,26]. In our own series of 22 cases of peritoneal shunting, 15 showed excellent and 7 cases good results. Hida et al., in the series mentioned earlier [14], gave the results of syringosubarachnoid (SS) shunts in 37 cases. With a mean 60-month follow-up, improvement was seen in 97% of patients; lower cranial nerve symptoms and ataxia were improved in 25%, motor weakness in 85%, sensory disturbance in 95%, and pain in 92%. Comparing the results obtained with FMD, relief of severe pain was better with the shunt operation; the syrinx decreased in size in 94% of the FMD group and 100% in the SS shunt patients. The average time for the syrinx to reduce in size was 6.3 weeks after FMD and 1.8 weeks after SS shunting. Hida concluded that

SS shunting resulted in more rapid improvement in clinical symptoms and radiological findings and that it may be superior to FMD as the initial treatment for syringomyelia associated with Chiari I malformation, especially with patients who have a large syrinx.

An essential factor in subarachnoid shunting is whether the pressure in the syrinx is higher than that in the subarachnoid space. Heiss et al. [1] at operation measured the pressures in the syrinx and the subarachnoid space. The pressure in the syrinx was 15 ± 5.8 mmHg and in the subarachnoid space 15.1 ± 4.7 mmHg, so that there was in fact no pressure gradient. The studies by Stoodley et al. [8,9] showed that there is normally a passage for the flow of fluid from the subarachnoid space into the perivascular space, through the interstitial space and into the central canal, so that pressure differences would tend to equalize. Again, Milhorat et al. [17] emphasized that a requirement of syrinx to subarachnoid space shunting was that the space, including the upper cervical theca, provided a competent path for CSF drainage. Such shunts are likely to fail if the CSF pathway rostral to the syrinx is blocked, and in such cases the use of subarachnoid shunts would be contraindicated. The best chance of reducing the pressure in the syrinx may therefore be to shunt the fluid to a low-pressure extraspinal site.

From the long-term point of view, there are still many problems with syrinx shunts that need to be solved. There are many reports that postoperatively some shunts fail to drain. The cause may be scarring of the subarachnoid space or arachnoiditis, particularly in the subarachnoid shunts, or malfunction of the shunting system [1,2,18,27,28].

In our group of patients, followed for a mean of 27 months, all patients showed an excellent or good result; there were no poor results and no recurrence of the syrinx. We believe that this is due to the use of the T-tube peritoneal shunt. It is not affected by subarachnoid scarring or arachnoiditis and, with no recurrence of the syrinx, evidently has remained patent. Nevertheless we believe that a longer-term follow-up is required. It is possible that in spite of the collapse of the syrinx neurological function may deteriorate because of astrocytic proliferation in the syrinx wall, axonal degeneration and demyelination, and perhaps spinal cord tethering.

Acknowledgment. We are grateful to Mr. Philip Wrightson, F.R.A.C.S., for help in preparing this report for publication.

References

1. Heiss JD, Patronas N, DeVroom HL, et al (1999) Elucidating the pathology of syringomyelia. J Neurosurg 91:553–562
2. Matsumoto T, Symon L (1989) Surgical management of syringomyelia: current results. Surg Neurol 25:131–136
3. Milhorat TH, Nobandegani F, Miller JI, et al (1993) Noncommunicating syringomyelia following occlusion of central canal in rats: experimental model and histological findings. J Neurosurg 78:274–279
4. Milhorat TH, Johnson RW, Milhorat RH, et al (1995) Clinicopathological correlations in syringomyelia using axial magnetic resonance imaging. Neurosurgery 37:206–213
5. Milhorat TH, Capocelli AL, Anzil AP, et al (1995) Pathological basis of spinal cord cavitation in syringomyelia: analysis of 105 autopsy cases. J Neurosurg 82:802–812

6. Milhorat TH, Capocelli AL, Kotzen RM, et al (1997) Intramedullary pressure in syringomyelia: clinical and pathophysiological correlates of syrinx distension. Neurosurgery 41:1102–1110
7. Oldfield EH, Muraszk K, Shawker TH, et al (1994) Pathophysiology of syringomyelia associated with Chiari malformation of the cerebellar tonsils: implications for diagnosis and treatment. J Neurosurg 80:3–15
8. Stoodley MA, Jones NR, Brown CJ (1996) Evidence for rapid flow from the subarachnoid space into the spinal cord central canal in the rat. Brain Res 707:155–164
9. Stoodley MA, Gutschmidt B, Jones NR (1999) Cerebrospinal fluid flow in an animal model of noncommunicating syringomyelia. Neurosurgery 41:1065–1076
10. Barbaro NM, Wilson CB, Gutin PH, et al (1984) Surgical treatment of syringomyelia. J Neurosurg 61:531–538
11. Batzdorf U (1988) Chiari I malformation with syringomyelia: evaluation of surgical therapy by magnetic resonance imaging. J Neurosurg 68:726–730
12. Erkan K, Unal F, Kiris T (1999) Terminal syringomyelia in association with the tethered cord syndrome. Neurosurgery 45:1351–1359
13. Faulhauer K, Loew K (1978) The surgical treatment of syringomyelia. Long term results. Acta Neurochir (Wien) 44:215–222
14. Hida K, Iwasaki Y, Koyanagi I, et al (1995) Surgical indication and results of foramen magnum decompression versus syringosubarachnoid shunting for syringomyelia associated with Chiari I malformation. Neurosurgery 37:673–679
15. Isu T, Iwasaki Y, Akino M (1990) Syringo-subarachnoid shunt for syringomyelia associated with Chiari malformation (type I). Acta Neurochir (Wien) 107:152–160
16. Isu T, Sasaki H, Takamura H, et al (1993) Foramen magnum decompression with removal of the outer layer of the dura as treatment for syringomyelia occurring with Chiari I malformation. Neurosurgery 33:844–849
17. Lesoin F, Petit H, Thomas CE, et al (1986) Use of the syringoperitoneal shunting in the treatment of syringomyelia. Surg Neurol 25:131–136
18. Milhorat TH, Johnson WD, Miller JI (1992) Syrinx shunt to posterior fossa cisterns (syringocisternostomy) for bypassing obstruction of upper cervical theca. J Neurosurg 77:871–874
19. Mushi I, Frim D, Stine-Reyes R, et al (2000) Effects of posterior fossa decompression with and without duraplasty on Chiari malformation-associated hydromyelia. Neurosurgery 46:1384–1390
20. Padovani R, Cavallo M, Gaist G (1989) Surgical treatment of syringomyelia: favourable results with syringosubarachnoid shunting. Surg Neurol 32:173–180
21. Peerless SJ, Durward QJ (1983) Management of syringomyelia: a pathophysiological approach. Clin Neurosurg 30:531–576
22. Tator CH, Meguro K, Rowed DW (1982) Favourable results with syringosubarachnoid shunt for treatment of syringomyelia. J Neurosurg 56:517–523
23. Tognetti F, Calbucci F (1993) Syringomyelia: syringo-subarachnoid shunt versus posterior fossa decompression. Acta Neurochir (Wien) 123:196–197
24. Vaguero J, Martinez R, Salazer J (1987) Syringo-subarachnoid shunt for treatment of syringomyelia. Acta Neurochir (Wien) 84:105–109
25. Williams B, Fahy G (1983) A critical appraisal of "terminal ventriculostomy" for the treatment of syringomyelia. J Neurosurg 58:188–197
26. Calenbergh FV, Bergh RVD (1987) Syringoperitoneal shunting: results and problems in a consecutive series. Acta Neurochir (Wien) 84:203–205
27. Wiedemayer H, Godde G, Stolke D (1987) Problems in the operative treatment of syringomyelia. Acta Neurochir (Wien) 84:207–209
28. Chakrabortty S, Tamaki N, Ehara K, et al (1997) Experimental syringomyelia: Late ultrastructural changes of spinal cord tissue and magnetic resonance imaging evaluation. Surg Neurol 48:246–254

Diagnosis and Treatment of Syringomyelia: Our Experience with 164 Cases

Toshiaki Abe, Yoshiji Okuda, Toshiro Hida, and Satoshi Tani

Summary. One hundred sixty-four cases of syringomyelia unrelated to tumor were reviewed to determine the correct diagnosis and the most appropriate surgical treatment. We found that foramen magnum decompression (FMD) was the most appropriate treatment for syringomyelia with Chiari malformation. FMD with fourth ventricle-subarachnoid shunt was also appropriate for syringomyelia with basal arachnoiditis. FMD with opening of the foramen Magendie was appropriate for syringomyelia with obstruction of the foramen Magendie. Establishment of a syringoperitoneal or syringosubrachnoid shunt was appropriate for syringomyelia with spinal arachnoiditis, depending on its location. Lumboperitoneal shunt was appropriate for idiopathic syringomyelia. Each treatment was equally successful in collapsing the syrinx; however, the postoperative clinical course differed with the associated lesion.

Key words. Syringomyelia, Chiari malformation, Foramen Magendie, Basal arachnoiditis, Spinal arachnoiditis

Introduction

Many theories have been proposed for the pathogenesis of syringomyelia [1–3]. Furthermore, many surgical treatments and technical variations are available to treat syringomyelia [4–6]. We performed a retrospective study of 164 consecutive patients with syringomyelia unrelated to tumor in whom the results of magnetic resonance imaging (MRI) had been used to make the correct diagnosis and determine the most appropriate surgical treatment.

Patients and Methods

On the basis of MRI and intraoperative findings, cases of syringomyelia were classified into five types according to the associated lesions: type 1, Chiari malformation; type 2, basal arachnoiditis; type 3, congenital obstruction of the foramen

Department of Neurosurgery, The Jikei University School of Medicine, 3-25-8 Nishi-Shinbashi, Minato-ku, Tokyo 105-8461, Japan

Magendie; type 4, spinal arachnoiditis; type 5, idiopathic. Our main goals in surgical treatment of syringomyelia are to correct abnormal cerebrospinal fluid (CSF) flow, which is almost always present in all types of syringomyelia, and to collapse the intraspinal syrinx. Whether the selected operative procedure had been appropriate was evaluated on the basis of the rate of syrinx collapse. In addition, the patient's neurological status and the size of the syrinx were routinely evaluated in each type of syringomyelia.

Results

Patient data are listed in Table 1. In patients with type 1 syringomyelia, MRI revealed that the herniated tonsils were wedge shaped and occupied the cisterna magna; the rostral end of the syrinx was conical, and the caudal part of the fourth ventricle had been obliterated. These findings suggested that the herniated tonsils compressed the brainstem and the spinal cord and mechanically obstructed the flow of CSF at the foramen magnum. Therefore, foramen magnum decompression (FMD) was selected to treat all cases of type 1 syringomyelia.

Postoperative MRI revealed that the syrinx had collapsed in 116 of 119 cases. In addition, the tip of the herniated tonsils was rounded and shifted upward, creating an enlargement of the subarachnoid space around the foramen magnum (Fig. 1). These MRI changes confirmed that FMD had successfully corrected the abnormal CSF flow. There were no operative complications except for transient worsening of pyramidal signs in both legs in a patient who had a marked basilar impression. The neurological status improved or stabilized after surgery in all patients except one patient with pain in both upper extremities.

All patients with type 2 syringomyelia had been born after a difficult labor, except for two patients who had a history of meningitis. MRI revealed that the cisterna magna was narrowed by scar tissue or herniated tonsils (Fig. 2). However, the tip of the tonsils was rounded and a cavity resembling the subarachnoid space was noted in the region of the cisterna magna. In addition, the upper end of the syrinx was rounded and the lower part of the fourth ventricle was well visualized. These MRI findings suggested that the foramen magnum was not mechanically obstructed by herniated tonsils but rather by arachnoid scarring due to arachnoiditis. The foramen Magendie, which was found at surgery to be obstructed owing to arachnoid scarring in all cases of type 2 syringomyelia, was opened after FMD. A shunt tube was placed between the fourth ventricle and the intact subarachnoid space around the spinal cord, usually at the

Table 1. Demographic data for 164 patients with syringomyelia classified into five types by associated lesions

	Type 1	Type 2	Type 3	Type 4	Type 5
No. of cases	119	17	3	20	5
Male/female	46:73	7:10	0:3	14:6	4:1
Age (mean) (years)	34.9	35.2	37.7	46.0	45.8
Follow-up (mean) (years)	5.6	9.8	7	4.1	5.8

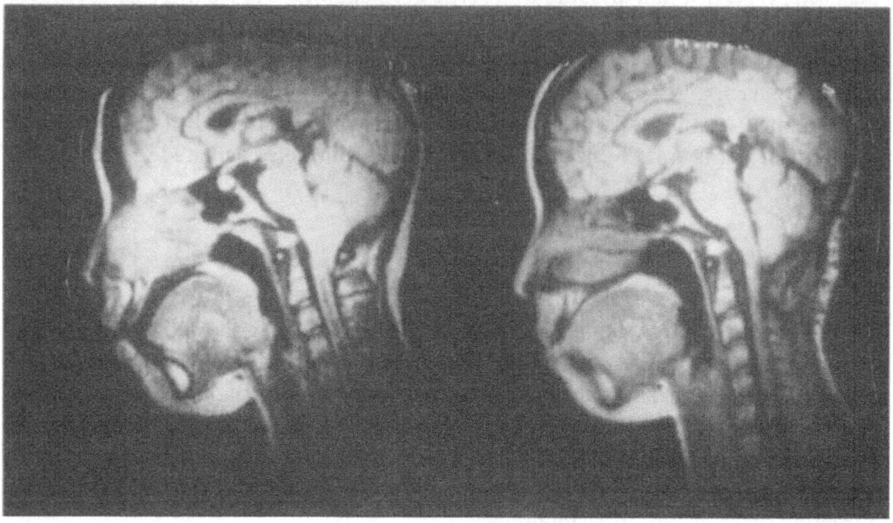

FIG. 1. Magnetic resonance imaging (MRI) of syringomyelia with Chiari malformation (type 1), before (*left*) and after (*right*) operation

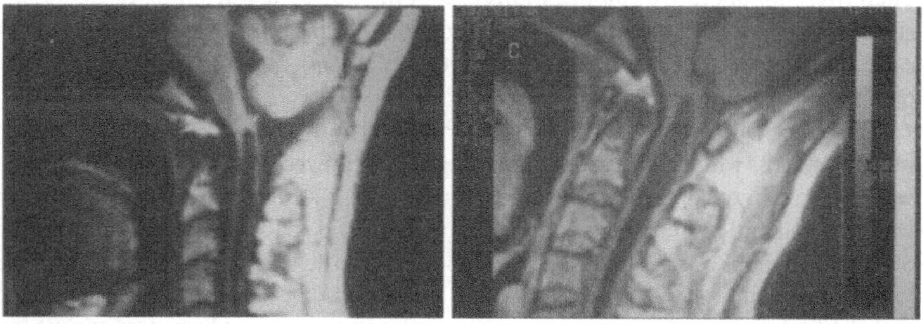

FIG. 2. MRI of syringomyelia with basal arachnoiditis (type 2), before (*left*) and after (*right*) operation

ventral side of the spinal subarachnoid space, to prevent reobstruction of the foramen Magendie. Postoperative MRI revealed that the syrinx had collapsed in 14 of 17 cases with upward shift of tonsils. Neurological deterioration was arrested with surgery in 60% of the patients but continued in 40% of patients.

In patients with type 3 syringomyelia, MRI revealed that the syrinx was directly connected with the fourth ventricle via a patent central canal in association with hydrocephalus in one of three cases (Fig. 3). The foramen Magendie, which was obstructed by a membrane with overlaying normal subarachnoid space in all cases, was opened to equalize the pressure between the ventricular system and the subarachnoid space. Postoperative MRI revealed that the syrinx had collapsed but the

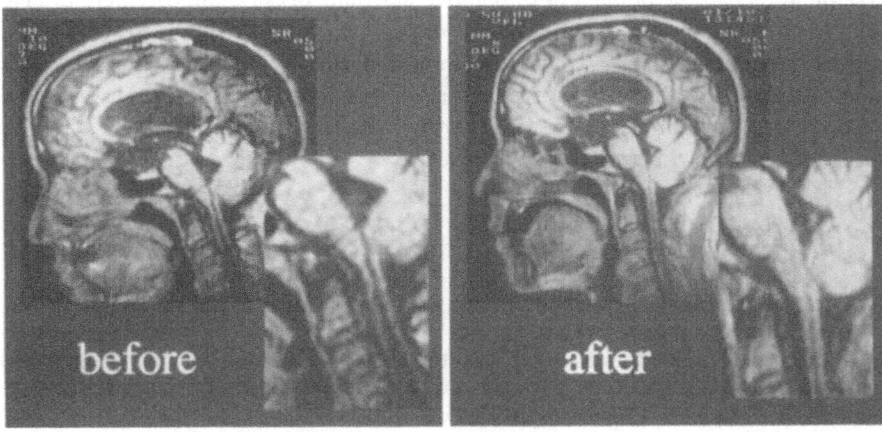

FIG. 3. MRI of syringomyelia with obstruction of the foramen Magendie (type 3) before operation (*left*) and after foramen magnum decompression (FMD) with obex plugging (*right*)

tonsils had not changed shape or position (Fig. 3). Clinically, neurological symptoms were stabilized after surgery in all patients.

In patients with type 4 syringomyelia, MRI revealed obliteration of the subarachnoid space around the spinal cord due to arachnoid scarring, a normal craniovertebral junction, and extension of the syrinx both rostrally and caudally from the site of scarring. A syringosubarachnoid shunt was established rostrally from the site of scarring when scarring was localized. When scarring was not localized, a syringoperitoneal shunt was established. The syrinx continuously collapsed in 66% of patients after the first operation, but a shunt obstruction was present in 34% of patients, who required a reoperation to collapse the syrinx. Clinically, extension of the neurological deficits to the upper extremities was prevented with surgery; however, paraplegia, which was a characteristic feature in patients with type 4 syringomyelia, progressed slowly after surgery in 27% of the patients. In patients with type 5 syringomyelia, associated lesions could not be found with myelography, MRI, or CSF flow studies using cine-MRI. Although both syringosubarachniod and lumboperitoneal shunts were effective for collapsing the syrinx, the lumboperitoneal shunt was considered more appropriate because the surgery was less invasive. The neurogical condition of all patients was stable after surgery.

Conclusion

Our surgical treatment, which had been selected on the basis of the results of MRI, successfully collapsed the syrinx without severe complications in most patients. However, after collapse of the syrinx, the postoperative clinical course differed in patients according to the associated lesion. Patients with syringomyelia with Chiari malformation had the best postoperative outcome. In contrast, the presence of arachnoiditis was the most unfavorable factor, and patients with syringomyelia with spinal arachnoiditis had the poorest postoperative outcome. Because improvement of neurological deficits was limited, the goal of surgical treatment should be to stabilize the patient's neurological status. Therefore, in all types of syringomyelia surgical treatment should be performed as soon as neurological symptoms start to progress. Furthermore, we hope that in the future we will encounter fewer patients with all the classic signs and symptoms of syringomyelia.

References

1. Gardner WJ, Angel J (1958) The mechanisim of syringomyelia and its surgical correction. Clin Neurosurg 6:131–140
2. Oldfield EH, Muraszko K, Shawker TH, et al (1994) Pathophysiology of syringomyelia assocoated with Chiari I malformation of the cerebellar tonsils. Implications for diagnosis and treatment. J Neurosurg 80:3–15
3. Williams B (1969) The distending force in the production of "communicating syringomyelia." Lancet II:189–193
4. Hida K, Iwasaki Y, Koyanagi I, et al (1995) Surgical indication and results of foramen magnum decompression versus syringosubarachnoid shunting for syringomyelia associated with Chiari I malformation. Neurosurgery 37:673–679
5. Milhorat TH, Johnson WD, Miller JI, et al (1992) Surgical treatment of syringomyelia based on magnetic resonance imaging criteria. Neurosurgery 31:231–245
6. Williams B (1993) Surgery for hindbrain related syringomyelia. Adv Tech Stand Neurosurg 20:107–164

Simple Expansive Suboccipital Cranioplasty Following Foramen Magnum Decompression for the Treatment of Syringomyelia Associated with Chiari I Malformation

Masakazu Takayasu, Toshihisa Nishizawa, and Jun Yoshida

Summary. We have done expansive suboccipital cranioplasty for the treatment of syringomyelia associated with Chiari malformation in 14 patients since 1992, based on the hypothesis that the bony covering may keep the cisterna magna enlarged and prevent postoperative restenosis by the scar tissue in addition to cosmetic advantage. We demonstrate our simple method for expansive suboccipital cranioplasty using a suboccipital bone flap and the favorable results. A free suboccipital bone flap was made from the rostral part by placing two to four burr holes and connecting them with a craniotome. The posterior marginal bone of the foramen magnum was removed piece by piece. Then, C1 wide laminectomy and dural plasty using a patch graft were done as usual. The suboccipital bone flap was placed more caudally to cover the foramen magnum after tailoring the shape of the flap to fit the bone window. The bone flaps were fixed with titanium miniplates. The rostral part of the cranial window was filled with bone chips obtained during craniotomy and the C1 laminectomy. Preoperative symptoms improved significantly except for persistent dysesthetic pain in two patients. Postoperative MRI showed ascent of the tonsils and disappearance or decrease of the syrinx in all patients. Our simple expansive suboccipital cranioplasty is an useful method for the treatment of syringomyelia associated with Chiari malformation.

Key words. Syringomyelia, Chiari malformation, Foramen magnum decompression, Cranioplasty

Introduction

A few methods for expansive suboccipital cranioplasty for the treatment of syringomyelia associated with Chiari malformation have been introduced [1,2]. The supposed advantages of cranioplasty over craniectomy are that the rigid bony frame may enlarge the cisterna magna better and may prevent postoperative restenosis by the scar tissue, in addition to the cosmetic advantage of cranioplasty. However, con-

Department of Neurosurgery, Nagoya University School of Medicine, 65 Tsurumai-cho, Showa-ku, Nagoya 466-8560, Japan

ventional methods for expansive cranioplasty are too complicated. We introduce a simple method for expansive suboccipital cranioplasty using a suboccipital bone flap and demonstrate the advantages of this method.

Materials and Methods

Operative Procedure

Because most patients have small posterior cranial fossae with thick internal occipital cristae, en bloc suboccipital craniotomy usually is not easy. Craniotomy is started by placing two or four burr holes, which are connected with a craniotome (Fig. 1). As the internal occipital crista of the occipital bone is well developed in most patients with Chiari malformation, the middle parts of both the rostal and caudal craniotomy lines are thinned using an air drill to accomplish craniotomy. The posterior marginal bone of the foramen magnum is carefully removed using air drills, a Kerrison punch, and a rongeur. The posterior arch of the C1 is also carefully resected until the maximum diameter of the C1 arch is exposed. When the tonsilar herniation is below the C2 level, the upper part of the C2 lamina is removed (partial laminectomy of C2 was performed in 5 of 14 patients).

A thick epidural fibrosis is usually located at the interlaminar space between the C1 and C2. The dura is opened in a Y-shaped fashion from the cranial to spinal direction, keeping the arachnoid membrane intact as much as possible. When arachnoiditis is not obvious at the dorsal part of the foramen magnum cistern, the arachnoid membrane is not opened and the dura is closed with a patch graft of Goatex dura, which

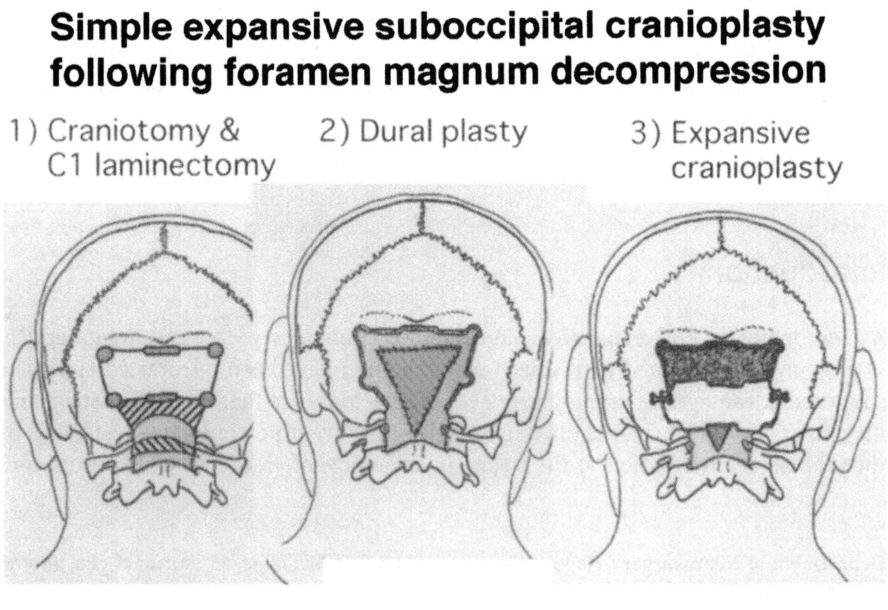

FIG. 1. Schematic drawing of each step for simple expansive cranioplasty

is sealed with fibrin glue. Then, expansive cranioplasty is done. The bone flap is tailored to fit the bone window. Because the internal crista of the occipital bone is usually thick, this part is removed. The flap was often placed in an inside-out fashion for better fitting (9 of 14 patients). The flap is positioned more caudally to cover the foramen magnum and fixed with titanium miniplates. In recent cases, the Gore-Tex dura is tacked to the center of the bone flap to expand the dorsal cisterna of the foramen magnum. The bone chips obtained during craniotomy are placed into the rostral open space of craniotomy and hardened with fibrin glue.

Patient Data

We have done expansive suboccipital cranioplasty for the treatment of syringomyelia associated with Chiari malformation in 14 patients since 1992. Among them, we analyzed 11 patients who were followed more than 1 year. There were 8 female and 3 male patients with a mean age of 29 years (13–41). The follow-up period was 13 months to 8 years. Preoperative clinical symptoms and signs in 11 patients were cranial nerve and cerebellar signs in 4, motor weakness in 4, sensory disturbance in 9, and intractable pain in 4 patients. Most of the patients had symptoms caused by syringomyelia such as sensory disturbance, while one-third of the patients (36%) displayed brainstem or cerebellar signs. The degree of tonsilar herniation and syringomyelia were evaluated by magnetic resonance imaging (MRI) in all cases. The tonsilar herniation was classified into five categories depending on the position of the tip of the tonsil, i.e., posterior fossa, foramen magnum, C1, C1–C2, and C2. The syringomyelia was also classified into five categories depending on the thickness of the syrinx, i.e., ballooned, thick, thin, linear, and non. Postoperative recovery of clinical symptoms and signs and radiological findings was evaluated periodically.

Results

The results of surgery were successful. There was no operative morbidity or mortality, and no major complications, including intractable subcutaneous cerebrospinal fluid (CSF) retention. Preoperative symptoms and signs improved significantly within a few weeks in all patients except for persisting dysesthetic pain in two patients. Improvement of neuroimaging was noted in all patients (Fig. 2). The position of the tonsilar tip was located between the C1 and C2 level preoperatively and ascended to the posterior fossa (73%) or foramen magnum (27%) postoperatively in all patients (Table 1). The size of the syrinx varied from ballooned type to linear thin type preoperatively (Table 2); it decreased to the linear type (64%) or disappeared completely (non, 36%). There was no recurrence of symptoms and signs or no deterioration of neuroimaging during the follow-up period in any patient (Fig. 2).

Discussion

Foramen magnum decompression has been the most effective and widely used procedure in treating syringomyelia associated with Chiari I malformation [3]. Although short-term effectiveness is good in the foramen magnum decompression procedures,

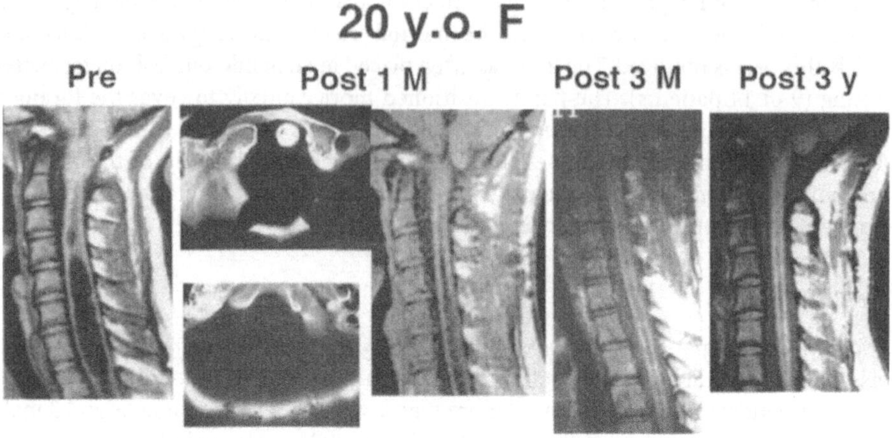

FIG. 2. Neuroimaging of a 20-year-old female patient showing significant ascent of the tonsil and decrease of the syrinx postoperatively on follow-up MRI

TABLE 1. The position of the tonsilar tip on MRI in 11 patients

	Number of patients	
Position of tonsilar tip	Preoperative	Postoperative
Posterior fossa	0	8
Foramen magnum	0	3
C1	7	0
C1–C2	2	0
C2	2	0

TABLE 2. The size of the syrinx on MRI in 11 patients

	Number of patients	
Syrinx size	Preoperative	Postoperative
Ballooned	3	0
Thick	6	0
Thin	1	0
Linear	1	7
Non	0	4

relapse of the symptoms has been reported in a significant proportion [4]. One cause of relapse may be restenosis of the dorsal cisterna of the foramen magnum. Therefore, the advantages of posterior fossa reconstruction have been advocated.

A method of posterior fossa reconstruction has been reported by Sahuquillo et al. in which the dural graft was tented to the fascial plane to avoid scarring after craniectomy and laminectomy [5]. However, the dorsal cistern of the foramen magnum should be more effectively held open with the bony frame, which method was reported by Sakamoto et al. [2]. The supposed advantages of expansive cranioplasty over craniectomy are that the rigid bony frame may enlarge the cisterna magna better and may prevent postoperative restenosis by the scar tissue, in addition to the cosmetic advantage. However, their method seems to be too complicated for a routine procedure, so we introduced a method for simple expansive suboccipital cranioplasty. The results of long-term follow-up were excellent. There was no relapse of symptoms and signs during the follow-up period. The tonsilar ascent and decrease in syrinx size were noted in all patients on MRI, and these favorable findings have been maintained on follow-up MRI.

Furthermore, the operated sites are kept in cosmetically good shape postoperatively in all patients without depression, which is often observed after suboccipital craniectomy. There was no intractable subcutaneous CSF retention, which may be another advantage.

References

1. Tokuno H, Hakuba A, Suzuki T, et al (1988) Operative treatment of Chiari malformation with syringomyelia. Acta Neurochir Suppl 43:22–25
2. Sakamoto H, Nishikawa M, Hakuba A, et al (1999) Expansive suboccipital cranioplasty for the treatment of syringomyelia associated with Chiari malforamtion. Acta Neurochir (Wien) 141:949–961
3. Oldfield EH, Muraszko K, Shawker TH, et al (1994) Pathophysiology of syringomyelia associated with Chiari I malforamtion. J Neurosurg 80:3–15
4. Paul KS, Lye RH, Strang FA, et al (1983) Arnold-Chiari malformation. J Neurosurg 58:183–187
5. Sahuquillo J, Rubio E, Poca M-A, et al (1994) Posterior fossa reconstruction: a surgical technique for the treatment of Chiari I malformation and Chiari I/syringomyelia complex: preliminary results and magnetic resonance imaging quantitative assessment of hindbrain migration. Neurosurgery 35:874–885

Surgical Treatment of Syringomyelia with Chiari Malformation Type I

KAZUTOSHI HIDA and YOSHINOBU IWASAKI

Summary. Several surgical procedures have been used for the treatment of syringomyelia associated with Chiari I malformation in our institute. The purpose of this paper is to evaluate the results of two major surgical procedures, foramen magnum decompression (FMD) and syringosubarachnoid (SS) shunting. The series consisted of 111 patients with syringomyelia associated with Chiari I malformation who were surgically treated. Their ages ranged from 3 to 59 years (median, 29 years). FMD was performed on 53 patients and SS shunting on 58 patients. The follow-up period ranged from 6 months to 18 years. The clinical and radiological outcomes were analyzed comparing the two groups. We principally performed FMD in patients with symptoms of Chiari I malformation or a small syrinx or both. We prefer to use SS shunting in patients with a large syrinx. Postoperative magnetic resonance imaging demonstrated that the syrinx had collapsed or decreased in size in 93% of the patients who underwent FMD and in 100% of the patients who underwent SS shunting. Neurological improvements were observed in 82% and in 97%, respectively, of the patients who underwent FMD and SS shunting. The average time for the syrinx to collapse was 5.6 weeks after surgery in the FMD group and 1.5 weeks in the SS shunting group. These results indicate that clinical symptoms and radiological findings improved much more quickly in the SS shunt group than in the FMD group.

Key words. Chiari malformation, Syringomyelia, Foramen magnum decompression, Syringosubarachnoid shunt

Introduction

The diagnosis of syringomyelia has been greatly facilitated by the introduction of magnetic resonance imaging (MRI). Many authors have reported the clinical and radiological characteristics of syringomyelia associated with various types of pathogenesis [1–11]. Chiari I malformation is the most common condition in syringomyelia patients. However, the selection of the type of surgery is still controversial [1–11]. We

Department of Neurosurgery, University of Hokkaido School of Medicine, North 15, West 7, Kita-ku, Sapporo 060-8638, Japan have treated 111 cases of syringomyelia with Chiari I malformation. In this study, we described our surgical option for syringomyelia with Chiari type I malformation and its surgical outcomes.

Materials and Methods

From 1982 to March 2000, 111 patients with syringomyelia associated with Chiari I malformation were treated in Hokkaido University Hospital and its affiliated hospitals. There were 36 males and 75 females; their age on admission ranged from 3 to 75 years, with a mean of 29 years. In all patients, syringomyelia was diagnosed using magnetic resonance imaging (MRI). Magnetic resonance images were obtained with a 1.5-T MRI system using a surface coil.

As an initial surgical procedure, foramen magnum decompression (FMD) was performed on 53 patients, and syringosubarachnoid (SS) shunting was performed on 58 patients. Selection of surgical procedures was based on the following principles: in patients with symptoms of Chiari I malformation, or small syrinx, we performed FMD; in patients who had a large syrinx, we preferred to use SS shunting.

Symptoms and Signs

Table 1 shows clinical signs and symptoms at admission. Lower cranial nerve palsy or nystagmus was observed in 17% of the patients. Motor weakness was found in 56% of the patients, sensory disturbance in 87%, pain in 41%, autonomic nerve disturbance in 16%, and scoliosis in 55%.

Surgical Selection

We primarily prefer to use an SS shunt in patients who have a large syrinx in the widened spinal cord. The large syrinx has paper-thin walls, particularly at the dorsal root entry zone, which made SS shunting safe. In patients with a small syrinx or those whose main symptoms are caused by Chiari malformation, we performed FMD. The details of our surgical technique have been reported elsewhere [4,7].

Surgical Outcome

The results of surgery were successful. There were no patients who suffered a major operative complication, and no deaths. The mean follow-up period was 65 months,

TABLE 1. Clinical signs on admission of syringomyelia with Chiari malformation

Sign	Number of patients	Percent
Cranial nerves	19/108	17
Motor weakness	62/111	56
Sensory disturbance	97/111	87
Pain	45/111	41
Autonomic nerve	18/111	16
Scoliosis	61/111	55

TABLE 2. Postoperative results of magnetic resonance imaging (MRI)

	Collapsed syrinx	Interval (weeks)	Mean (weeks)
FMD	47/50 (94%)	2–24	5.6
SS shunt	58/58 (100%)	0.5–4	1.5

FMD, foramen magnum decompression; SS, syringosubarachnoid.

TABLE 3. Postoperative results of FMD

Factor	Number	Improved	Unchanged	Worsened
Cranial nerve	10	5 (50%)	5 (50)	0
Motor weakness	22	14 (64%)	7 (32%)	1 (5%)
Sensory disturbance	38	29 (76%)	9 (24%)	0
Pain	15	9 (60%)	6 (42%)	0

TABLE 4. Postoperative results of SS shunt

	Number	Improved	Unchanged	Worsened
Cranial nerve	8	2 (25%)	6 (75%)	0
Motor weakness	36	31 (86%)	5 (14%)	0
Sensory disturbance	50	45 (90%)	5 (10%)	0
Pain	18	16 (89%)	2 (11%)	0

ranging from 6 months to 17 years. Postoperative MRI revealed the syrinx decreased in size in 94% (50 of 53 patients) of the FMD group and 100% (58 of 58 patients) of the SS shunt group (Table 2). Neurological improvements were observed in 82% and in 97% of the patients who underwent FMD and SS shunting, respectively (Tables 3, 4). In the FMD group, improvement of the lower cranial nerve and ataxia was observed in 50% of the patients, of motor weakness in 64%, of sensory disturbance in 76%, and of pain 60%. In the SS shunt group, improvement of the lower cranial nerve and ataxia was observed in 25% of the patients, of motor weakness in 86%, of sensory disturbance in 90%, and of pain 89%.

However, secondary surgery was necessary in 3 of 53 patients in the FMD group and 9 of 58 patients who underwent SS shunting. In the FMD group, these patients were treated with the use of SS shunting. In the SS shunt group, they were revised by SS shunting in 1 patient, by FMD in 4 patients, and by both FMD and SS shunting in 4 patients.

Discussion

Several surgical procedures have been performed for the treatment of syringomyelia associated with Chiari I malformation, including FMD with or without obex plugging [2,3,5,6], SS shunting [4,7,8,9], syringoperitoneal shunting [1], and thecoperitoneal shunting [10,11]. As for the selection of surgical procedure, we prefer to use SS shunting in patients who have a large syrinx in the widened spinal cord, and we perform FMD in patients with symptoms of Chiari I malformation or a small syrinx [4].

FMD is now a widely accepted surgical procedure because it can restore cerebrospinal fluid (CSF) circulation at the foramen magnum. However, even FMD with dural plasty has a possibility of the following postsurgical complications: aseptic meningitis, meningitis, pseudomeningocele, and CSF fluid collection in the operative wound [2,5]. We also observed temporary meningitis in 2 of 21 patients (10%) on whom dural plasty had been performed. Recently, FMD with removal of the layer of dura was reported to avoid such complications. However, FMD may not be an ideal treatment for patients with a rapid progression due to syrinx because it take much more time than does the SS shunt.

The SS shunt is one of the major surgical treatments for syringomyelia with Chiari malformation. It is also a safe and effective treatment. Some have reported the disadvantages of the SS shunt. Additionally, the main criticism for SS shunting is that it is not able to improve the CSF pathways around the foramen magnum. However, the SS shunt group in our series showed decreased syrinx size even after a long follow-up period.

Conclusion

Both surgical procedures, FMD and SS shunting, are efficient, but should be selected on the basis of preoperative clinical and radiological findings. The SS shunt group improved in both clinical symptoms and radiological findings in a much shorter time than did those in the FMD group.

References

1. Barbaro NM, Wilson CB, Gutin PH, Edwards MSB (1984) Surgical treatment of syringomyelia: favorable results with syringoperitoneal shunting. J Neurosurg 61:531–538
2. Batzdorf U (1988) Chiari I malformation with syringomyelia. J Neurosurg 68:726–730
3. Foster JB (1991) Neurology of syringomyelia. In: Batzdorf U (ed) Syringomyelia: current concepts in diagnosis and treatment. Williams & Wilkins, Baltimore, pp 91–115
4. Hida K, Iwasaki Y, Izumi K, et al (1995) Surgical indication and results of foramen magnum decompression versus syringosubarachnoid shunting for syringomyelia associated with Chiari I malformation. Neurosurgery 37(4):673–679
5. Hoffman HJ, Neill J, Crone KR, et al (1987) Hydrosyringomyelia and its management in childhood. Neurosurgery 21:347–351
6. Isu T, Sasaki H, Takamura H, Kobayashi N (1993) Foramen magnum decompression with removal of the outer layer of the dura as treatment for syringomyelia occurring with Chiari I malformation. Neurosurgery 33(5):844–850
7. Iwasaki Y, Hida K, Koyanagi I, Abe H (2000) Reevaluation of syringosubarachnoid shunt for syringomyelia with Chiari malformation. Neurosurgery 46(2):407–413
8. Padovani R, Cavallo M, Gaist G (1989) Surgical treatment of syringomyelia: favorable results with syringosubarachnoid shunting. Surg Neurol 32:173–180

9. Rhoton AL Jr (1976) Microsurgery of Arnold–Chiari malformation in adults with and without hydromyelia. J Neurosurg 45:473–483
10. Vassilouthis J, Papandreou A, Anagnostaras S, Pappas J (1993) Thecoperitoneal shunt for syringomyelia: Report of three cases. Neurosurgery 33:324–328
11. Vengsarkar US, Panchal VG, Tripathi PD, et al (1991) Percutaneous thecoperitoneal shunt for syringomyelia. Report of three cases. J Neurosurg 74:827–831

Surgical Results of Two Types of Foramen Magnum Decompression for Syringomyelia

Shinji Imae, Yasuhiko Nishimura, and Toru Itakura

Summary. We evaluated the surgical outcomes between two types of foramen magnum decompression (FMD), dural plasty with a Gore-Tex sheet and removal of the outer layer of the dura mater, for patients with syringomyelia associated with Chiari type 1 malformation. In the plasty group and the outer layer group there were 12 and 9 cases, respectively. Effects following surgical treatment were evaluated by assessing the volume of syrinx cavity on sagittal T_1-weighted magnetic resonance imaging (MRI) and neurological symptoms. The ratio in the area of the syrinx and spinal cord (S-C ratio) on preoperative and postoperative sagittal T_1-weighted MRI were measured by means of computer (reduction rate). With regards to neurological symptoms, the recovery rate of the neurological cervical spine scale (NCSS, in Japan) was used. The reduction rates of the plasty group and the outer layer group were 52.1% and 41.5%, respectively, but there was no significant difference between the two groups. The recovery rate of the patients of the outer group was significantly poorer than that of the patients with plasty; 2 cases in the plasty group and 1 case in the outer group required a second surgery. However, all these patients showed a decrease in the size of syrinx and recovery of symptoms. Both the plasty and the outer layer groups demonstrated good results, but we must investigate further to determine which method is better.

Key words. Syringomyelia, Foramen magnum decompression, Chiari type I malformation MRI, Complications

Introduction

Foramen magnum decompression (FMD) of syringomyelia associated with Chiari type I malformation has not yet been standardized. No one procedure has always proven successful, leading to the development of many alternative procedures [1–7]. For the past 5 years, we have randomly performed two types of FMD: dural plasty with a Gore-Tex sheet and removal of the outer layer of the dura mater. We evaluated

---

Department of Neurological Surgery, Wakayama Medical University, 811-1 Kimiidera, Wakayama 641-0012, Japan

the surgical outcome between these two types of FMD. In this study, we describe the surgical results and the reports of three cases that required a second operation.

Materials and Methods

Twenty-one patients with syringomyelia associated with Chiari type I malformation, which were diagnosed with magnetic resonance imaging (MRI), underwent dural plasty with a Gore-Tex sheet or removal of the outer layer of the dura mater. There were 12 cases in the plasty group and 9 cases in the outer group; 11 men and 10 women, ranging from 15 to 56 (mean, 32.5) years of age. The mean follow-up periods were, respectively, 2.1 and 2.3 years and the mean duration of symptoms was 3.8 and 4.5 years. There were no significant differences between the two groups.

The two surgical procedures were as follows. In the case of dural plasty, a 4-cm midline skin incision within the hairline was made and a suboccipital craniectomy was performed to a point at which the lateral edge of the foramen magnum could be confirmed. The extent was approximately 4 cm in the transverse direction and 3 cm in the vertical direction. All patients underwent an approximately 2-cm-wide C1 laminectomy but none of them received C2 laminectomy even if the level of tonsillar herniation was C2. A Y-shaped dural incision was made and the dura mater was covered with a Gore-Tex sheet having a thickness of 0.3 mm. In the case of removal of the outer layer, the extent of suboccipital craniectomy and C1 laminectomy were the same as that of dural plasty, and the outer layer of dura mater including the epidural band was removed to a point at which tonsil pulsation could be seen transparently.

Evaluation of the effects following surgical treatment was performed on the volume of the syrinx cavity on sagittal T_1-weighted MRI and neurological symptoms. The ratio in the area of the syrinx and spinal cord (S-C ratio) on preoperative and postoperative sagittal T_1-weighted MRI were measured by means of a computer [8]. With regards to evaluation of neurological symptoms, the recovery rate of the neurological cervical spine scale was used [9].

Results

The reduction rates of the plasty group and the outer layer group was 52.1% and 41.5%, respectively, but there was no significant difference between the two groups (Fig. 1A). The recovery rates of the plasty group and outer group were 49.6% and 34.1%, respectively. The recovery rate of the outer group was significantly poorer than that of the patients in the plasty group (Fig. 1B); two cases in the plasty group and one case in the outer group required a second operation. However, after this second operation all these patients showed a decrease in syrinx size and considerable recovery of symptoms. Descriptions of these three cases follow.

Case Reports

The first case is a 14-year-old boy. MRI showed syringomyelia associated with Chiari type I malformation (Fig. 2, left). Two months after dural plasty, the syrinx was remarkably reduced; however, there was much subcutaneous cerebrospinal fluid collection in

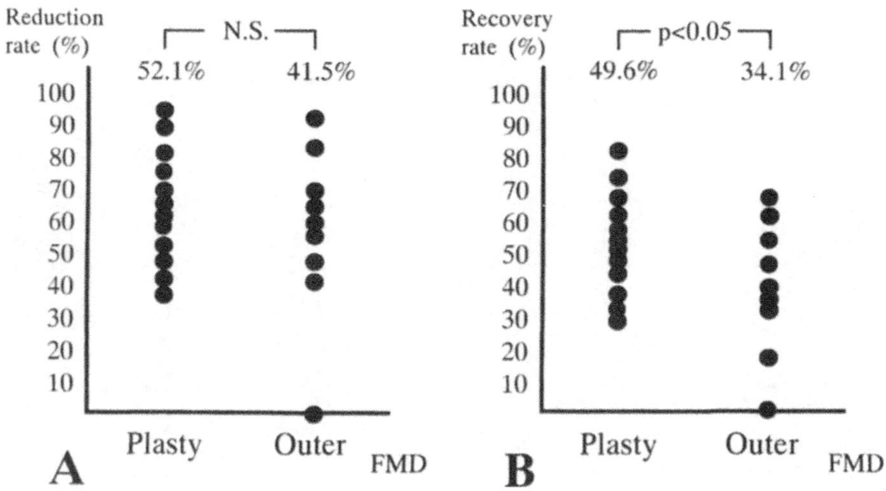

Fig. 1A,B. Comparison of surgical outcomes between plasty group and removal of outer membrane group. **A** Reduction rate. **B** Recovery rate. *NS*, not significant; *FMD*, foramen magnum decompression

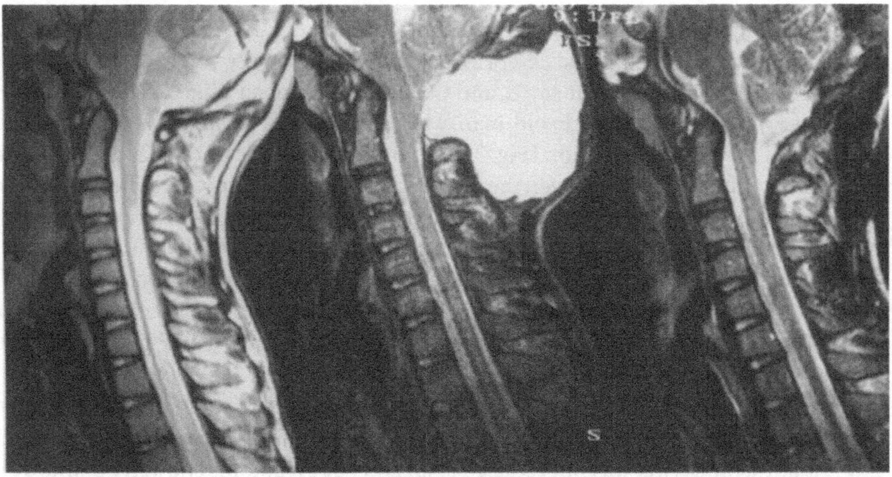

Fig. 2. Case 1. Sagittal T_2-weighted magnetic resonance (MR) imaging. *Left*: preoperative image shows a syrinx from C2 to T3 associated with Chiari type I malformation. *Center*: postoperative image shows a large collection of cerebrospinal fluid (CSF) in the suboccipital space. *Right*: postreoperative image demonstrates complete collapse of the syrinx and no CSF leakage

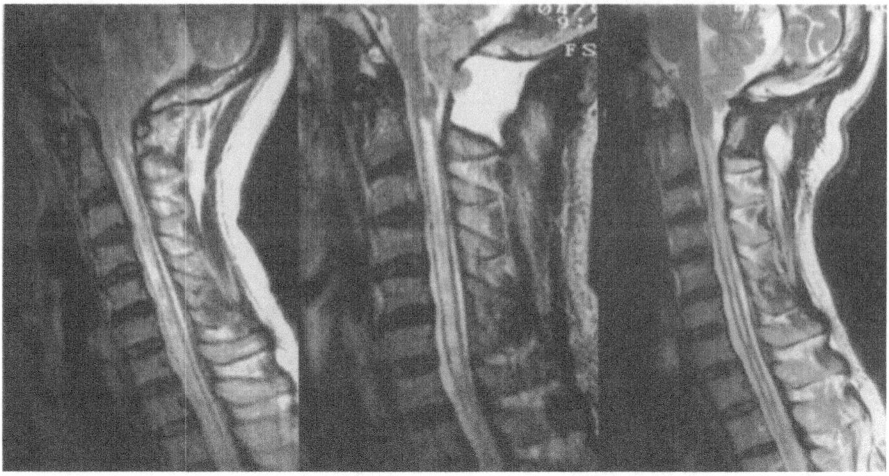

FIG. 3. Case 2. Sagittal T_2-weighted MR imaging. *Left*: preoperative image shows a syrinx from C2 to T2 associated with Chiari type I malformation. *Center*: postoperative image shows a small collection of CSF in the suboccipital space and posterior protrusion of the cerebellar tonsil. *Right*: postreoperative image demonstrates considerable reduction of the syrinx and no CSF leakage

the suboccipital area. Two months later, the patient complained of severe headaches and MRI demonstrated an enlarged cerebrospinal fluid (CSF) space (Fig. 2, center). Repair surgery of the fistula was performed, and CSF leakage stopped (Fig. 2, right).

The second case is a 46-year-old man. MRI also showed syringomyelia associated with Chiari type I malformation (Fig. 3, left). One month after dural plasty, the syrinx was remarkably reduced; however, there was slight subcutaneous CSF collection in the suboccipital area. Four months later, the patient complained of vertigo with nystagmus. MRI showed tonsil extrusion to the posterior through the Gore-Tex sheet (Fig. 3, center). During the second surgery, sheet flattening and extrusion of tonsil were confirmed. Therefore, the site of suture between the Gore-Tex sheet and the dura mater was reinforced with the fascia of the suboccipital muscle (Fig. 3, right). No further problems were experienced.

The third case is a 50-year-old woman. MRI also showed syringomyelia associated with Chiari type I malformation (Fig. 4, left). Ten months after removal of the outer layer of dura, the syrinx was not reduced at all and her symptoms showed no improvement. MRI demonstrated an adhesive change between the inner layer of dura mater and the suboccipital muscles (Fig. 4, center), so dural plasty with a Gore-Tex suture was performed. The site of suture between the Gore-Tex sheet and dura mater was reinforced with fascia of the suboccipital muscle. Six months after dural plasty, the syrinx was remarkably reduced (Fig. 4, right).

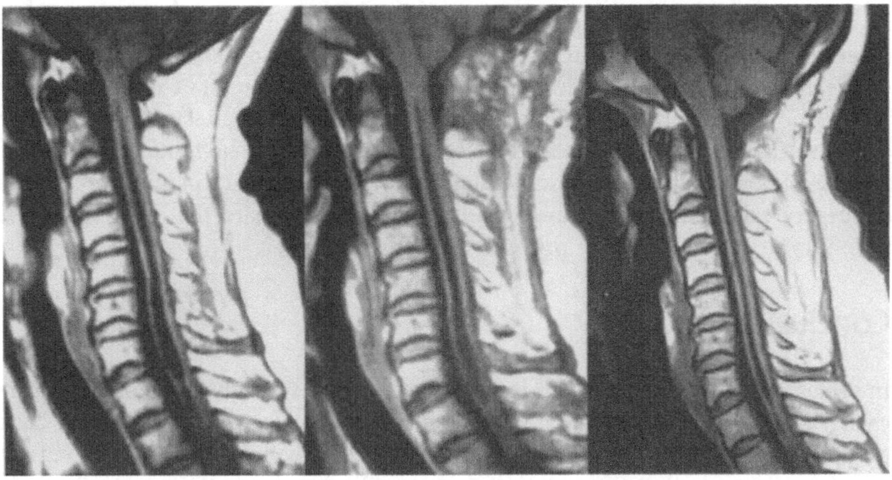

FIG. 4. Case 3. Sagittal T_1-weighted MR imaging. *Left*: preoperative image shows a syrinx from C2 to T2 associated with Chiari type I malformation. *Center*: postoperative image shows adhesive change between the inner layer of dura mater and suboccipital muscles and no effect of surgical decompression. *Right*: postreoperative image demonstrates considerable reduction of the syrinx and no adhesive change

Discussion

Many surgical procedures have been recommended for the treatment of syringomyelia associated with Chiari type I malformation, but none has yet been standardized. Currently, suboccipital craniectomy or cranioplasty and C1 or C2 laminectomy (FMD) are the most frequently used procedures; however, no one procedure of FMD has proven always successful, leading to the development of a number of alternative procedures [2–7,9,10].

In 1993, Isu et al. [2] advocated that FMD dividing the outer layer of the dura mater is sufficient because circulatory disturbance of the CSF is corrected at the level of the foramen magnum. This procedure may be less invasive than that of any other FMD. Moreover, the most favorable point of this procedure is that artificial sheets are not needed. On the other hand, the question remains whether this procedure will suffice for all syringomyelia associated with Chiari type I malformation. To resolve that question, we have randomly performed dural plasty with Gore-Tex sheet or removal of the outer layer of the dura mater for the past 5 years. There was no significant difference in reduction rate between the plasty group and the outer group. The recovery rate of the patients in the outer group was significantly poorer than that of the patients in the plasty group. Because there were no significant differences in any parameters between the two groups, it may be possible that Gore-Tex plasty was more effective than removal of the outer layer in the degree of decompression.

However, the rate of second operation in the plasty group was much higher than that of the outer group. The most frequent cause of failure in the plasty group was CSF leakage. The Gore-Tex sheet has no affinity for surrounding tissue including the dura mater and arachnoid membrane. Although for surgical decompression it might be very useful, its disadvantage in lack of affinity required us to repair CSF leakage several times. We had never experienced the necessity to do a second operation for CSF leakage until lyophilized dura mater, which nowadays cannot be used because of the risk of viral infection, was replaced by Gore-Tex. Therefore, it is necessary for the site of suture between the Gore-Tex sheet and dura mater to be reinforced with the fascia of suboccipital muscle or something else. With these results in mind, both types of surgery exhibit advantages and disadvantages. Therefore, further investigation is necessary to determine which procedure is better.

Conclusion

In evaluation of the effects of surgical treatment on the subsequent volume of syrinx cavity, there were no significant differences between the plasty group and outer layer group. With regards to neurological symptoms, the recovery rate of the outer group was significantly poorer than that of the plasty group. On the other hand, the rate of second operation in plasty group was much higher than that of the outer group. Therefore, as noted, further investigation to determine which method is better remains necessary.

References

1. Batzdorf U (1988) Chiari I malformation with syringomyelia. J Neurosurg 68:726–730
2. Isu T, Sasaki H, Kobayashi N, et al (1993) Foramen magnum decompression with removal of the outer layer of the dura as treatment for syringomyelia occurring with Chiari I malformation. Neurosurgery 33:845–850
3. Morgan D, Williams B (1992) Syringobulbia: a surgical appraisal. J Neurol Neurosurg Psychiatry 55:1132–1141
4. Pillay PK, Awad IA, Little JR, et al (1991) Symptomatic Chiari malformation in adults: a new classification based on magnetic resonance imaging with clinical and prognostic significance. Neurosurgery 28:639–645
5. Pollack IF, Pang D, Krieger D, et al (1992) Outcome following hindbrain decompression of symptomatic Chiari malformations in children previously treated with myelomeningocele closure and shunts. J Neurosurg 77:881–888
6. Raftopoulos C, Sanchez A, Brotchi J, et al (1993) Hydrosyringomyelia-Chiari 1 complex. Prospective evaluation of a modified foramen magnum decompression procedure: preliminary results. Surg Neurol 39:163–169
7. Sahuquillo J, Rodriguez-Baea A, Cervera C, et al (1994) Posterior fossa reconstruction: a surgical technique for the treatment of Chiari 1 malformation and Chiari 1/syringomyelia complex. Preliminary results and magnetic resonance imaging quantitative assessment of hindbrain migration. Neurosurgery 35:874–885
8. Fujii K, Natori Y, Fukui M, et al (1991) Management of syringomyelia associated with Chiari malformation: comparative study of syrinx size and symptoms by magnetic resonance imaging. Surg Neurol 36:281–285
9. Imae S, Ozaki F, Itakura T, et al (1997) Clinical evaluation of the outcome and the method of surgical decompression for syringomyelia associated with Chiari type 1 malformation. Int Cong Neurol Surg 11:1375–1379
10. Dubby JM, Williams B (1991) Hindbrain migration after decompression for hindbrain hernia: a quantitative assessment using MRI. Br J Neurosurg 5:141–152

Operative Results of Syringomyelia with Reference to Patients Who Required Multiple Treatments

Makoto Senoo, Hiroshi Takahashi, Makoto Taniguchi, Katsuhisa Ide, Naoko Tanaka, and Yoshibumi Okada

Summary. We report a retrospective study of 37 patients with syringomyelia who underwent surgical treatment. The patients were classified into three groups: (1) Chiari I malformations (27 patients), (2) extramedullary compressive lesions (5 patients), and (3) arachnoiditis (5 patients). A total of 46 surgeries were performed on 37 patients. Of the 27 Chiari I patients, 14 patients were treated by our standard procedure, posterior fossa decompression (PFD) and laminectomy with duraplasty. Good results were achieved in 9 patients (64%). However, the 2 patients primarily treated by syringosubarachnoid (SS) shunt alone had a recurrence of symptoms and needed further treatment. In all 5 patients with extramedullary compressive lesions, excellent results were achieved with simple excision of the compressive lesion or SS shunt. Five patients associated with arachnoiditis were initially treated by SS shunt, syringoperitoneal (SP) shunt, or syringotomy. However, 4 of them suffered recurrences and needed further treatment. Good results were sustained in 2 of the 5 patients treated by ventriculoperitoneal (VP) shunt or lumboperitoneal (LP) shunt.

Key words. Syringomyelia, Chiari I malformations, Arachnoiditis, Posterior fossa decompression, Shunt

Introduction

In this study, we retrospectively review 37 syringomyelia patients who were surgically treated, especially focusing on those patients who underwent multiple surgeries.

Method

Patients and Surgical Treatments

A total of 37 patients who underwent surgical treatment for progressive symptoms of syringomyelia between March 1982 and January 2000 at Tokyo Metropolitan Neuro-

Department of Neurosurgery, Tokyo Metropolitan Neurological Hospital, 2-6-1 Musashidai, Fuchu, Tokyo 183-0042, Japan

logical Hospital were evaluated. In this study, patients with syrinxes associated with intramedullary tumor were excluded. There were 15 male and 21 female patients ranging in age from 15 to 75 years (mean age, 45 years), and they were classified into three groups. Of the 37 subjects, 27 patients were associated with Chiari I malformations, and 5 patients had extramedullary compressive lesions. The remaining 5 patients exhibited arachnoiditis. A total of 46 surgeries were performed on the 37 patients.

Chiari Malformation I

Over the period covered in our study, we utilized a variety of treatment methods according to the state of the patient. In the 27 Chiari I patients, 24 patients (89%) were treated by posterior fossa decompression (PFD) and 23 of them (96%) additionally underwent simultaneous laminectomy of C1 or C1–C2. Of the 24 patients, duraplasty was performed in 17 cases (71%), and the syringosubarachnoid (SS) shunt was employed in 4 cases (17%). Of the remaining 3 patients, 2 received an SS shunt and 1 patient underwent a ventriculoperitoneal (VP) shunt. In recent years, we have chosen PFD as the primary treatment of Chiari I malformations, and in most cases we have included duraplasty and laminectomy of C1 or C1–C2.

In the PFD procedure, we make a wide craniectomy of the occipital bone to allow a sufficient decompression of the cisterna magna. In earlier patients, we dissected the arachnoid membrane, trying to open the foramen of Magendie. However, we currently take care not to injure the arachnoid membrane, thereby avoiding secondary arachnoiditis.

Extramedullary Compressive Lesions

Five cases of syrigomyelia were associated with extramedullary compressive lesions: arachnoid cyst, cervical canal stenosis, ossification of the thoratic yellow ligament, achondroplasia, and atlantaxial dislocation. In such cases, the pathogenesis of the syrinx formation is considered to be a chronic spinal cord compression; therefore, at that time, simple decompression of the responsible lesions was performed in four patients. In the fifth case, an atlantoaxial dislocation, the syrinx was treated by insertion of an SS shunt.

Arachnoiditis

Five patients had syringomyelia associated with arachnoiditis. Three of them had meningitis, and the remaining two were postsubarachnoid hemorrhage patients. Of the three meningitis patients, two patients were treated by syringoperitoneal (SP) shunts and one patient underwent syringotomy. The two subarachnoid hemorrhage (SAH) patients initially underwent SS shunt insertion.

Results

Chiari Malformation I

Of our 27 patients, 14 patients (52%) showed clinical improvement after the first treatment with the syrinx diminishing or being eliminated. Nine patients (33%) remained unchanged, and 1 patient (4%) became worse after surgery. The remaining 3 patients (11%) suffered a recurrence and needed further treatment.

It is noteworthy that both cases initially treated with SS shunt had to undergo a second operation. Of the total, 14 patients (52%) were treated by our standard procedure, PFD and C1 or C1–C2 with duraplasty. Of the 14 patients, 9 patients (64%) experienced long-lasting clinical and radiological improvement with this standard technique.

Extramedullary Compressive Lesions

The postoperative course of the patients in this group was excellent. All five patients had symptomatic relief soon after the operation, with radiological improvement of the syrinx. There were no recurrent patients, and no further treatments were required in this group.

Arachnoiditis

A total of 11 operations were performed on 5 patients. Of these, 4 patients needed further treatment, and 2 of them reported a long-lasting relief of symptoms. Even though each of the 5 patients received short-term relief of the symptoms, none of them experienced long-term relief without further treatment.

One meningitis patient (case 1) was initially treated by SP shunt. Her symptoms diminished for a time but subsequently returned. Two months later, we had to exchange the SP shunt for a syringosubarachnoid (SS) shunt. Despite this, her clinical symptoms did not improve, and a third operation was performed employing a VP shunt; this was also not successful. It was not until a lumboperitoneal (LP) shunt was inserted that a more favorable result was achieved.

A good outcome was also attained in one of the SAH patients (case 2). She had undergone an operation for a ruptured aneurysm 5 years previously, and her hydrocephalus had been controlled by an LP shunt. As we considered that the condition of her syrinx seemed to be related to hydrocephalus, we reinserted a new LP shunt. We also added an SS shunt to complete the primary procedure. Unfortunately, the improvement was only temporary, so we implanted a VP shunt, which proved effective.

Two patients remained clinically unchanged postoperatively. One of the meningitis patients did not show any clinical improvement after the SP shunt, despite radiological improvement. The second meningitis patient was additionally treated by a VP shunt after a failed thoratic syringotomy, which also did not relieve her symptoms.

One patient suffered a complication while undergoing syrinx treatment. A 64-year-old man after spinal SAH was treated by a VP shunt after a failed SS shunt. Two months later, a computed tomography (CT) scan revealed right chronic subdural hematoma, and we had to remove the VP shunt and drain the hematoma.

Discussion

Syringomyelia may occur in association with many pathological conditions, such as malformations, tumors, trauma, infection, and many compressive diseases. Even though the pathogenesis and mechanism of syrinx formation still remain unclear, this unique and complex state of the spinal cord is presumably brought about by an abnormal pressure gradient of local cerebrospinal fluid (CSF) flow. With the introduction of magnetic resonance imaging, providing us with refined delineation of the state of the syrinx and CSF flow, new evidence [1,2] has been reported that is contradictory to the conventional hypothesis proposed by Gardner [3] and Williams [4].

In the treatment of syrinx occurring with Chiari I malformations, two fundamental procedures are in common use, PFD and various types of shunts. In this series, 64% of the patients who underwent our standard procedure demonstrated a decrease in syrinx size and good long-term outcome. Conversely, the 2 patients treated by SS shunt alone suffered relapses. Considering this result, we propose that Chiari I malformations should be primarily treated by PFD with duraplasty, and that other shuntings should be used additionally only when the residual syrinx is considered to be the cause of the remaining symptom after the initial operation [2,5]. We also suggest that decompression should be wide enough to release the CSF flow obstruction at the foramen magnum. Moreover, care must be taken when opening the dura to avoid injuring the arachnoid membrane, thereby causing secondary arachnoiditis [5].

Extramedullary compressive lesions also lead to syringomyelia. Following the clinical course of this group, good results were acquired in all five patients soon after the operation with good radiological improvement. Furthermore, there were no recurrent patients, which strongly indicates that decompressive surgery of the responsible lesions is most suitable for the treatment of this type of syrinx.

Syringomyelia occurring with arachnoiditis seems to be the most difficult condition to treat. The high recurrence rate of 80% in this study demonstrates the difficulty involved in treatment. Of the five syringomyelia patients, we implanted SS or SP [6,7] shunts in four patients as an initial procedure. In all cases, the effects were only temporary. Long-lasting clinical relief was sustained in only two patients who were treated by VP or LP shunts [1,8]. Case 1 somehow achieved clinical improvement with an LP shunt after three failed shunt operations. In case 2, a VP shunt was found to be effective, presumably because the subject had hydrocephalus, even though the communication between the fourth ventricle and central canal was radiologically unclear. These two cases indicate that a VP shunt may be useful in patients with hydrocephalus, and LP shunts also seem to have a potential to reduce the CSF inflow from the subarachnoid space to the syrinx cavities.

These results tend to support the hypothesis that CSF can in fact communicate between the subarachnoid space and central canal via the spinal cord [2]. Consequently, we would suggest considering the utilization of these shunts for intractable cases with arachnoiditis [9]. We also recommend, for those patients showing symptomatic signs of syringomyelia, that surgical treatment should be initiated as early as possible to avoid irreversible cord injury. This recommendation also applies to recurrent cases.

References

1. Milhorat TH, Johnson WD, Miller JI, et al (1992) Surgical treatment of syringomyelia based on magnetic resonance imaging criteria. Neurosurgery 31:231–245
2. Oldfield EH, Muraszko K, Shawker TH, et al (1994) Pathophysiology of syringomyelia associated with Chiari I malformation of the cerebellar tonsils. Implications for diagnosis and treatment. J Neurosurg 80:3–5
3. Gardner WJ (1977) Hydrodynamics factors in Dandy-Walker and Arnord-Chiari malformations. Childs Brain 3:200–212
4. Williams B (1969) The distending force in the production of "communicating syringomyelia." Lancet 2:189–193
5. Pillay PK, Awad IA, Little JR, Hahn JF (1991) Symptomatic Chiari malformation in adults: a classification based on magnetic resonance imaging with clinical and prognostic significance. Neurosurgery 28:639–645
6. Tator CH, Meguro K, Rowed DW (1982) Favorable results with syringosubarachnoid shunts for treatment of syringomyelia. J Neurosurg 56(4):517–523
7. Williams B, Page N (1987) Surgical treatment of syringomyelia with syringopleural shunting. Br J Neurosurg 1(1):63–80
8. Park TS, Cail W, Broaddus WC, Walker MG (1989) Lumboperitoneal shunt combined with myelotomy for treatment of syringohydromyelia. J Neurosurg 70:712–727
9. Sgouros S, Williams B (1995) A critical appraisal of drainage in syringomyelia. J Neurosurg 82:1–10

Variation of Foramen Magnum Decompression for the Treatment of Syringomyelia Determined by Intraoperative CSF Flow Dynamics Study

Yoshiji Okuda, Toshiro Hida, Akira Isoshima, Hiroyasu Nagashima, Satoshi Tani, and Toshiaki Abe

Summary. Foramen magnum decompression (FMD) is commonly performed for the treatment of Chiari type I-related syringomyelia. However, because no objective evaluation of cerebrospinal fluid (CSF) dynamics has been introduced to estimate the effect of FMD, many technical variations of FMD have been proposed. We reported previously that pressure/volume index (PVI) and CSF outflow resistance (Ro) calculated by the formula of Marmarou et al. were reliable indicators for the effects of FMD from the hydrodynamic point of view. This year, we measured PVI and Ro in another 8 patients (total, 21 patients) with Chiari type I malformation-related syringomyelia. To determine the extension of FMD, PVI and Ro were monitored during FMD in four stages: preoperation, after bone removal, after removal of the outer layer of the dura, and after dural plasty. CSF circulation improved in all 21 cases, and PVI and Ro were normalized. Postoperative MRI also showed a size reduction of the syrinx. Evaluation performed during surgery showed that bone removal alone was insufficient; 1 case showed improvement after removal of the outer layer of the dura but the remaining 5 cases required dural plasty. In conclusion, the measurement of PVI and Ro during operation is effective for determining the extent of decompression and is important for carrying out minimally invasive surgery.

Key words. Syringomyelia, Chiari malformation, Cerebrospinal fluid (CSF), Foramen magnum decompression (FMD), Pressure volume index (PVI)

Introduction

Various surgical procedures have been proposed to treat syringomyelia-related Chiari malformation. Nevertheless, at present, it is generally accepted that foramen magnum decompression is a safe and effective treatment for improving cerebrospinal fluid circulation disruption at the craniocervical junction. Even though foramen magnum decompression is being performed at many institutions, the extent of osteotomy and handling of the dura mater vary from one institution to the next because there are no

Department of Neurosurgery, The Jikei University School of Medicine, 3-25-8 Nishi-Shinbashi, Minato-ku, Tokyo 105-8461, Japan

established methods to objectively assess its effectiveness. Consequently, we measured shifts in the pressure-relieving function of the craniospinal lumen (pressure/volume index, PVI) and cerebrospinal fluid (CSF) outflow resistance (Ro) [1,2] before and after surgery to quantify the effect of foramen magnum decompression on CSF circulation [3]. Furthermore, the effectiveness of decompression was ascertained by measuring PVI and Ro at various stages of surgery, and the degree of improvement in CSF circulation was analyzed to ascertain whether these parameters would be useful in determining a surgical field size and selecting an appropriate surgical procedure.

Subjects

Over a 5-year period between 1994 and 1998, a total of 21 patients (5 male and 16 female) with Chiari I malformation underwent foramen magnum decompression for the treatment of syringomyelia, and their CSF circulation was quantitatively assessed before and after surgery. Also, CSF pressure was monitored during surgery in 6 of these patients, 2 men and 4 women whose average age was 25.8 years (range, 20–32 years).

Methods

PVI and Ro were measured before and after foramen magnum decompression as follows. First, each patient was asked to lie on their side; a lumbar puncture needle was inserted into the lumbar subarachnoid cavity and connected to a pressure transducer. Through the use of a computer, CSF pressure waveforms were recorded after injecting physiological saline. Then, according to the bolus injection method proposed by Marmarou and colleagues [4], PVI and Ro were calculated using the following equations:

$$PVI = \Delta V / \log(P_P / P_o)$$

$$R_o = t2 \cdot (PVI) \cdot \log[P_2 (P_P - P_o) / P_2 - P_o]$$

PVI and Ro were measured before and after surgery while resting the patient's neck at three different positions (neutral, flexed, and extended). PVI represents the amount of volume load required to increase the CSF pressure tenfold and thus is a parameter governing the ability of the craniospinal lumen to relieve pressure. Ro represents the level of resistance for the absorption of physiological saline (bolus injection) from the subarachnoid cavity to the venous system and thus is a parameter of the patency of CSF circulation pathways. The reference values for PVI and Ro in healthy adults are greater than 25 ml and less than 3 mmHg/ml/min, respectively [5].

Also, CSF pressure was monitored during surgery by positioning each patient on their side under general anesthesia and inserting a vinyl tube (internal diameter, 1.0 mm) in the lumbar subarachnoid cavity to continuously monitor CSF pressure. PVI and Ro were calculated as described at various stages of surgery: before and after osteotomy, after outer membranectomy, and after dural plasty.

Results

Shifts in PVI and Ro and the degree of improvement in these parameters before and after surgery were assessed in 21 patients with Chiari malformation-related syringomyelia while resting the neck in three positions (neutral, flexed, and extended). The results showed that the degree of improvement in CSF pressure was poorest (68.9%) and its actual measurement was lowest (22.68 ml) when the neck was in the flexed position. These findings suggest that if the levels of PVI and Ro reach target values when the neck is flexed during surgery, then CSF circulation could be improved at any position. Also, when CSF circulation disruption improved after surgery, PVI and Ro were normalized for all neck positions. The degree of improvement in PVI and Ro, on average, was 78.1% and 31.27%, respectively (Table 1).

Table 2 shows the mean PVI and Ro for the six patients in whom these parameters were measured at the various stages of surgery. Except for one patient, dural plasty was performed because osteotomy and outer membranectomy were not sufficient in normalizing PVI and Ro levels. Duraplasty was not done in one patient because PVI was 20.83 ml and Ro was 3.32 mmHg/ml/min following outer membranectomy; these numbers were close to the reference values established for the flexed position. In every patient who underwent duraplasty, magnetic resonance imaging (MRI) showed a reduction in the size of syringomyelia within 3 months of surgery (Fig. 1), and in the patient who underwent outer membranectomy, MRI showed a reduction in the size of syringomyelia 10 months after surgery (Fig. 2).

The next section concerns a patient in whom the size of foramen magnum decompression was determined by intraoperatively monitoring CSF circulation. Before exposing the occipital bone, PVI and Ro were calculated for the first time

TABLE 1. Preoperative and postoperative pressure/volume index (PVI) and cerebrospinal fluid outflow resistance (Ro)

	PVI (ml)		Ro (mmHg/ml/min)	
Position ($n = 21$)	Pre	Post	Pre	Post
Neutral	19.70	32.16 (86.8%)	4.50	2.73 (34.7%)
Extension	17.38	29.12 (78.3%)	4.14	2.63 (30.6%)
Flexion	17.20	22.68 (68.9%)	4.88	3.59 (28.5%)
Average of PVI and Ro values	18.10	30.21	4.51	2.95
Average of improved rate	78.1%		31.27%	

TABLE 2. Average PVI and Ro values during each stage of operation

Stage ($n = 6$)	PVI (ml)	Ro (mmHg/ml/min)
Preoperation	14.09	9.08
Postcraniectomy	16.81	5.82
Post outer membranectomy	19.28	4.84
Post dural plasty	24.29	2.77

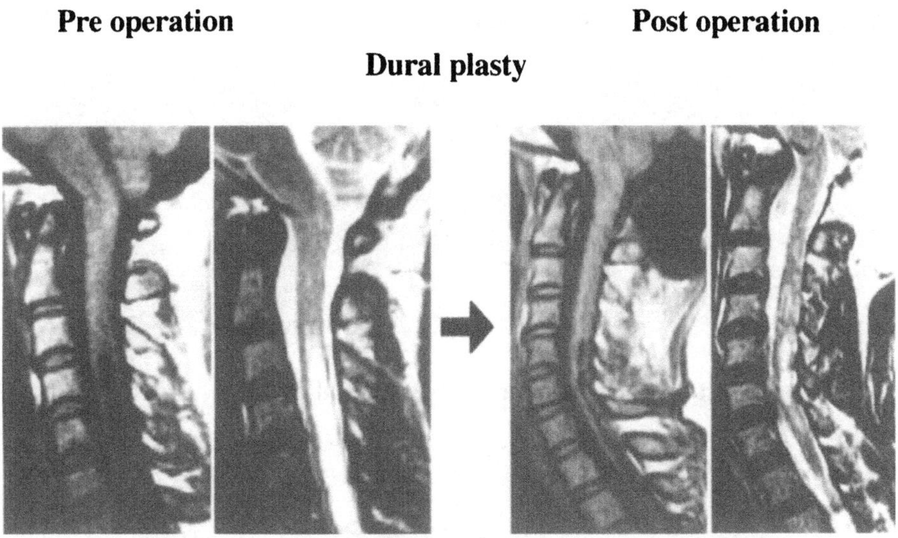

FIG. 1. Pre- and postoperative magnetic resonance imaging (MRI) in a case of dural plasty

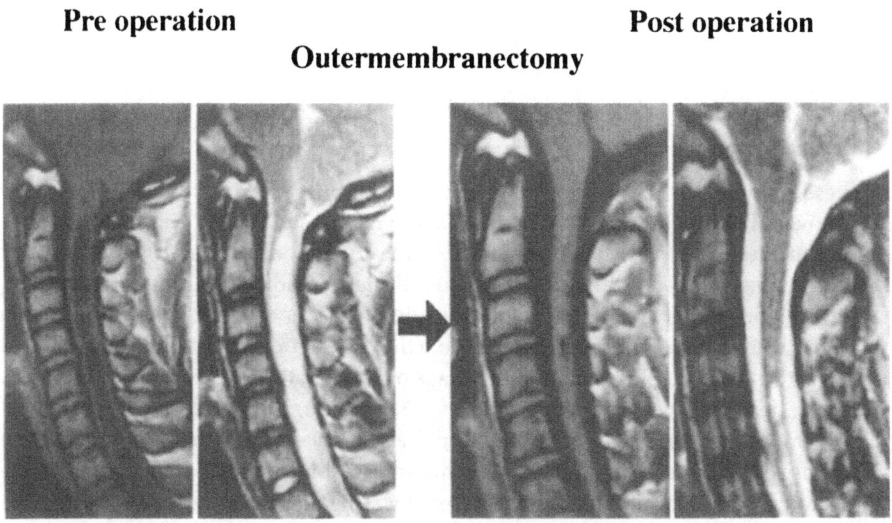

FIG. 2. Pre- and postoperative MRI in a case of outer membranectomy

(Fig. 3, preoperative). In this patient, PVI was 16.80 and Ro was 6.45; thus, these numbers deviated significantly from their respective reference values (PVI greater than 25 ml and Ro less than 3 mmHg/ml/min). Next, while utilizing the inferior nuchal line as a guideline, osteotomy of the occipital bone and then C1 laminectomy were performed (see Fig. 3, after craniectomy). During this procedure, the C1 arch and the lateral bone of the foramen magnum region were removed. At this time, a second measurement was taken: PVI was 18.97 and Ro was 5.18.

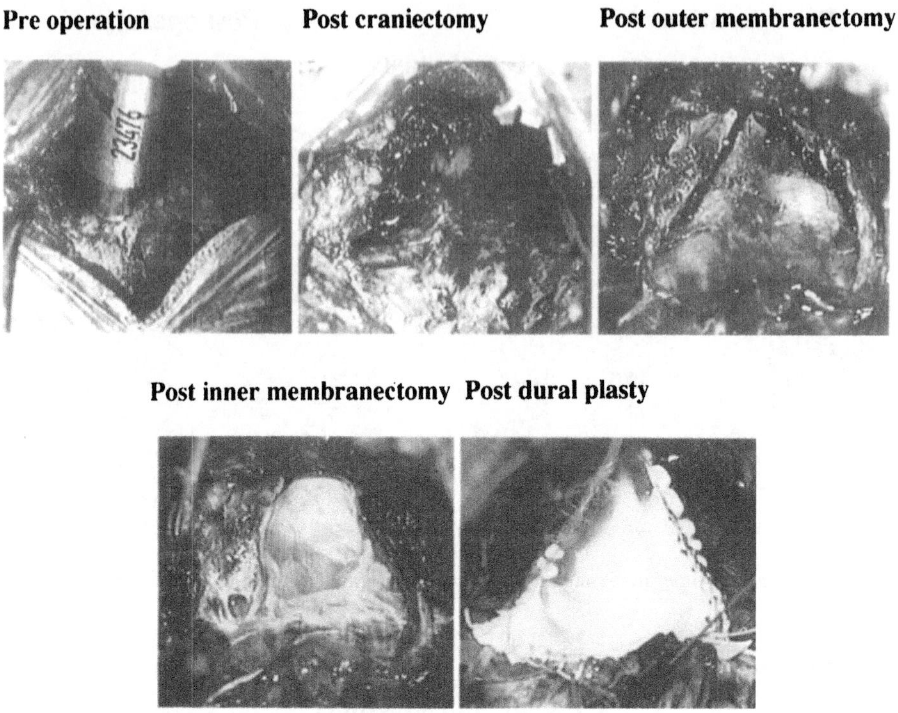

FIG. 3. Intraoperative photograph of each stage

These parameters showed improvement, but because they were not within their respective reference values, outer membranectomy was performed (Fig. 3, after outer membranectomy). A "Y" incision was made on the outer membrane, and when the outer membrane was removed sufficiently to expose the lateral side of the foramen magnum, a pulsating cerebellar tonsil that had descended from its original position was seen through a thin inner membrane. At this time, a third measurement was taken. If PVI and Ro are within the reference values at this stage of surgery, the surgical wound is closed. In this patient, PVI was 19.14 and Ro was 4.38. Although these parameters showed improvement, because they were not within the reference values, the inner membrane was removed without damaging the arachnoid membrane (Fig. 3, after inner membranectomy). A fourth and final measurement was taken at this stage of surgery; PVI was 24.49 and Ro 2.79. Because both parameters were outside their respective reference values, it was clear that PVI and Ro would not normalize without duraplasty. As a result, duraplasty was performed using a Gore-Tex membrane and Gore-Tex sutures (see Fig. 3, after duraplasty). Finally, a fibrin sealant was used to close the surgical wound.

Discussion

There are various theories on the mechanism of onset and progression of syringomyelia-related Chiari I malformation, but the effect of CSF circulation in the foramen magnum on the pathophysiology of syringomyelia-related Chiari I malformation has yet to be fully elucidated. However, when a strangulated cerebellar tonsil in the foramen magnum disrupts the CSF circulation in the craniocervical junction, a large pressure gradient difference between the cranial and spinal cavities is certain to play a role in cavitation.

To resolve this type of CSF circulation disruption, foramen magnum decompression is performed. The results of long-term observations on foramen magnum decompression have proven its effectiveness. Nevertheless, there is no established method to objectively assess the degree of improvement in cerebrospinal fluid circulation. The results of the present study showed that measuring PVI and Ro before and after surgery could quantify the degree of improvement in CSF circulation. In the future, it will be necessary to investigate the severity of circulation disruption based on preoperative data and to determine the relationship between changes in the results of diagnostic imaging and the degree of postoperative improvement.

Foramen magnum decompression is performed to improve CSF circulation, but the size of the surgical field and surgical techniques vary from one medical institution to the next (Fig. 4). When we perform foramen magnum decompression [6–8], the size of craniectomy on the occipital bone is comparable to the size of foramen magnum (width, 3 cm; height, 3–4 cm), and the C1 arch is also removed. Yamaura and colleagues [9,10] have reported that CSF circulation disruption showed greater improvement when the lateral margin of the occipital bone was removed to enlarge the foramen magnum. Hakuba and colleagues [11–13] emphasized the importance of foramen magnum decompression combined with expansive suboccipital cranioplasty using such bone as the ilium, because the volume of the posterior cranial fossa of Chiari

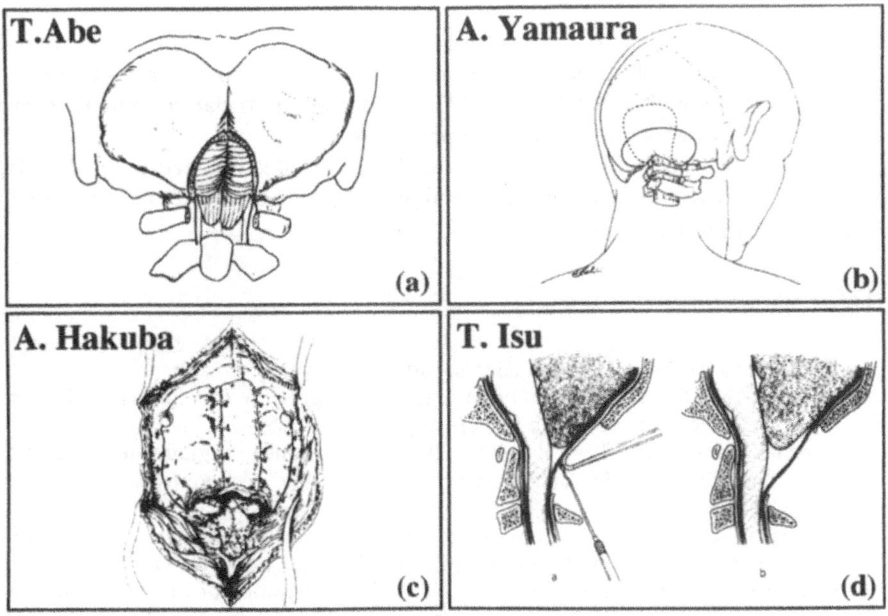

FIG. 4a–d. Variations of foramen magnum decompression (FMD)

malformation patients is significantly smaller than that of healthy individuals. Nonetheless, the results of the present study showed that CSF circulation could be improved when the size of osteotomy on the occipital bone was about the size of the horizontal diameter of the foramen magnum. Furthermore, we believe that if excessive craniectomy were performed, the cerebellar hemisphere could cause the cerebellum to descend, thus compressing the medulla oblongata.

So far as handling of the dura mater is concerned, Isu and colleagues [14,15] successfully treated syringomyelia by making an incision and removing the outer membrane without duraplasty utilizing Gore-Tex materials. In fact, every one of our surgical procedures is done in the epidural space, thus increasing the risk of such postoperative complications as liquid retention in the epidural space, or meningitis. Hence, the method of Isu and colleagues is less invasive, but their procedures are not easy to perform. Also, the characteristics of the dura mater vary from one patient to the next, and the degree of venous sinus development near the foramen magnum limits its indications.

Duraplasty was not performed in one of the six patients in whom CSF circulation was monitored during surgery because the levels of PVI and Ro were close to their respective reference values. In this patient, somewhat more time was required for the size of the syringomyelia to decrease (10 months after surgery) when compared to the five patients who underwent duraplasty. Our findings suggest that intraoperative measurement of PVI and Ro would be clinically useful in deciding whether to perform duraplasty.

Conclusions

1. PVI and Ro were measured before and after surgery in 21 patients with syringomyelia-related Chiari malformation. The results showed that, on average, PVI and Ro improved 78.1% and 31.27%, respectively, thus clarifying that the level of these parameters normalizes postoperatively.
2. Intraoperative measurement of PVI and Ro is an effective method in deciding the size of decompression and is useful and important in selecting a minimally invasive surgical procedure.

References

1. Goto F, et al (1983) ICP & brain edema. Yodosha, Tokyo, pp 63–76
2. Wachi A, Tsuji O, Sato K, et al (1993) Lumbar CSF pressure monitoring for external spinal cord decompression. Jpn J Neurosurg (Tokyo) 2:226–231
3. Okuda Y, Tani S, Abe T, et al (1998) Efficacy of foramen magnum decompression upon the CSF dynamics of Chiari type 1 associated syringomyelia. Spinal Surg 12(2):169–176
4. Marmarou A, Shapiro K, LaMorgese J (1975) Compartmental analysis of compliance and outflow resistance of the cerebrospinal fluid system. J Neurosurg 43:523–534
5. Shapiro K, Marmarou A, Shulaman K (1980) Characterization of clinical CSF dynamics and neural axis compliance using the pressure-volume index. Ann Neurol 7:508–514
6. Abe T (1992) Operative procedure for syringomyelia associated with Chiari malformation. Spine Spinal 5(9):659–663

7. Abe T (1995) Pathogenesis and surgical treatment of syringomyelia. No Shinkei Geka 23:759–766
8. Abe T, Okuda Y, Tani S, et al (1995) Surgical treatment of syringomyelia. Clin Neurol 35:1406–1408
9. Yamaura A (1992) Surgical technique for Chiari malformation 1 associated with syringomyelia: foramen magnum decompression with lateral extention. Spine Spinal 5(9):665–670
10. Yamaura A, Ozawa Y, Arai S, et al (1996) Analysis of syringomyelia in children, associated with Chiari type 1 malformation. Nerv Syst Child 21:307–313
11. Hakuba A, Tokunou N, Nishimura S, et al (1988) Surgical treatment of syringomyelia. Spine Spinal Cord 1:227–234
12. Hakuba A, Tokunou N, Nishimura S, et al (1990) Surgical treatment of syringomyelia associated with Chiari malformation. Spinal Surg 4:69–76
13. Sakamoto H, Nishikawa M, Hakuba A, et al (1994) Surgical treatment of syringomyelia associated with Chiari malformation. Spinal Surg 8:1–6
14. Isu T (1992) Surgical treatment of Chiari malformation: foramen magnum decompression combined with dissection and removal of outer layer of the dura mater. Spine Spinal 5(9):671–676
15. Isu T, Sasaki H, Takamura H, et al (1993) Foramen magnum decompression with removal of the outer layer of the dura as treatment for syringomyelia occurring with Chiari I malformation. Neurosurgery 33(5):844–849

Surgical Treatment of Syringomyelia Associated with Chiari I Malformation: Advantage of Cranioplasty Using Hydroxyapatite Implants

YASUNOBU ITOH, NAOYUKI KUWAHARA, YOSHITAKA HIRANO, TOSHIO SASAJIMA, AKIRA SUZUKI, and KAZUO MIZOI

Summary. Suboccipital craniectomy (SOC) for the treatment of syringomyelia associated with Chiari I malformation has been routinely performed to improve clinical symptoms. A retrospective study was conducted of eight patients who underwent SOC followed by cranioplasty with hydroxyapatite (HA) implants. Neurological impairments and radiological findings based on magnetic resonance imaging (MRI) were assessed preoperatively and at a mean 13.3-month follow-up. The six female and two male patients ranged in age from 9 to 66 years (mean, 41.4 years). Each patient exhibited varying degrees of sensory discomfort of the extremities. Computed tomography study in one case with an intramedullary lesion revealed a cerebrospinal fluid (CSF) density, and the patient was diagnosed with syringomyelia. Operations were performed through SOC and upper cervical laminectomies. Duraplasty using Gore-Tex or resection of the outer layer of the dura was selected under intraoperative ultrasound echography. Subsequently, the decompressed foramen magnum was covered with a curved plate of HA and tenting sutures of the dura were added. Neurological impairments improved in five of eight patients and persisted in three cases. Postoperative MRI showed diminution in the size of the syrinx and the ascent of the cerebellar tonsils in seven of eight cases. Three-dimensional computed tomography (3D-CT) in some patients revealed bone fusion of HA with the adjacent occipital bone within 6 months after surgery. In conclusion, the findings in this study showed HA cranioplasty has the advantage of early securement of the retrotonsillar subarachnoid space and preclusion of epidural CSF retention.

Key words. Syringomyelia, Chiari I malformation, Cranioplasty, Hydroxyapatite, Three-dimensional computed tomography

Introduction

A variety of surgical treatments have been proposed for syringomyelia associated with Chiari I malformation [1]. Gardner and Angel initially recommended a suboccipital craniectomy (SOC) and cervical laminectomy to decompress the malformation and

---

Department of Neurosurgery, Akita University School of Medicine, 1-1-1 Hondo, Akita 010-8543, Japan

subsequent plugging of the obex with a small piece of muscle [2]. They subsequently reported that most of the patients treated in this fashion later developed progressive neurological deficits. Plugging the obex increases the chance of damaging the hypoglossal and vagal nuclei that are located at the level of the obex near the rostral end of the central canal [1]. The most effective treatment for syringomyelia with Chiari malformation seems to be SOC, upper cervical laminectomy, and duraplasty with fascia or Gore-Tex to decompress the Chiari malformation, combined with drainage of the syrinx through the dorsal root entry zone into the subarachnoid space [1].

Resection of the outer layer of the dura has been adopted as an alternative method for duraplasty [3]. Expansive suboccipital cranioplasty has also proposed as an alternative procedure for SOC [4]. A retrospective study was conducted of eight patients who underwent SOC followed by cranioplasty with hydroxyapatite (HA) implants.

Patients and Methods

Eight patients with syringomyelia with Chiari I malformation who underwent SOC followed by cranioplasty with HA implants during the past 19 months were reviewed. Diagnosis was based on physical, neurological, and neuroradiological examinations using magnetic resonance imaging (MRI) including phase-contrast cine-MRI and three-dimensional computed tomography (3D-CT).

Results

Table 1 is a summary of eight cases with cranioplasty using HA. The six female and two male patients ranged in age from 9 to 66 years. The mean term of illness was 40 months, ranging from 3 months to 15 years. The most frequent complaint on admission was dysesthesia in the unilateral upper extremity. The other complaints were nuchal pain or dullness in three cases and hearing loss in one case.

MRI revealed tonsillar herniation (seven cases to C1 level; one case to C2 level) and syrinx (seven cases at cervicothoracic level; one case at cervical level) in all patients (Fig. 1A). Phase-contrast cine-MRI showed the absence of cerebrospinal fluid (CSF) flow in the retrotonsillar subarachnoid space and to-and-fro movement within the syrinx in seven cases.

In the operation, we performed foramen magnum decompression with C1 laminectomy (seven cases), and C1 and C2 upper dome laminectomies (one case). Duraplasty using Gore-Tex membrane (W.L. Gore & Associates, Flagstaff, Az, USA) was performed in three cases and resection of the outer layer of the dura was performed in five cases. Subsequently, cranioplasty using HA implants (Asahi Optical, Tokyo, Japan) was performed in all cases and tenting sutures of the dura to the implants were also added.

On follow-up neurological status, five patients improved and three patients remained unchanged. Postoperative MRI revealed the collapse or diminution of the syrinx in seven patients during the follow-up period (Fig. 1B). HA was removed in case 4 because of an epidural abscess, and no further neurological deterioration was

TABLE 1. Clinical summary of eight cases with cranioplasty

Case	Age/sex	Symptoms	Radiological findings	Operation	Outcome (follow-up)
1	9/F	3-month history of left hearing loss	Tonsillar herniation and syrinx (C5–T1)	FMD, C1 and C2 upper dome laminectomies, resection of outer layer of dura	No change (19 months)
2	66/F	15-year history of dysesthetic pain of left UE and gait disturbance	Tonsillar herniation and syrinx (C1–T2)	FMD, C1 laminectomy, dural plasty (Gore-Tex)	Good recovery (18 months)
3	33/F	4-month history of nuchal pain stiffness of bilateral fingers	Tonsillar herniation and syrinx (C3–T5)	FMD, C1 laminectomy, dural plasty (Gore-Tex)	Good recovery (16 months)
4	61/F	5-year history of motor weakness of bilateral hands and sensory disturbance of bilateral LEs	Tonsillar herniation and syrinx (C2–T11)	FMD, C1 laminectomy, dural plasty (Gore-Tex)	Epidural abscess, no change (16 months)
5	38/F	5-month history of nuchal pain and stiffness and dysesthesia of bilateral UEs	Tonsillar herniation and syrinx (C3–T2)	FMD, C1 laminectomy, resection of outer layer of dura	Good recovery (13 months)
6	17/M	3-month history of nuchal dullness	Tonsillar herniation and syrinx (C1–C2)	FMD, C1 laminectomy, resection of outer layer of dura	Good recovery (9 months)
7	61/F	6-month history of stiffness and dysesthesia of bilateral UEs	Tonsillar herniation and syrinx (C1–T2)	FMD, C1 laminectomy, resection of outer layer of dura	Good recovery (8 months)
8	46/M	5-year history of dysesthetic pain of bilateral UEs	Tonsillar herniation and syrinx (C1–T2)	FMD, C1 laminectomy, resection of outer layer of dura	No change (7 months)

UE, upper extremity; LE, lower extremity; FMD, foramen magnum decompression.

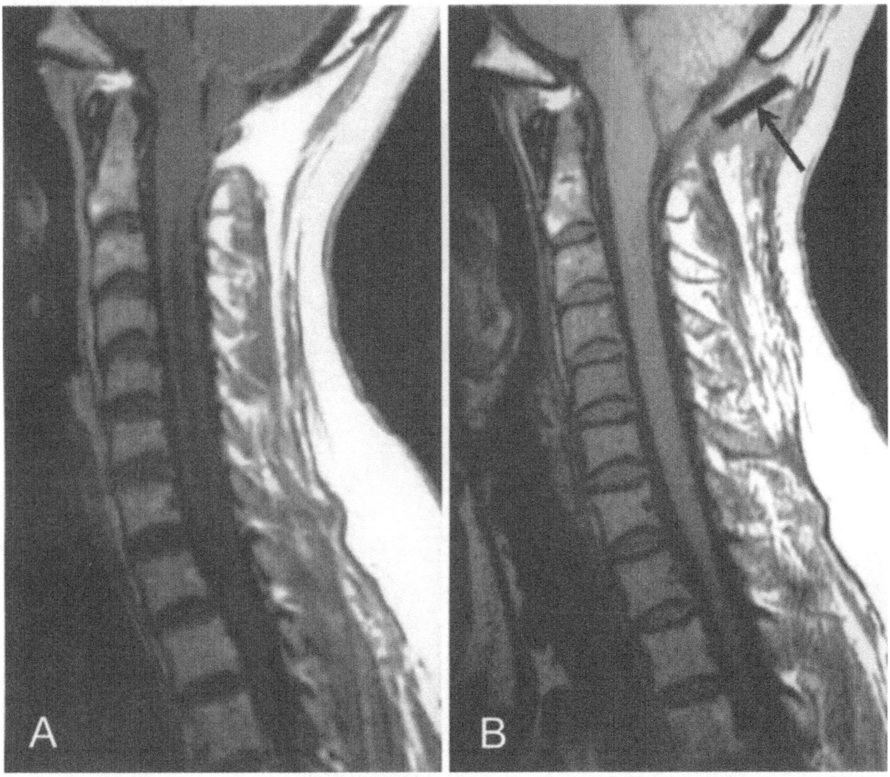

Fig. 1. **A** Sagittal section of preoperative magnetic resonance imaging (MRI) in case 5. **B** Postoperative MRI in case 5. *Arrow* indicates hydroxyapatite (HA) implant

noted on follow-up. Although the hearing loss in case 1 did not improve, improvement of the audiogram was noted. 3D-CT revealed that the HA implant was integrated with the adjacent occipital bone within 6 months after surgery (Fig. 2).

Discussion

SOC, upper cervical laminectomy, and duraplasty, combined with a syrinx-subarachnoid shunting operation, have been used as surgical treatment for syringomyelia associated with Chiari I malformation. A variety of other additional procedures have also been proposed for this condition. Resection of the outer layer of the thickened dura mater (dural band) at the craniovertebral junction can be replaced with duraplasty with Gore-Tex in patients without arachnoid adhesions [3]. The same procedure performed in five cases in our series confirmed acceptable pulsation of herniated tonsils under intraoperative ultrasound echography.

Expansive suboccipital cranioplasty that involves enlarging the small posterior fossa to obtain a sufficient flow of CSF has been reported to show significant improve-

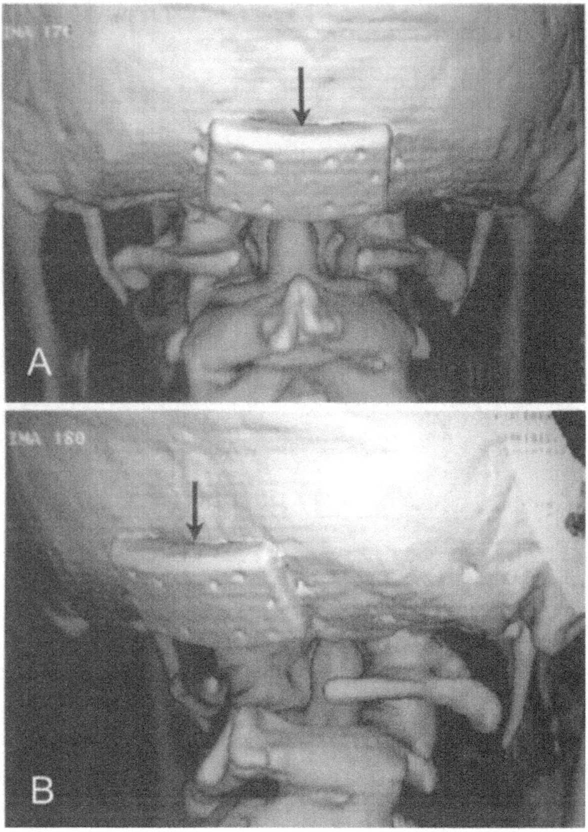

FIG. 2A,B. Posterior view (A) and right posterior view (B) of three-dimensional computed tomography in case 5. *Arrows* indicate HA

ment of the CSF flow at the major cistern and of symptoms [4]. Because continuative bone flaps for expansive suboccipital cranioplasty can be absorbed in the long term [3], this procedure remains controversial [5]. We used a synthetic HA as a substitute for autologous bone grafts in cranioplasty. HA is a hydroxyl compound of calcium phosphate and is the main constituent of the naturally occurring bone matrix. The biocompatibility of this material is well established [6] and the usage of HA implants is technically easy; the combination of tenting sutures of the dura can also inhibit the retention of CSF at epidural space after surgery. A sufficient subarachnoid space for CSF flow can be obtained at an early stage after operation, although long-term observation remains necessary.

References

1. Rhoton AL, Hamilton AJ (1999) Chiari malformation and syringomyelia. In: Benzel EC (ed) Spine Surgery. Churchill Livingstone, New York, pp 793–812
2. Gardner WJ, Angel J (1959) The mechanism of syringomyelia and its surgical correction. Clin Neurosurg 6:131–140

3. Nakamura N, Iwasaki Y, Hida K, et al (2000) Dural band pathology in syringomyelia with Chiari I malformation. Neuropathology 20:38–43
4. Sakamoto H, Nishikawa M, Hakuba A, et al (1999) Expansive suboccipital cranioplasty for the treatment of syringomyelia associated with Chiri malformation. Acta Neurochir (Wien) 141:949–960
5. Takahashi T, Suzaki N, Sawamura S, et al (1997) Surgical treatment of Chiari malformation. Spine Spinal Cord 10:711–718
6. Kim P, Wakai S, Matsuo S, et al (1998) Bisegmental cervical interbody fusion using hydroxyapatite implants: surgical results and long-term observation in 70 cases. J Neurosurg 88:21–27

Intractable Syringomyelia: Study of Reoperation Cases

Toshiro Hida, Yoshiji Okuda, Akira Isoshima, Satoshi Tani, and Toshiaki Abe

Summary. From a long-term evaluation, we report several cases of syringomyelia in which the shrinkage was unsatisfactory, or syrinx enlargement was noted, causing worsening of symptoms and necessitating reoperation. By analysis of these cases, we discuss the possible methods to prevent and treat such cases. We report here 12 reoperative cases in which the primary surgery was performed elsewhere and 10 cases from our own department, a total of 22 cases. We discuss the possible cause and therapy of recurring syrinx enlargement by chronological study of radiologic and operative findings. Of the 164 cases of syringomyelia that we experienced, there were 13 cases of reoperation in those who had Chiari malformation; in 5 of these, syringo-subarachnoid (S-S) shunt obstruction was noted, in 3 cases, foramen magnum decompression (FMD) was insufficient, and in 4, calcification or scar tissue formed around the foramen magnum following FMD. In 1 case, bone removal of the skull base was excessive, causing the lower cerebellum to fall through the foramen magnum with resulting cerebrospinal fluid (CSF) flow disturbance. In our department, there were only 2 cases in which post-FMD scar formation was noted in Chiari malformation. Basal arachnoiditis was seen in 1 case of 16, foramen of Magendie obstruction in 1 of 2 cases, and spinal arachnoiditis in 6 of 14 cases. Of these, 5 spinal arachnoiditis cases and 1 basal arachnoiditis case were initially operated on at our department. We present several significant cases.

Key words. Intractable, Syringomyelia, Reoperation, Surgical treatment

Introduction

Recent advances in therapeutic methods [1] have made possible the shrinkage of the syrinx in the majority of cases of syringomyelia [2–4]. However, in a long-term evaluation, we have seen several cases in which the shrinkage was unsatisfactory or syrinx enlargement was noted, causing worsening of symptoms and necessitating reoperation. By analysis of these cases, we discuss the possible methods to prevent and treat such cases.

Department of Neurosurgery, The Jikei University School of Medicine, 3-19-18 Nishi-Shinbashi, Minato-ku, Tokyo 105-8471, Japan

Methods

We have observed 12 reoperative cases in which the primary surgery was performed elsewhere and 10 cases from our own department, a total of 22 cases. We discuss the possible cause and therapy of recurring enlargement by chronological study of the radiologic and operative findings.

Results

Table 1 shows the causes of the 164 cases of syringomyelia that we experienced and the reoperative cases. There were 13 cases of reoperation in those who had Chiari malformation; in 5 syringosubarachnoid (S-S) shunt obstruction was noted, in 3, foramen magnum decompression (FMD) was insufficient, and in 4, calcification or scar tissue formed around the foramen magnum following FMD. In 1 case, bone removal of the skull base was excessive, causing the lower cerebellum to fall through the foramen magnum with resulting cerebrospinal fluid (CSF) flow disturbance. There were only 3 cases in our department in which post-FMD scar formation was noted in Chiari malformation.

Obstruction of the foramen of Magendie was seen in 1 of 2 cases, spinal arachnoiditis in 7 of 20 cases, and basal arachnoiditis in 1 of 17 cases. Of these, 5 cases of spinal arachnoiditis and 1 case of basal arachnoiditis were initially operated on at our department. We present here several significant cases.

Case 1 is a 53-year-old woman with syringomyelia with Chiari malformation (Fig. 1) whose S-S shunt had been performed elsewhere. Postoperatively, reenlarge-

TABLE 1. Syringomyelia: 164 cases and causes of reoperation

Type	Number of cases	Causes of reoperation	Number of reoperations	Primary operation at our department
Chiari malformation	119	Shunt malfunction	5 cases	
		Incomplete bone removal	3 cases	
		Calcification of dura	1 case	
		Scar formation of foramen magnum	3 cases	3 cases (2.5%)
		Excess removal of occipital bone	1 case	
Total:			13 cases	
Obstruction of foramen Magendie	3	Foramen of Magendie not opened	1 case	
Spinal arachnoiditis	20	Shunt malfunction	7 cases	6 cases (30.0%)
Basal arachnoiditis	17	Shunt malfunction	1 case	1 case (5.9%)
Idiopathic	5		None	
Total:	164		22 cases (13.4%)	10 cases (6.1%)

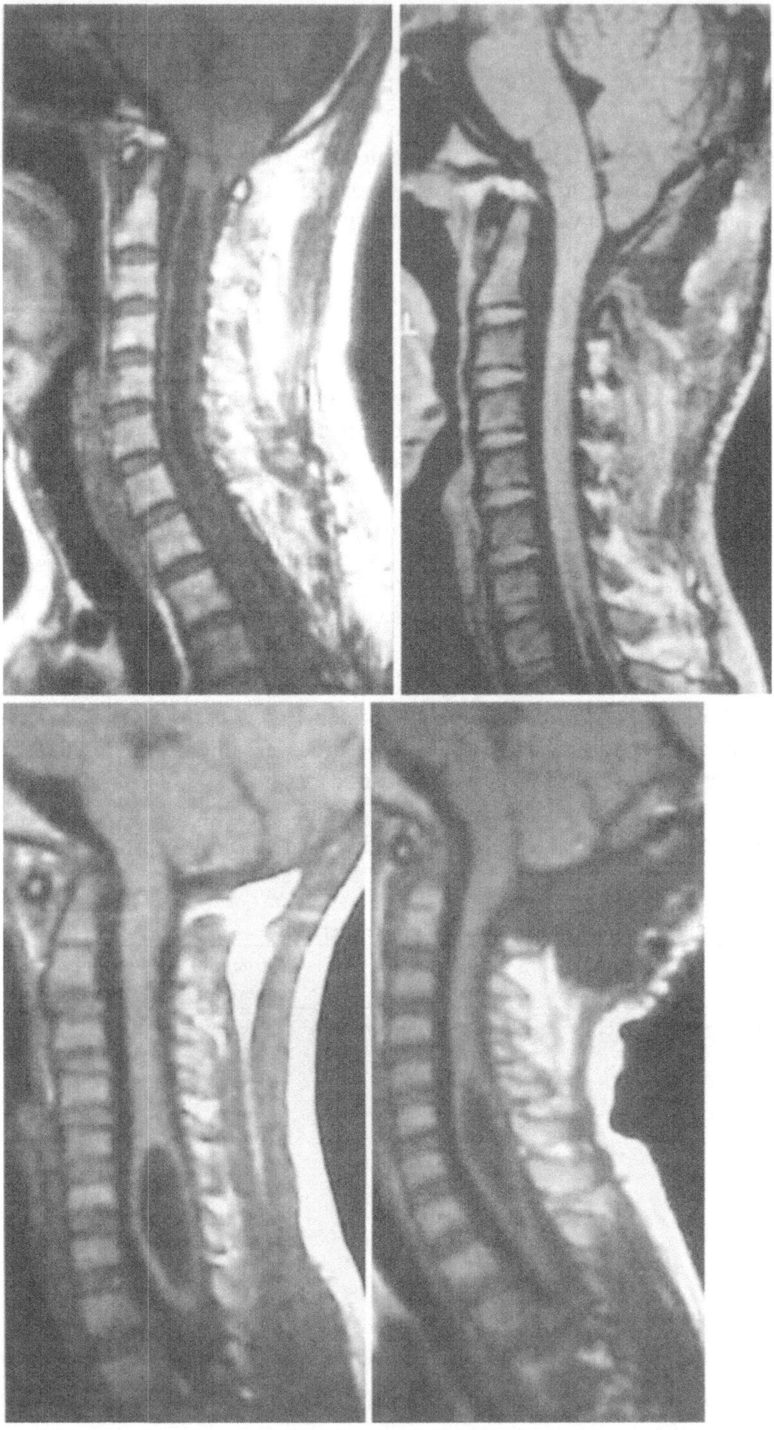

FIG. 1. *Upper left*: preoperative magnetic resonance imaging (MRI) of case 1. *Upper right*: postoperative MRI of case 1. *Lower left*: preoperative MRI of case 2. *Lower right*: postoperative MRI of case 2

a,b 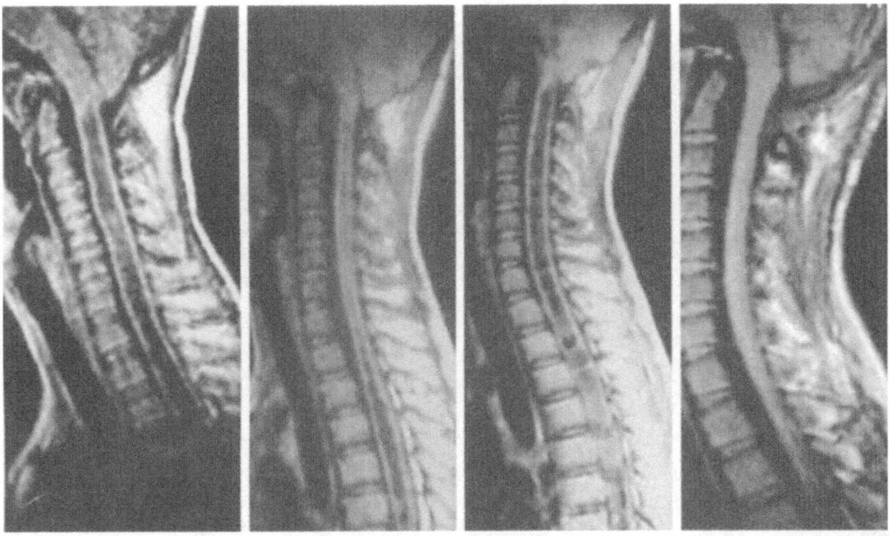 c,d

Fig. 2a–d. MRI of case 3. **a** Preoperative MRI. **b** Postoperative MRI; foramen magnum decompression (FMD) without dural plasty. **c** MRI shows regrowth of syrinx. **d** Postoperative view of FMD with dural plasty shows successful decompression of foramen magnum and marked decrease in size of syrinx

ment of the syrinx was noted; FMD was performed at our department, and subsequently shrinkage was noted.

Case 2 is a 14-year-old girl with Chiari malformation who underwent FMD without dural plasty elsewhere (see Fig. 1). The syrinx shrunk, but reenlargement after dural calcification narrowed the foramen. FMD and dural plasty were performed and the syrinx shrunk.

Case 3 is a 7-year-old girl with scoliosis and Chiari I (Fig. 2). She was the case for which reoperation was needed after FMD was performed at our department. Two years after FMD and dural plasty, scar tissue formation was noted at the foramen, as well as reenlargement of the syrinx. Scar tissue dissection and dural plasty with Gore-Tex was performed, resulting in syrinx shrinkage.

Case 4 is a 32-year-old woman with syringomyelia caused by congenital foramen of Magendie obstruction (Fig. 3). FMD was performed elsewhere, but because the foramen of Magendie was untouched the syrinx shrinkage was insufficient. Obstructive hydrocephalus and syrinx enlargement were noted, and ventricular drainage was performed followed by opening of the foramen of Magendie. Syrinx shrinkage was noted afterward.

Case 5 is a 42-year-old man with syringomyelia caused by spinal arachnoiditis (see Fig. 3). A syringoperitoneal (S-P) shunt was performed but obstruction caused reenlargement. S-P shunt reconstruction was effective.

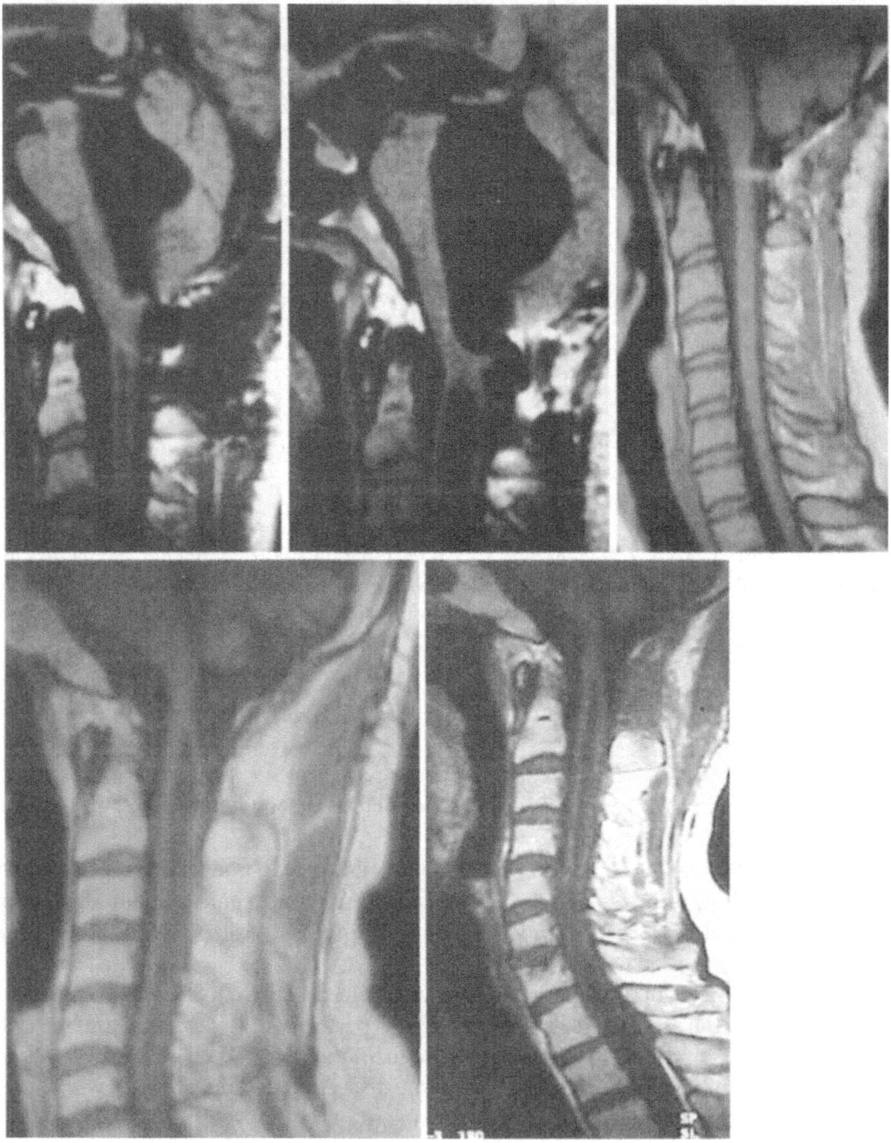

Fig. 3. *Upper left*: preoperative MRI of case 4. *Upper center*: post-FIMD MRI of case 4. *Upper right*: postoperative MRI of case 4. *Lower left*: preoperative MRI of case 5. *Lower right*: postoperative MRI of case 5

Table 2. Surgical strategy for cases requiring reoperation

Type	Primary operation	Cause	Method of reoperation
Chiari malformation	S-S shunt	Shunt malfunction	FMD
	FMD	Incomplete bone removal	FMD
		Calcification of dura	FMD
		Scar formation of foramen magnum	FMD
		Excess removal of occipital bone	S-C shunt
Obstruction of foramen Magendie	FMD	Foramen of Magendie not opened	Opening of foramen Magendie
Spinal arachnoiditis	S-S shunt or S-P shunt	Shunt malfunction	S-P or S-S shunt
Basal arachnoidits	S-S shunt	Shunt malfunction	4th vent.-S shunt

S-S shunt, syringosubarachnoid shunt; FMD, foramen magnum decompression; S-C shunt, syringocisternal shunt; S-P shunt, syringoperitoneal shunt; 4th vent.-S shunt, 4th ventricle–subarachnoid shunt.

Discussion

At our facility, we perform FMD for Chiari I malformation. The method involves the removal of a piece of the occipital bone, 3 by 3 cm in size, C1 laminectomy, and dural plasty using Gore-Tex. We now monitor CSF pressure intraoperatively, and if sufficient improvement is noted, dural plasty is not performed. Of the 119 FMD cases in our facility there were only 3 pediatric cases (2.5%) in which reenlargement was noted because of scar tissue of the foramen magnum. We believe reoperation of the 8 post-FMD recurrent cases from other institutions could have been prevented with our methods.

Obstruction of the shunt following S-S shunt for Chiari malformation is a complication seen more often than following FMD. Thus, our methods may prevent reenlargement. For spinal arachnoiditis, we perform an S-P or S-S shunt. However, recurrence following S-P shunt is common; we believe the length of the shunt tube should be kept short.

We summarize the therapeutic options for recurrence cases in our facility in Table 2. In recurrent cases caused by obstruction of the S-S shunt, FMD is performed. If spinal arachnoiditis due to the S-S shunt is suspected, FMD with an S-S shunt or a syringocisternal (S-C) shunt is performed. In S-P shunt obstruction in spinal arachnoiditis, S-P shunt reconstruction is performed. Finally, a 4th ventricle-S shunt is performed for basal arachnoiditis cases [5].

Conclusions

The most common reason that cases need reoperation is that of shunt malfunction. Shunt construction should not be the primary choice. In pediatric cases, calcification and scarring of the dura may occur following FMD. Thus, dural plasty is favorable. It is necessary to confirm that the CSF flow [6] has been improved after FMD by means of radiologic evaluation or CSF pressure studies.

References

1. Oldfield EH, Muraszko K, Shawker TH, et al (1994) Pathophysiology of syringomyelia associated with Chiari I malformation of the cerebellar tonsil. Implications for diagnosis and treatment. J Neurosurg 80:3–15
2. Hida K, Iwasaki Y, Koyanagi I, Sawamura Y (1995) Surgical indication and results of foramen magnum decompression versus syringosubarachnoid shunting for syringomyelia with Chiari I malformation. Neurosurgery 37:673–679
3. Isu T, Sasaki H, Takamura H, Kobayasi N (1993) Foramen magnum decompression with removal of the outer layer of the dura as treatment for syringomyelia occurring with Chiari I malformation. Neurosurgery 33:845–850
4. Barbaro NM, Wilson CB, Guitin PH, Edwards MSB (1984) Surgical treatment of syringomyelia. Favorable results with syringoperitoneal shunting. J Neurosurg 61:531–538
5. Williams B (1969) The distending force in the production of "communicating syringomyelia." Lancet II:189–193
6. Okuda Y, Isoshima A, Nagashima H, Abe T, et al (1998) Efficacy of foramen magnum decompression upon the CSF dynamics of Chiari type I-associated syringomyelia. Spinal Surg 12(2):169–176

5. Syringomyelia Associated with Chiari II Malformation

Hydromyelia and the Chiari II Malformation

David G. McLone and Frank LaMarca

Key words. Myelomeningocele, Spinal dysraphism, Syringomyelia

Introduction

It is the Chiari malformation that makes the child with spina bifida different from all the other children whom we see with other spinal cord lesions. The child with traumatic paraplegia or the child with a lipoma usually has problems restricted to the bladder and bowel or weakness in the lower extremities. I am not trying to minimize those, and I know that they present significant problems in society, but the Chiari malformation inflicts additional significant difficulties on the child. The Chiari malformation will kill 15%–20% of the children who have it before they reach the age of 20. It will render some 25% of the afflicted children permanently dependent, and 90% of them will have hydrocephalus and all the associated complications and revisions. Almost all these children have abnormal respiratory problems, and their blood gases are not normal. Vocal cord paralysis is present in one-third of the children, as are gastric reflux, apnea, and learning disabilities. As we work with these children, we find that the majority have some degree of attention deficit disorder (ADD). Hydromyelia is a direct result of this malformation.

For many years people from different disciplines, both pathologists and anatomists, have attempted to link the myelomeningocele to this hindbrain malformation [1–4] Many theories have been postulated, the simplest of which is that because the spinal cord is tethered at the bottom, it pulls the hindbrain out of the back of the skull [2]. There are others who postulated that the embryo has hydrocephalus, that the hydrocephalus blows open the back so that the back actually reopens instead of never closing [3,4], and the force of the hydrocephalus then pushes the posterior fossa content down into the upper cervical spine.

The amazing thing about the deformity is that in our series of 100 cases, which have been followed since 1975, in spite of the pancerebral abnormality many children have normal intelligence [5,6] and participate normally in society, and in a percentage of patients we anticipate independence. As is well known, in a Chiari malformation, a

Children's Memorial Hospital, 2300 Children's Plaza, #28, Chicago, IL 60614, USA portion of the cerebellum, usually the vermis but sometimes the tonsils, is herniated through the foramen magnum down into the cervical spine. What is often not realized is that there is also upward herniation [7,8]; the cerebellum is herniating upward out of the posterior fossa into the middle fossa. This is not a simple herniation through the foramen magnum, but a pancranial abnormality of the skull and brain: there is *lukenschadel* of the skull; to many gyri, ectopic gray matter; degrees of dysgenesis and in some cases agenesis of the corpus callosum; the massa intermedia in the third ventricle is huge; there is deficit in the tentorium; in some of these children, the tentorium is almost absent, there is extremely small posterior fossa, and in some children there is almost no posterior fossa; there is scalping at the base of the skull and a very enlarged foramen magnum. In spite of the gross deformity, the brain generates normal intelligence and is compatible with independent living for the majority of these children. Magnetic resonance imaging (MRI) shows these deformities and allows one to determine where the fourth ventricle is and the extent of the deformity and to know that there are many other things that can occur. The question has been, are these malformations related to the myelomeningocele, or are they caused by some genetic defect, or by some metabolic defect in the embryo that affects the entire nervous system? This is a possibility, but such a defect would have to affect all the germ layers because we know that the skull is abnormal and the nervous system is abnormal, so it would be a very unusual defect.

Theories about the cause of this malformation have been advanced by several people including Marin-Padilla [9], Penfield and Coburn [10], and Daniel and Strich [11]; the one that is accepted by most people is that of Padget [3,4]. The problem with Padget's theory is that hydrocephalus is necessary to generate the force to push the brain down into the brainstem. However, we know that there is not just downward herniation, but also upward herniation, and that makes it unlikely that hydrocephalus is the generating force. Figure 1 is an example of a midsecond-trimester spontaneously aborted fetus. The fetus has a marked Chiari malformation in the posterior fossa and absolutely no hydrocephalus. In a very good piece of work done by a Japanese neurosurgeon, Osaka et al. [12] studied a group of aborted fetuses and showed quite clearly that the Chiari malformation was present in spite of the fact that there was no evidence of hydrocephalus. The Chiari malformation precedes hydro-

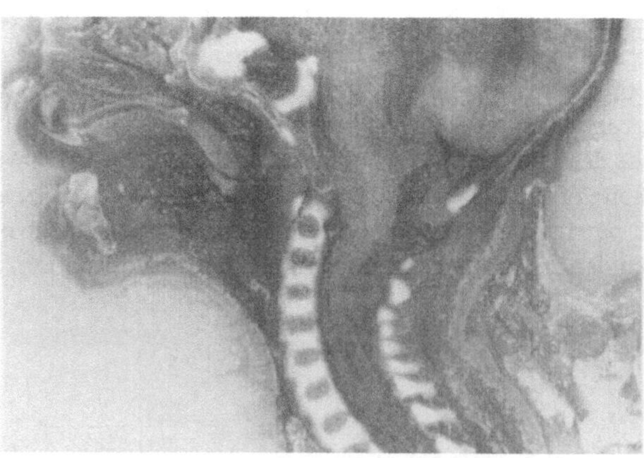

FIG. 1. Midsecond trimester with a myelomeningocele and severe Chiari II malformation without hydrocephalus. Note that the lower brainstem and most of the cerebellum are in the upper cervical canal and the posterior fossa is extremely small

cephalus and we will show quite clearly that hydrocephalus is the result of the Chiari malformation, not the cause.

An interesting experiment was done by Desmond and Schoenwolf [13] in which they observed developing chick embryos and showed that the hollow neurotube, the myelocele, goes from the head end of the embryo all the way to the posterior portion. If this tube is filled with a dye, it can be seen that it closes spontaneously from the cervical to the spine portion (Fig. 2); this is called occlusion. The occlusion is a critical event that allows the cerebral hemispheres to distend. However, if there is an open myelomeningocele at the bottom when occlusion is complete, after about 48 h, and the neural tube reopens, all the fluid runs through the open myelomeningocele and the cerebral hemispheres are decompressed. There is cartilage on either side, surrounding the posterior fossa. The posterior fossa is already determined and is solid; it is already in a cartilaginous box (Fig. 3). What determines the size of this box is the distending force, which occurs during occlusion. If that force is not there, the posterior fossa will be small. There will be not only cerebral deformities from the collapse of the mantle, but also a very small posterior fossa, which will lead to a Chiari malformation. Thus, it is the decompression of these vesicles (the embryonic ventricles, if you will) during primary neurulation that leads to the Chiari malformation. The neural tube is left open so that the fluid can pass out and decompress the head of the embryo. In the embryo with a myelomeningocele, there is no room for the anticipated cerebellum and there is a herniation of the contents of the posterior fossa into the upper cervical spine. The critical step is the loss of the volumetric expansion that the embryo needs to anticipate the development of the elements in the posterior fossa.

The embryological development of the Chiari II permanently links the ventri cular system and the center canal of the spinal cord. It is unusual to see a newborn child with a myelomeningocele with a hydromyelia; only with the onset of rapidly progressive hydrocephalus or a shunt malfunction does hydromyelia develop (Fig. 4). Unfortunately, the shunt malfunction may not be overt and only with the appearance of scoliosis or deterioration in lower extremity motor functions will the hydromyelia be found on a MRI. Prompt revision of the shunt often leads to reversal of the hydromyelia and resolution or stabilization of the neurological deficit.

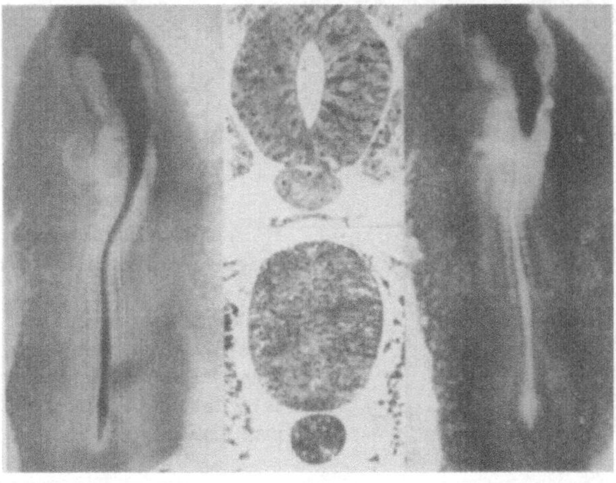

FIG. 2. Desmond and Schoenwolf's chick embryo experiment. Dye fills the entire neurocele on the *left*. An open neurocele is shown in the *upper center*. With occlusion, the neurocele closes (*middle bottom*) and the dye is excluded from the spinal neurocele (*right side*)

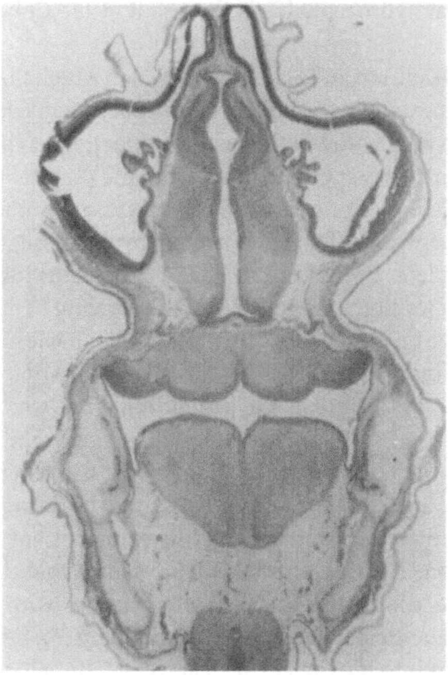

FIG. 3. Human embryo at about 35 days shows the large space surrounding the brainstem available for the brain stem to grow into. Note the posterior fossa is enclosed in cartilage

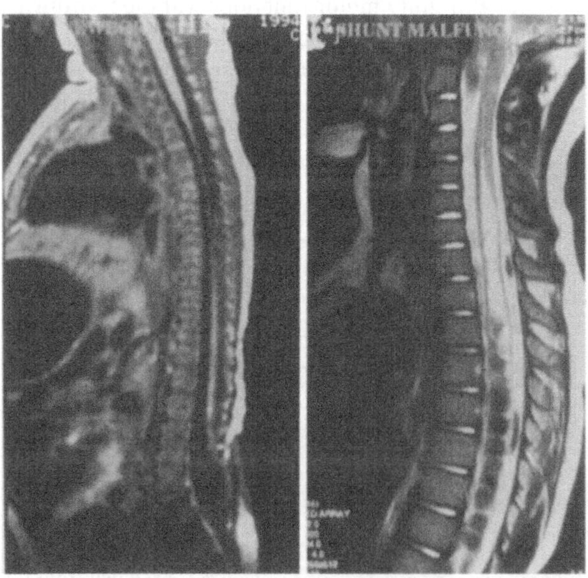

FIG. 4. Magnetic resonance imaging (MRI) on a newborn child with a myelomeningocele and shunted hydrocephalus (*left*). *Right*: MRI on the same child at the time of the first shunt malfunction

Cavitating lesions of the spinal cord in children with spina bifida and Chiari type II malformation have been referred to us as hydromyelia, syringomyelia, and also hydrosyringomyelia [14–17]. Although the term syringomyelia is commonly used to describe a progressive degenerative or invasive lesion of the spinal cord resulting in the accumulation of liquid within the parenchyma, the term hydromyelia reflects an alteration of the cerebrospinal fluid (CSF) circulation within the spinal cord that results in the accumulation of CSF within the central spinal canal and its dilation. This is the pathological mechanism believed to determine a cavitating lesion in most children with myelomeningocele and Chiari type II malformation [18].

Not all children with an abnormal dilation of the central spinal canal are candidates for treatment, and it has not been proven that all children with hydromyelia will become symptomatic. Surgical intervention appears to be indicated for only those children who present with clinical deterioration. The classical deterioration of the hydrosyringomyelic syndrome consists of a dissociative sensory loss (relative sparing of light touch and perception) in a "capelike" distribution with upper extremity weakness of a lower motoneuron type and lower extremity weakness of an upper motoneuron type [19]. However, the actual clinical presentation may differ greatly and can include, either alone or in various combinations, weakness, sensory loss, pain, gait abnormality, scoliosis, and changes in bladder and bowel function. The determination of such conditions is, unfortunately, quite difficult in small children, especially if they are already affected by a complex malformation such as myelomeningocele. The possibility of a shunt malfunction or a tethered cord further complicates the diagnosis.

In the literature, various types of surgical procedures have been proposed for the treatment of hydromyelia in children, and a wide variety of results have been reported for each type of operation [14,20–24]. On the other hand, a specific series of indications regarding a precise therapeutic approach for treating children with hydromyelia associated with myelomeningocele and Chiari type II malformation has never been clearly stated.

Case Study Series

In a study of 1195 patients followed in the Multidisciplinary Spina Bifida Clinic at Children's Memorial Hospital in Chicago, we established the incidence of symptomatic hydromyelia in the spina bifida population with Chiari type II malformation. The patterns, clinical presentation, and eventually the relationships between symptoms and radiographic characteristics of the lesion and the strategies of treatment that were found to be the most effective emerged. The final goal was to determine a protocol for optimal management of this pathology in patients specifically affected by spina bifida and the Chiari type II malformation.

Our study encompassed 588 male and 607 female patients; their age ranged from newborn to 25 years of age. In the past 8 years, magnetic resonance imaging (MRI) studies have been obtained in every patient who presented with clinical deterioration during their follow-up. A total of 231 MRIs of the spine were obtained in children with myelomeningocele and Chiari II malformation who also presented with neurological deterioration. Hydromyelia was found in 112 (48.5%) of the 231 spina bifida patients who underwent a spine MRI study for progressive neurological deterioration. The remaining 199 patients did not present any abnormal dilations of the spinal central canal.

The level of spinal defect, the presence of hydrocephalus, the age at onset of symptoms, and the characteristics of the presenting symptoms were recorded to search for eventual correlation with the pathology. Patient symptoms that led to requesting the MRI study were classified into three groups. In group I, stridor, vocal cord paresis, swallowing difficulties, neck rigidity, and upper extremity symptoms (pain, muscle weakness, spasticity) were dominant. The patients in group II presented predominately with altered bladder and bowel functions or lower extremity abnormalities. Group III was composed of patients with mixed group I and II symptomatology, scoliosis, or a type of symptomatology that was not clearly dominant. All patients had repair of their myelomeningocele within 72h after birth. All patients had hydrocephalus that was treated with a ventriculoperitoneal shunt in infancy. All patients had a Chiari type II malformation on MRI studies.

The pathological cavities of the spinal cord were categorized into two types according to the MRI findings: (1) segmental hydromyelia that involved only isolated longitudinal portions of the central spinal canal, and (2) holocord hydromyelia, in which the central spinal canal was enlarged in its entirety (Fig. 5). The former was subdivided further into high-level (cervical or cerviothoracic) and low-level (thoracic or

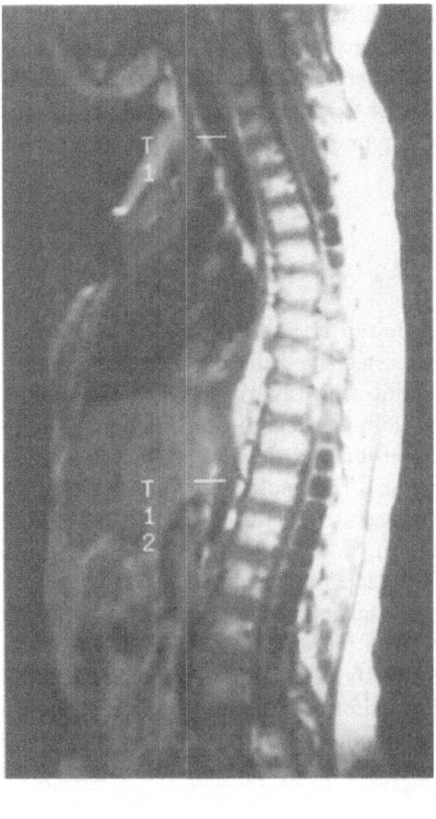

Fig. 5. MRI of a child with a myelomeningocele and Chiari II malformation with holocord hydromyelia

thoracolumbar) segmental hydromyelia. The hydromyelic cavities were also subdivided into three groups according to the degree of dilation: (1) those with a dystrophic spinal cord presenting an enlarged central canal (usually occupying less than approximately one third of the total spinal cord diameter and a small spinal cord paranchyema with a well-represented CSF space); (2) those defined as moderate hydromyelia with a diameter between one third and one half the diameter of the spinal cord; and (3) hydromyelia associated with a distended spinal cord resulting from the dramatically enlarged central cavity with thinning of the spinal cord parenchyma, in which often "haustral-like" septations were also present.

In patients with dystrophic spinal cords or moderate hydromyelia (hydromyelia dilation of type 1 and 2), after the shunt was determined to be functioning, no surgical intervention aimed at reducing the size of the pathologic cavity was undertaken. On the other hand, patients were considered to have severe hydromyelia when a type 3 dilation was observed on MRI and progressive clinical deterioration was present. In cases with severe hydromyelia, surgery was indicated. Of the 112 children with spina bifida and hydromyelia, 45 patients met this criteria, 19 girls and 26 boys.

Generally, the same therapy protocol was followed for all patients, although some variations in the protocol occurred because of the specific needs of the patients and the occasional differences in the surgeon's preference for one type of procedure over another. The first step in management was to assess correct function of the CSF shunting device. Ventricular size was analyzed on CT scans or MRI and the integrity of the shunting system was determined by radiographic studies. Shunt malfunction was excluded when functioning shunt was observed at surgery or through a shunt tap. The latter was carried out by inserting a needle into the shunt system's reservoir that permitted CSF aspiration and showed that the intracranial pressure was normal within its limits. If shunt malfunction was diagnosed, a ventriculoperitoneal shunt revision (VPSR) only was carried out.

Treatment

If the need for VPSR has been ruled out or if it had failed to resolve or improve the patients's condition, a tethered cord release (TCR) procedure, a hydromyelia-pleural shunt (HP1S) placement, or a posterior cervical decompression (PCD) were considered as the next step in treatment on the basis of symptomatology. The surgical procedures were considered unsuccesful if the patients did not show stabilization or improvement generally within a few weeks to months after the operation; this period of observation obviously could vary in relation to the given clinical conditions of the patient. However, the main goal of surgery was to obtain at least a stabilization of the progression of symptoms.

In the case of patients with hydromyelia and group I symptoms, a PCD was indicated, especially if MRI showed occlusion of the foramen magnum secondary to herniation of the cerebellar elements and the brainstem, typical of the Chiari II malformation. For those with group II symptomatology, TCR was carried out. Patients with group III symptoms underwent HP1S placement. Only one child in this latter group underwent TCR simultaneously with a VPSR that proved to be unsuccesful; subsequently, a successful HP1S insertion was carried out for this child.

In the case of segmental hydromyelia, PCD was indicated for patients with group I symptomatology and TCR for patients with group II and III symptoms. Two patients with group II symptoms varied from the protocol; one underwent an initial HP1S insertion and the other an initial PCD with fenestration of the hydrpmyelic cavity. Both cases were without success. Another child with group III symptoms initially underwent a succesful HP1S insertion.

The procedure for TCR has been previously described [25]. PCD was done through a classic cervical laminectomy from C1 down to the level just below the cerebrellar hernitaion with the creation of an adequate subarachnoid space, usually obtained through duraplasty. No plugging of the obex or manipulation of the nervous tissue was carried out. HP1S procedures were performed in the lateral decubitus position through a midline "pinhole" myelotomy using a CO_2 laser with placement of a Spetzler catheter into the hydromyelia cavity that was then tunneled under the skin to a separate incision in the midaxial line for insertion of the catheter into the pleural cavity.

Representation of symptoms caused by hydromyelia was considered as a recurrence when new onset occurred at least 2 years after the last successful treatment. In the case of hydromyelia recurrence, the type of hydromyelia was taken into consideration and the same protocols followed. Obviously, the possibility of a HP1S malfunction was taken into consideration in children in whom a HP1S was initially inserted. In the case in which a patient had already undergone a PCD, another type of intervention (HP1S or TCR) was preferred. The average postoperative follow-up period was 6.9 years (range, 1.3–11.3 years). No patient was lost to follow-up during this period. Postoperative MRIs were obtained in 23 cases. All patients continued to be clinically evaluated every 3 months in the first postoperative year and on a yearly basis thereafter.

Of the 112 children who presented with hydromyelia on MRI studies, the average age of the onset of the symptomatology leading to the necessity for the MRI investigation was 4.7 years (range, 6 months to 10.5 years). Thirty-two children presented with hydromyelia secondary to a dystrophic spinal cord, 39 with a holocord hydromyelia and 41 with a segmental hydromyelia. Of the latter, 11 were high level and 28 were low level. Of the 39 patients with holocord hydromyelia, 13 were of moderate dilation and 26 were severe. Of the 41 patients with segmental hydromyelia, 22 were of moderate dilation and 19 were severe (10, high level; 9, low level). Symptoms that proved to be progressive and persistent in nature were found in all 45 children with severely dilated hydromyelia. These patients went on to have treatment for the hydromyelia. Of the 45 patients with spina bifida who underwent treatment for hydromyelia, 15 (5 high-level segmental; 10 holocord) had group I symptoms, 18 (3 high-level segmental; 8 low-level segmental; 7 holocord) had group II symptoms, and the remaining 12 (2 high-level segmental; 1 low-level segmental; 9 holocord) had group III symptoms.

The level of myelomeningocele in these 45 patients was thoracic in 3 cases, thoracolumbar in 7 cases, lumbar in 21 cases, and lumbosacral in 13 cases. All the children treated for hydromyelia had hydrocephalus that was initially treated at the mean age of 11 days (range, 1 day to 7.7 years). Sixteen children never needed a shunt revision before MRI detection of the hydromyelia. Eight children underwent one shunt revision before hydromyelia diagnosis; 6 underwent two revisions and 15 needed three or more. Ventricular size was larger than normal in 6 patients at the time hydromyelia was diagnosed. Four of these children had a holocord hydromyelia and 2 a segmental hydromyelia. Ventricular size was considered within normal limits in 27 children, of whom 17 presented with a holocord hydromyelia and 10 with segmental hydromyelia. Of these 27 children, 8 were found to have a shunt malfunction although ventricular enlargement was not present. Cerebral ventricles were actually small in size or slit in 12 children, of whom 5 had a holocord hydromyelia and 7 a segmental hydromyelia. Of these patients with slit ventricles, 3 had a shunt malfunction at the time of diagnosis.

Postoperative MRIs appeared to be obtained randomly in our series, according to the surgeon or physician who had followed up the patient. Postoperative MRIs were obtained in 23 cases (17 with holocord hydromyelia and 6 with segmental hydromyelia). Of the 17 children with holocord hydromyelia, the hydromyelic cavity was reduced in size in 14 cases and unvaried in 3. All these patients had successful surgery, except 2 who did not improve. Both the latter cases had reduced hydromyelic cavities on the postoperative MRI studies. Of the 6 children with segmental hydromyelia, 4 showed smaller-sized hydromyelic cavities on MRI studies and 2 had stable hydromyelia. All these children improved after surgery.

Patients with Holocord Hydromyelia

The mean age at onset of symptoms for this group of patients was 4.4 years (range, 6 months to 10.5 years). Of the 26 patients with severe holocord hydromyelia, a total of 36 surgical procedures were initially carried out. An additional 9 procedures were carried out on 7 patients who experienced recurrence of symptomatic hydromyelia at least 2 years after initial treatment. Eleven patients initially underwent a revision of the ventriculoperitoneal shunt system because of shunt malfunction. Seven of these children benefited from shunt revision; in 4 cases VPSR failed to improve clinical status. The latter subsequently went on to have further treatment.

In 15 cases, VPSR was not indicated. Six of these children had group I symptoms. They underwent PCD followed by improvement in 3 cases, while 2 children went on to require further surgical treatment and 1 worsened progressively. One of 3 children who did not appear to benefit from the PCD required a VPSR because of a new onset of shunt malfunction after the PCD was carried out. The procedure was subsequently carried out with success. The other children underwent HP1S placement, after which improvement was observed. In the child who worsened postoperatively, progressive deterioration started once the PCD was carried out. The shunt malfunction was missed because a shunt tap was not carried out and the cerebral ventricles appeared normal on CT scans, which led to an intraoperative complication at the time of decompression. The child had an immediate reoperation to obtain ventricular drainage. This complication severely compromised the child.

Five children who had group II symptoms underwent TCR because of a confusing mixed type of symptomatology. Improvement was observed in all five cases. One of these children, however, had undergone a prior unsuccessful VPSR; in this child, it was decided to perform a PCD procedure simultaneously with the TCR. The remaining eight children had group III symptoms. Three of these children had undergone a TCR, also with no improvement, before a HP1S was placed with success. The other five children underwent HP1S placement; three improved and two did not. These latter two children subsequently underwent PCD with improvement.

In the holocord hydromyelia group, 12 VPSR procedures were carried out, of which 8 were successful in resolving the symptomatology and the remaining 4 were not. Nine PCD procedures were carried out, of which 6 were successful and 3 failed. Nine HP1S insertion procedures were carried out, of which 7 resulted in success and 2 did not. Six TCR procedures were carried out, of which 5 were successful and 1 was not.

Patients with Segmental Hydromyelia

The mean age at onset of symptoms for this group of patients was 5.3 years (range, 3.4–10 years). Of the 19 cases with severe hydromyelia, a total of 28 procedures were carried out initially and a further 4 procedures were carried out on 4 of these patients who presented with recurrence. Eight children (5 with high-level and 3 with low-level segmental hydromyelia) initially underwent VPSR. In all but 1 (high-level segmental hydromyelia), VSPR failed to improve the symptomatology, determining a need for further treatment. Of the 7 cases that did not benefit from VPSR and the remaining 11 (5 high-level and 6 low-level segmental hydromyelia) who did not present with shunt malfunction, only 4 (all high-level segmental hydromyelia who initially underwent VPSR) presented with group I symptomatology. These 4 children subsequently underwent PCD with improvement.

Eleven children (3 with high-level and 8 with low-level segmental hydromyelia) had group II symptoms. These children, except for 2, underwent TCR. The 9 children of this group who underwent TCR all improved. The remaining 2 children in this group had group III symptoms; 1 underwent PCD and the other had a HP1S placed (both had high-level segmental hydromyelia). Two of these children underwent TCR with good results. The remaining children had a severely extended cervicothoracic hydromyelia and underwent HP1S placement that was successful.

In total, eight VPSRs were carried out, of which seven failed to resolve the symptoms. Five PCDs were carried out that were successful in four cases and unsuccessful in one case. Thirteen TCR procedures were carried out and all were successful. Two HP1Ss were inserted, of which one led to clinical improvement and the other did not.

Patients with Recurrence of Hydromyelia

Eleven children had a recurrence; 7 had a holocord hydromyelia and 4 a segmental hydromyelia. Of the 7 with holocord hydromyelia, 1 presented with a malfunction of the HP1S that was revised with subsequent improvement in the patients' conditions. Of the remaining 6 children, 3 presented with group II symptoms. These patients underwent TCR with improvement. The other 3 patients with holocord hydromyelia presented with group I symptoms: 2 patients were treated with PCD, of which 1 improved and 1 did not, and 1 patient had already undergone an initial PCD. This latter patient was treated with HP1S placement, carried out simultaneously with TCR, and improved. The child who did not benefit from PCD subsequently underwent HP1S placement and also improved. Of the 4 children with segmental hydromyelia, 1 needed a VPSR that was carried out with success. The remaining 3 children presented with type II symptomatology and were treated successfully with TCR.

Discussion

The radiological incidence of hydromyelia in patients with spina bifida who present symptoms suggestive of deterioration in our series was close to 50%. To calculate the overall radiological incidence of hydromyelia in spina bifida patients, it would be necessary to obtain a MRI screening examination of every child at regular intervals. One study carried out on 160 children showed a radiological incidence of 19% [16]. If one were to consider the most accepted theories regarding the pathogenesis of hydromyelia proposed by Williams [18], Gardner [26], or Oldfield et al. [27], it becomes evident why hydromyelia would be more common in spina bifida patients than in others. In fact, in these children the Chiari II malformation, hydrocephalus, and tethered cord favor the formation of a fluid accumulation within the spinal cord. On the other hand, the level of myelomeningocele does not seem to effect the incidence of hydromyelia. In our series, there was no significant correlation between the level of myelomeningocele and the presence or the extent of the hydromyelic cavity.

There was a significant correlation between the location of the hydromyelic cavity in the spinal cord and the type of presenting symptomatology. Of the children with segmental hydromyelia, all those with group I symptoms had the lesion in the cervical region, whereas 82% of those with group II symptoms presented with a low-level hydromyelic cavity. On the other hand, the different types of symptoms seemed to be evenly distributed in the children with holocord hydromyelia. Furthermore, in our study all the children with progressive and persistent symptoms who underwent surgical treatment had a severely dilated hydromyelia.

There was no statistically significant correlation between the outcome and changes in the size of the hydromyelic cavity after surgery. However, more than 51% of the patients had a postoperative MRI. To our knowledge, there is no evidence in the literature that proves that clinical improvement after treatment of hydromyelia is necessarily related to a reduction in size of the hydromyelia itself. In fact, both children in our series with postoperative MRI studies, who did not clinically improve after treatment, actually showed a reduction in the degree of dilation of the hydromyelic cavity. Furthermore, two (10%) of the children who did not improve showed no variation in the degree of dilation of the hydromyelia. However, we also found a reduction in size of the hydromyelia in 90% of patients who improved postoperatively. Other authors have reported similar findings [28,29]. Unfortunately, we are unable to make any significant conclusions regarding the correlation between the radiologic and clinical outcome at this time.

Conclusions

It has been generally accepted that hydromyelia is the result of an abnormality in CSF dynamics. Based on the different methods of treatment proposed, such as PCD, fenestration of the hydromyelic cavity, hydropleural, and hydroperitoneal or hydrosubarachnoid shunts [14,17,20–24], various theories have been postulated that try to explain the exact pathogenesis of this lesion [18,26]. However, although many studies have approached the treatment of hydromyelia, very few consider the treatment of the child specifically born with a myelomeningocele [17]. We believe that the complexity of this malformation present a particular difficulty in choosing the type of therapy the most adequate for the patient. In addition, the not yet clear nature of the lesion and its natural history further contribute to this difficulty.

This retrospective study was therefor carried out to determine a sequence that is optimal management of children with spina bifida and hydromyelia. It was possible to identify a pattern of treatment that led to good results. The sequence of optimal management is shown in Figs. 4 and 5 for holocord, segmental, and recurrent hydromyelia, respectively. The patients in our series who were not treated following these patterns had, for the most part, a poorer outcome or a more complicated therapeutic course.

Treatment of holocord hydromyelia, as well as segmental hydromyelia, should always start by determining the correct function of the ventriculoperitoneal shunt. Shunt malfunction is known to be able to mimic symptoms that are more characteristics of other types of pathology, such as tethered cord and the Chiari type II malformation [14]. In our series, all children had an associated hydrocephalus treated in infancy. A total of 42% of the patients underwent VPSR for shunt malfunction. Of these children, 8 (42%) of 19 did not require further surgery. Only 13% of the 8 children with segmental hydromyelia benefited from the VPSR, while 64% of the patients with holocord hydromyelia benefited. It would seem that children with holocord hydromyelia have a better chance of resolving symptoms with a VPSR.

Of the 19 children who initially underwent a VPSR because the shunt was not functioning, ventricular size was increased in only 32% of them on neuroimaging studies as compared to baseline. Ventricles were stable in 53% and actually smaller, with a "slitlike" shape, in the remaining 15%. Therefore, ventricular size was not a good indicator of shunt malfunction in these children. When a shunt tap cannot be carried out or the results of the tap are dubious, a VPSR is indicated to assure shunt patency. In our series, the only case that worsened after surgical intervention resulting in a poor outcome was that of the child who presented with normal ventricles on CT scans and did not undergo an initial shunt tap or VPSR before the PCD procedure.

It is interesting to note how many of the children with hydromyelia had associated small ventricles: 12 of 45 (27%). Ventricular dilation at the time of diagnosis did not appear to be significantly correlated with the extent of the hydromyelia, nor was the number of VPSRs before the diagnosis of hydromyelia correlated with the type of hydromyelia.

Once correct shunt function is determined or VPSR is found to be ineffective in resolving symptoms, the next step in management is based on the type of hydromyelia: holocord or segmental. Simultaneously, the type of symptomatology is to be considered in choosing the correct therapy. In the case of holocord or cervical segmental hydromyelia with group I symptoms, a PCD is indicated. Of the six children with this type of symptomatology and holocord hydromyelia who underwent PCD in our series, three improved and three did not. All four children with segmental hydromyelia presenting with group I symptoms benefited from PCD. However, of the children who did not improve, one presented with a shunt malfunction immediately following PCD and another actually required a VPSR later that may have saved the patient the PCD procedure. Therefore excluding these two children, PCD appears to be correctly indicated in cases of hydromyelia with group I symptoms, as 88% of the cases had a good outcome. Excluding the cases mentioned, only one child with holocord hydromyelia did not benefit from a PCD procedure and later underwent HP1S placement with good results.

In patients with group II symptoms, TCR is indicated. All patients with holocord or segmental hydromyelia and group II symptoms eventually underwent TCR with good outcome. The majority of the cases (69%) had a segmental lesion, and half the children had a low-level segmental hydromyelia. TCR appeared to be the most effective procedure in the case of segmental hydromyelia with type-II symptomatology. Two patients in our series with group II symptoms did not undergo this procedure initially; one had a PCD procedure initially and the other a HP1S placement. They did not improve and subsequently underwent TCR with improvement.

With regard to patients with mixed-type or group III symptomatology, a different therapeutic approach is preferred for children with holocord lesion as compared to those with segmental hydromyelia. In children with holocord lesion and group III symptoms, a HP1S insertion is indicated. This procedure provided good results in 75% of our cases. One child in this group did not benefit from a TCR procedure initially and was successfully treated with a HP1S placement. In the two cases in which the HP1S did not resolve the symptoms, a subsequent PCD operation proved to be very effective.

On the other hand, a TCR operation is indicated for the children with segmental hydromyelia, especially for those with low-level hydromyelia limited to three or four levels. This procedure has been found to be effective by other authors for cases with these characteristics [30]. However, in one child in our series with group III symptoms and a very extended cervicothoracic hydromyelic cavity (C4–T10), a HP1S was inserted with a successful outcome. All the other children in the group underwent TCR with success.

When multiloculated hydromyelic cavities are present or cavities separated by what appears to be a normal spinal cord are observed, the therapeutic approach remains the same as that stated for single lesions, although it would be less advisable to insert a HP1S. Regarding the recurrence of symptomatology 2 years after successful treatment, in our institution these cases were considered just as a new onset of symptomatic hydromyelia. However, the possibility of HP1S malfunction and past PCD operations were taken into consideration when planning possible therapeutic interventions.

Hydromyelia associated with a myelomeningocele and Chiari type II malformation constitutes a serious threat to the child's neurological stability. Unfortunately, no one type of surgery can guarantee a good outcome. However, the extent of the hydromyelia and the type of symptoms with which it presents are good indications for deciding with surgical procedure is most likely to be successful. Furthermore, the fact that one type of procedure fails to resolve the symptoms means only that another type of treatment must be sought. When we followed the sequences of optimal management that

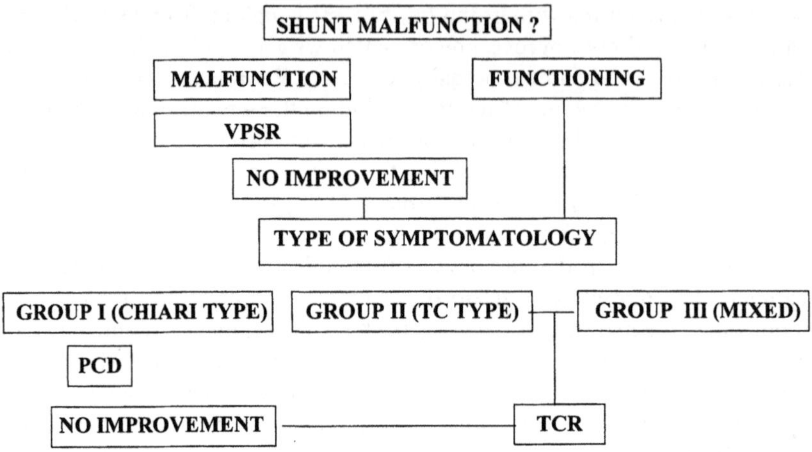

FIG. 6. Flow chart 1

we have proposed in flow chart 1 (Fig. 6), most of the patients obtained improvement in their symptoms.

Children are determined to be candidates for treatment on the basis of their clinical status and MRI findings. However, the presence of the accumulation of CSF within the spinal cord does not necessarily lead to neurological deterioration. For this reason, we believe that MRI studies are indicated only in cases of children with deterioration of their clinical status and not on a routine screening basis. However, we now perform a neuroradiological baseline MRI on all infants. Furthermore, follow-up MRIs are ordered only when there is reason to believe that therapy has failed or that the hydromyelia has recurred.

References

1. Barry A, Patten BM, Stewart BH (1957) Possible factors in the development of the Arnold-Chiari malformation. J Neurosurg 14:285–301
2. Lichtenstein BW (1942) Distant neuroanatomic complications of spina bifida (spinal dysraphism): hydrocephalus, Arnold-Chiari deformity, stenosis of the aqueduct of Sylvius, etc.: pathogenesis and pathology. Arch Neurol Psychiatry 47:185
3. Padget DH (1972) Development of so-called dysraphism, with embryologic evidence of clinical Arnold-Chiari and Dandy-Walker malformations. John Hopkins Med J 130:127
4. Padget DH, Lindenberg R (1972) Inverse cerebellum morphogenetically related to Dandy-Walker and Arnold-Chiari syndromes: bizarre malformed brain with occipital encephalocele. John Hopkins Med J 131:228
5. McLone DG, Knepper PA (1989) The cause of Chiari II malformations: a unified theory. Pediatr Neurosurg 15:1
6. McLone DG, Raimondi AJ, Sommers MW (1981) The results of early treatment of 100 consecutive newborns with myelomeningocele. Proceedings of the VIII Congress of the European Society for Pediatric Neurosurgery. Z Kinder Chir 2:115
7. Chiari H (1891) Uber Veranderungen des Kleinhirns infolge von Hydrocephalie des Grosshirns. Dtsch Med Wochenschr 17:1172

8. Chiari H (1895) Uber Veranderungen des Kleinhirns, der Pons und der Medulla oblongata infolge von congenitaler Hydrocephalie des Grosshirns. Denkschr Akad Wiss 63:71
9. Marin-Padilla M, Marin-Padilla TM (1981) Morphogenesis of experimentally induced Arnold-Chiari malformation. J Neurol Sci 50:29
10. Penfield W, Coburn DF (1935) Arnold-Chiari malformation and its operative treatment. Arch Neurol Psychiatry 40:328
11. Daniel PM, Strich SJ (1958) Some observations on the congenital deformity of the central nervous system known as the Arnold-Chiari malformation. J Neuropathol Exp Neurol 17:255
12. Osaka K, Matsumoto S, Tanimura T (1978) Myeloschisis in early human embryos. Childs Brain 4:347
13. Desmond ME, Schoenwolf G (1985) Timing and positioning of occlusion of the spinal neurocele in the chick embryo. J Comp Neurol 235:479
14. Milhorat TH, Johnson WD, Miller JI, Bergland RM, Hollenberg-Sher J (1992) Surgical treatment of syringomyleia based on magnetic resonance imaging criteria. Neurosurgery 31:231–245
15. Pojunas K, Williams Al, Daniels DL, Haughton VM (1984) Syringomyelia and hydromyelia: magnetic resonance evaluation. Radiology 153:679–683
16. Schwartz M, Voth D, Just M, Ermeert JA (1993) Form and incidence of hydro- and syringomyelia in spinal dysraphia in MRI. Acta Neurochir (Wien) 123:178
17. Wisoff JH, Epstein F (1989) Management of hydromyelia. Neurosurgery 25:562–571
18. Williams B (1993) Pathogenesis of syringomyelia. Acta Neurochir (Wien) 123:159–165
19. Adams RD, Victor M (1989) Principles of neurology, 4th edn. McGraw-Hill, New York
20. Hoffman HJ, Neill J, Crone KR, Hendrick B, Humphreys RP (1987) Hydrosyringomyelia and its management in childhood. Neurosurgery 21:347–351
21. Matsumoto T, Symn L (1989) Syringomyelia: current results. Surg Neurol 32:258–265
22. Tator CH, Meguro K, Rowed DW (1982) Favorable results with syringosubarachnoid shunts for the treatment of syringomyelia. J Neurosurg 56:347–351
23. Tognetti F, Calbucci F (1993) Syringomyelia: syringo-subarachnoid shunt versus posterior fossa decompression. Acta Neurochir (Wien) 123:196–197
24. Vaquero J, Martinez R, Arias A (1990) Syringomyelia-Chiari complex: magnetic resonance imaging and clinical evaluation of surgical treatment. J Neurosurg 73:64–68
25. McLone DG, Naidich TP (1989) The tethered spinal cord. In: McLaurin RL, Schut L, Venes JL, Epstein F (eds) Pediatric neurosurgery, 2nd edn. Saunders, Philadelphia, pp 71–96
26. Gardner WJ (1965) Hydrodynamic mechanism of syringomyelia: its relationship to myelocele. J Neurol Neurosurg Psychiatry 28:247–259
27. Oldfield EH, Muraszko K, Shawker TH, Patronas NJ (1994) Pathophysiology of syringomyelia associated with Chiari I malformation of the cerebellar tonsils. Implications for diagnosis and treatment. J Neurosurg 80:3–15
28. Firsching R, Sanker P (1993) MRI follow-up in syringomyelia. Observations from twelve cases. Acta Neurochir (Wien) 123:206–207
29. Van Calnbergh F, Van den Bergh R (1993) Syringo-peritoneal shunting: results and problems in a consecutive series. Acta Neurochir (Wien) 123:203–205
30. Hardwidge C, Williams B (1992) Spina Bifida and Syringomyelia. Child's Nerv Syst 8:173

Spectrum and Treatment Strategy of Neonatal Hydromyelia with Myelomeningocele (MMC)

Hiromi Sato and Noriko Sato

Summary. Neonatal hydromyelia with myelomeningocele (MMC) detected on neuroimages at birth has raised current issues about its management. However, little has been documented on its clinical spectrum and management remains unclear. The authors reviewed 12 cases of neonatal hydromyelia diagnosed in 38 consecutive patients with open MMC, attempting to obtain a rational therapeutic strategy. Results were analyzed in comparison with those of 19 nonneonatal hydromyelia cases. All but 4 neonatal cases of hydromyelia were large; all were associated with myeloschisis and advanced hydrocephalus. Two patients were overlapped with diastematomyelia. Seven patients showed a vermian shift up to the spinal level C4–C5. Four presented intractable symptomatic Chiari malformation. After MMC repair and ventricular shunting, 5 syrinx progressed and 2 were reduced to a slit. Two of 10 progressed syrinx were reduced by osseous craniocervical decompression (CCD). Syringospinal subarachnoid (SS) shunting, which was applied for the large syrinx after CCD, collapsed 2 syrinx and reduced 2. Syrinx of nonneonatal cord tethering-related hydromyelia remained collapsed for a maximum of 10 years after untethering and SS shunting. Our data suggest that the neonatal hydromyelia–MMC complex is not rare but poses a difficult issue concerning management. SS shunting assures the early reduction of the large syrinx with MMC. However, it is invasive for the immature spinal cord. Syrinx shunting should be preserved for the large and progressive syrinx refractory to MMC repair, ventricular shunting, or CVJD, which might eliminate the deteriorating factors. The authors propose a stepwise protocol for the management of neonatal hydromyelia with MMC.

Key words. Hydromyelia, Neonates, MMC, Dysraphism, Management

Introduction

A diverse pathomechanism, which operates in the developing spinal cord, leaves the management of pediatric hydromyelia with myelomeningocele (MMC) in dispute. The introduction of magnetic resonance imaging (MRI) diagnosis called attention on

---

Department of Neurosurgey, Shizuoka Children's Hospital, 860 Urushiyama, Shizuoka 420-8660, Japan

neonatal hydromyelia. However, its spectrum remains veiled. On the other hand, the current therapeutic attitude demands less invasive modalities. In this regard, we evaluate the clinical spectrum and discuss the surgical strategy of neonatal hydromyelia with MMC, focusing on its dynamic changes.

Patients and Methods

Between May 1983 and June 2000, 90 patients with MMC were surveyed by MRI or computed tomography (CT). Since 1993, neonates with MMC were surveyed by MRI. Of 38 neonates with MMC, 12 patients were associated with hydromyelia of various sizes. Neonatal hydromyelia was defined as hydromyelia diagnosed on MR images during 24 h after birth and before the repair of MMC. The size of the syrinx was evaluated based on the axial, sagittal, and coronal images. A syrinx was defined as large if the syrinx/cord ratio was ≥70% and extended over four vertebral segments. After repairing of MMC and shunting of the hydrocephalus, neonatal hydromyelia was followed up both by clinical exams and by MR images. The follow-up period ranged between 3 and 76 months. In one patient with holocord syrinx, the syrinx was explored by a thin-caliber endoscope to detect the destructive alterations of the spinal cord. The clinical features were compared with that of nonneonatally diagnosed MMC with hydromyelia.

Management Protocol

For all neonatal hydromyelia, a wait-and-see policy was applied at least for 4 months after repair and ventriculoperitoneal (VP) shunting at birth. For the management of hydromyelia, a stepwise protocol was designed for those with a large syrinx under the condition of a successfully controlled hydrocephalus (Fig. 1). Taking invasiveness against the premature spinal cord into consideration, the direct syrinx diversion (syringospinal subarachnoid shunt, SS) was preserved as for the final procedure. For a large and progressive syrinx seen on MRI, craniocervical decompression (CCD) was applied, referring to the deterioration of clinical symptoms and signs and the pathogenesis, before the final SS shunt. Efficacy of treatment was evaluated at least 3 months after each procedure.

CCD Procedures

After removing the dural band, which is always tough (Fig. 2, left upper), the outer layer of the dura was extensively but cautiously peeled off from just below the lower margin of the posterior lip of the foramen magnum to the upper cervical region (Fig. 2, left, lower). Without exception, the thinned-out dura bulges out, even though some remain tight without regaining dural pulsation. For those refractory patients, dural opening is indicated. Dissection of the thickened arachnoid and mobilization of the distorted lower vermis (Fig. 2, right upper) exposes the flattened obex (Fig. 2, lower). To avoid further invasiveness, no other manipulations including obex plugging and vermis resection are applied. The opened dura is patched with an ultrathin Gore-Tex sheet, and the dural decompression is completed.

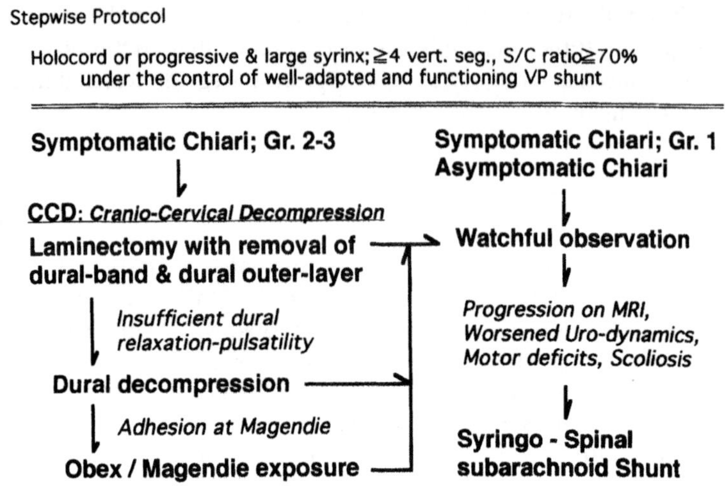

FIG. 1. Proposed stepwise protocol designed for the management of neonatal hydromyelia with myelomeningocele (MMC). A large syrinx under a successfully controlled hydrocephalus is a candidate. Wait-and-see policy is applied for the small or slitlike syrinx

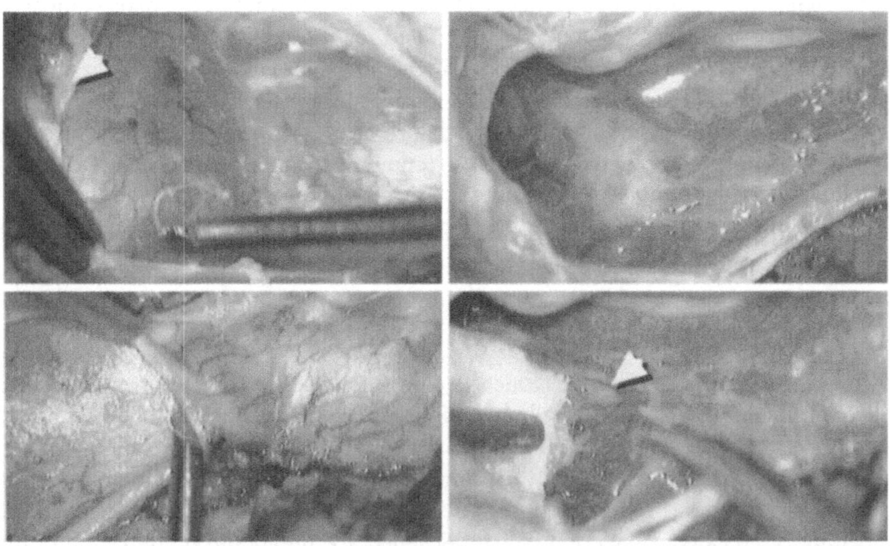

FIG. 2. Procedures of craniocervical decompression (CCD). Following the removal of the thick dural band, the outer membrane of dura is cautiously peeled off (*left upper* and *right lower*; *arrowhead*, exposed obex). Shifted lower vermis is covered with thickened arachnoid. Distorted vermis is hypoplastic and hypervascularized

SS Shunt

A syringospinal subarachnoid (SS) shunt catheter for neonates and early infants is not commercially available. At present, the cardiac catheter of Pudenz' infantile ventriculoatrial system is suitable as a one-way shunt tube with thin caliber. Shunting immediately collapses the syrinx. Further procedures of shunting using osteoplastic laminotomy have been described previously [1].

Results

The incidence of neonatal hydromyelia was 31% (Fig. 3a). Gestational age at birth ranged between 32 and 40 weeks; females were common (83%). All were myeloschisis with advanced hydrocephalus. Two neonates were associated with diastematomyelia; two had a holocord syrinx at birth (Fig. 4); and 70% had a large syrinx at birth. Among 31 hydromeylia with MMC, 19 hydromyelia were diagnosed later than neonatal period (Fig. 3b). Of 19 patients, 5 patients presented as symptomatic tethered cord, which were diagnosed at a mean age of 5.7 years. Fourteen patients with hydromyelia were diagnosed on follow-up MRI at mean age 6.2 years.

Signs and Symptoms

For all neonatal hydromyelia, a wait-and-see policy was applied for at least 4 months after repair and VP shunting at birth. During this follow-up period, worsening of Chiari type II signs and urodynamics was noticed in 60%. On MRI, syrinx progressed in 42%. However, no definitive correlation between syrinx progression and neurological deterioration was detected (Table 1).

Features of Syrinx

As compared with the posttoddler's symptomatic cord tethering-related hydromyelia, the large syrinx showed a remarkably higher level of motor deficit than that of the spinal defect (see Fig. 3a). Mean span in vertebral level between the uppermost motor deficit and the spinal defect was 3.7 vertebral segments in the holocord syrinx and 1.6 vertebral segments in others, which suggested a correlation between the extent of the syrinx and the severity of the motor deficit. Although the vermian shift was more severe (mean lowermost vertebral level, C3–C6) than those diagnosed postneonatally (Fig. 3a,b), all showed the postshunted reduction. There were two prenatally completed holocord syrinx (Fig. 3); one of two diastematomyelia was associated with diplomyelia and syrinx, which extended into both the split cords (Fig. 3a).

Postrepaired and post-VP-shunted progression was detected in five, which comprised 42% (Table 2). In one of them, a postshunted isolated fourth ventricle was defined as the deteriorating factor (Fig. 5). MR images of the post-SS-shunted hydromyelia with MMC were classified into two groups: the well-reconstituted spinal cords (Fig. 6) and the hypoplastic spinal cords (Fig. 7). Endoscopic view disclosed dorsally dominated destructive alterations in the rostral end of the syrinx (Fig. 8).

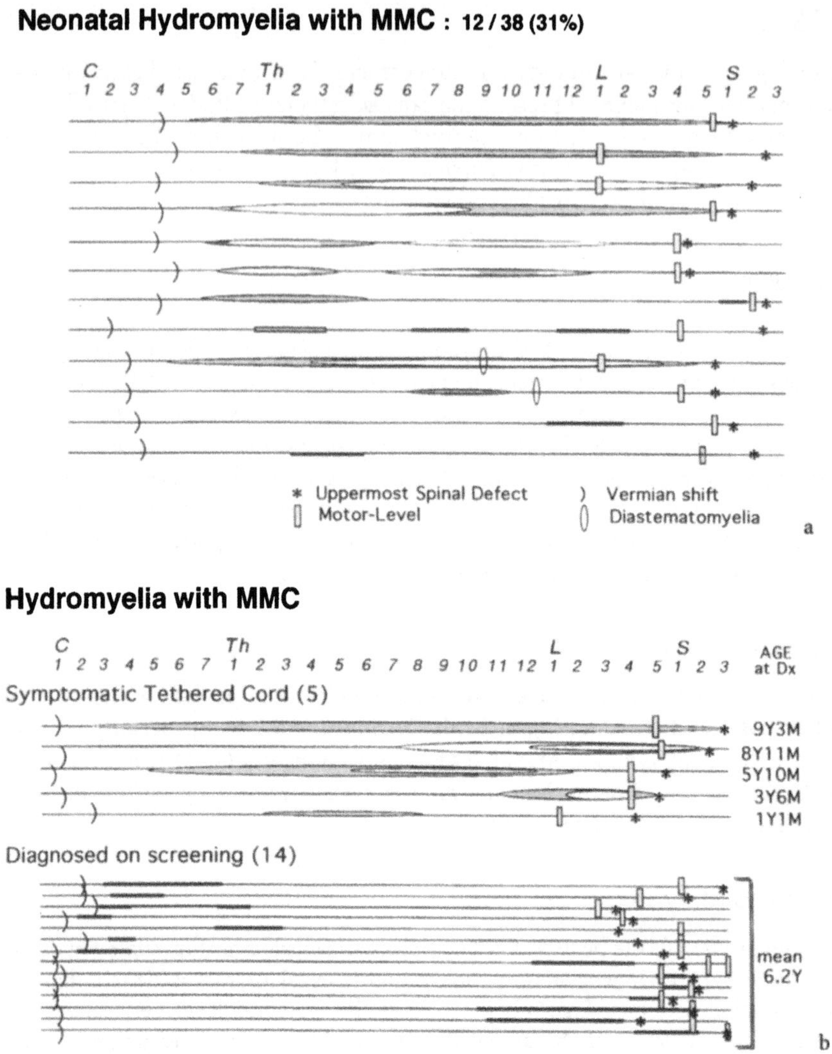

FIG. 3. **a** Summarized features of neonatal hydromyelia with MMC. Progression of syrinx after repair of MMC and VP shunting is indicated by the change of color of spindle (syrinx) from *white* to *gray*. **b** Summarized features of nonneonatally diagnosed hydromyelia with MMC

Outcome

To ameliorate the likely deteriorating factors, various procedures referred to the designed protocol were applied on an individual basis. SS shunting was undertaken for half of neonatal hydromyelia as the final procedure. All patients are alive; two have been under intensive care due to failure to thrive and have required intermittent oxygen supply as a result of the tracheostomied condition.

Compared with the satisfactory result of the symptomatic tethered cord group [1] in posttoddlers, the outcome of neonatal hydromyelia is limited. Evaluation of uro-

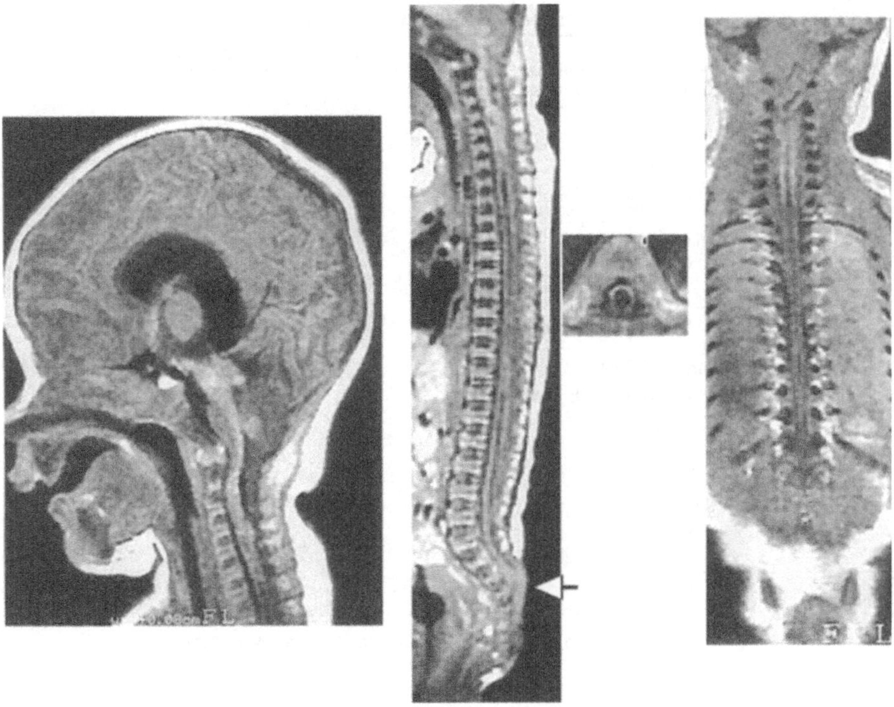

FIG. 4. Prenatally completed holocord syrinx with sacral myeloschisis (*arrowhead*). This patient was transferred as intrauterine-diagnosed hydrocephalus at 36 gestational weeks. The uppermost spinal defect level was S2. However, motor deficit level was L1. Craniocervical decompression (CCD) with obex exposure reduced the syrinx, which supported the prenatally isolated central canal as a hypothetical mechanism

dynamics and muscle power revealed improvement in 25% and stabilization in 60%. However, worsening was recorded in 10%. As for syrinx size, collapse or reduction was attained in 70%. A hypoplastic cord, which remains underdeveloped, resulted in two of three collapsed syrinx (Table 3).

Discussion

Our neonatal survey disclosed the incidence of hydromyelia with MMC at birth. Peach [2] reported the incidence of neonatal hydromyelia or hydromyelia at birth as 20% (4/20). However, neonatal hydromyelia has been rarely reported [3], even after the advent of CT and MRI, and its clinical spectrum is obscure. No data are available on the incidence of hydromeylia in neonates with MMC.

The incidence of hydromyelia on MRI after MMC repair is reported to be 27% [4]. Others reported that it ranged from 19% to 28% [4–7]. Our MRI survey showed relatively high incidence (31%) in neonates with MMC. However, reduction to a slitlike

TABLE 1. Signs, symptoms, and MRI changes after neonatal ventriculoperitoneal (VP) shunt and repair

	n	Worsened
Chiari II, apnea monitoring		
None	3	
Grade 1	4	7 (58%)
Grade 2	3	
Grade 3	2	
Urodynamics		
VUR under IC Grade ≦2	6	
Grade ≧3	4	7 (58%)
Overflow incontinence	2	
Motor deficits		
Above L1 (UE involved)	3 (2)	4 (33%)
Below L1	9	
Scoliosis	3	3 (25%)
Syrinx		
Progressed	5	
Stable	5	5 (42%)
Reduced	2	

$n = 12$; follow-up at 4 months–22 months (mean, 14 months).

TABLE 2. Procedures applied for neonatal hydromyelia and the spinal cord tethering-related hydromyelia with myelomeningocele (MMC)

Outcome	Neonatal hydromyelia ($n = 10$)	Symptomatic tethered cord ($n = 5$)
Follow-up period	3 months–6 years 4 months	2–9 years
Age at syrinx-directed operation	3 months–1 year 11 months	3–9 years
CCD	2	—
VP revision, CCD, obex exposure	1	—
CCD, Obex exposure → fourth VP shunt	1	—
CCD → SS Shunt	5	—
SS shunt plus diastematomyelia repair/untethering	1	3
Untethering plus syringostomy	—	2
Mortality	0	0

syrinx was noticed in two, and the incidence of nonslit hydromyelia decreased to 26% in the follow-up period of 4 to 22 months.

Neonatal hydromeylia with MMC is not rare. The significant incidence of hydromeylia in neonates with MMC dictates the neurosurgical implication. With the advent of perinatal and infantile care, the mortality of MMC has decreased and improvement of long-term morbidity has become the current agenda. In this regard, we should recognize the clinical implications of neonatal syringomyelia more than we did previously.

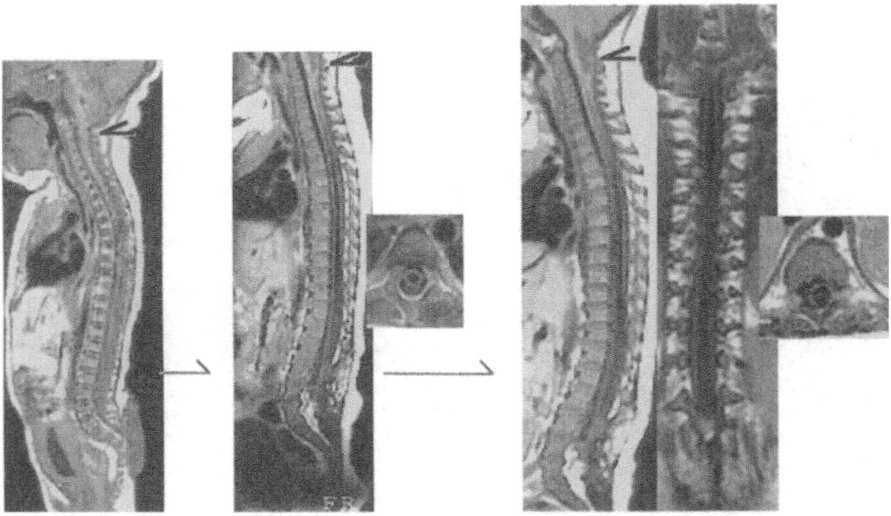

FIG. 5. Postnatally formed holocord syrinx along with the postshunted isolated fourth ventricle. This full-term newborn was associated with isolated fourth ventricle after VP shunting at birth. Large hydromyelia at birth progressed, and holocord syrinx was completed 9 months after the repair of MMC and ventriculoperitoneal (VP) shunting (*center*). *Right*: at 12 months of age. CCD with fourth VP shunting collapsed syrinx. Transobex CSF influx was confirmed by the direct filling of syrinx by the contrast material introduced into the fourth ventricle

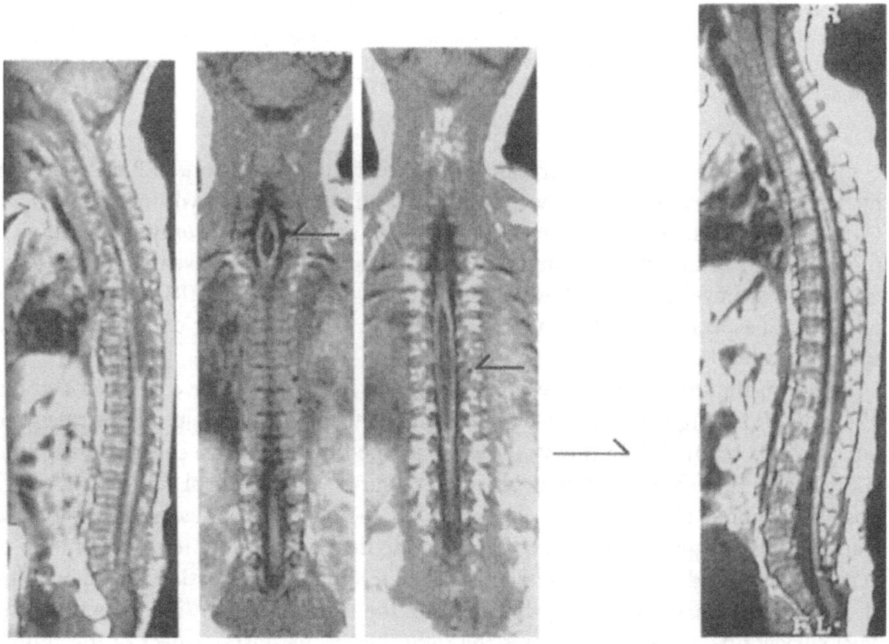

FIG. 6. Neonatal hydromyelia that showed progression after repair and VP shunting. The fully reconstituted spinal cord was visualized on MRI at 6 months after the osseous craniocervical decompression (*right*)

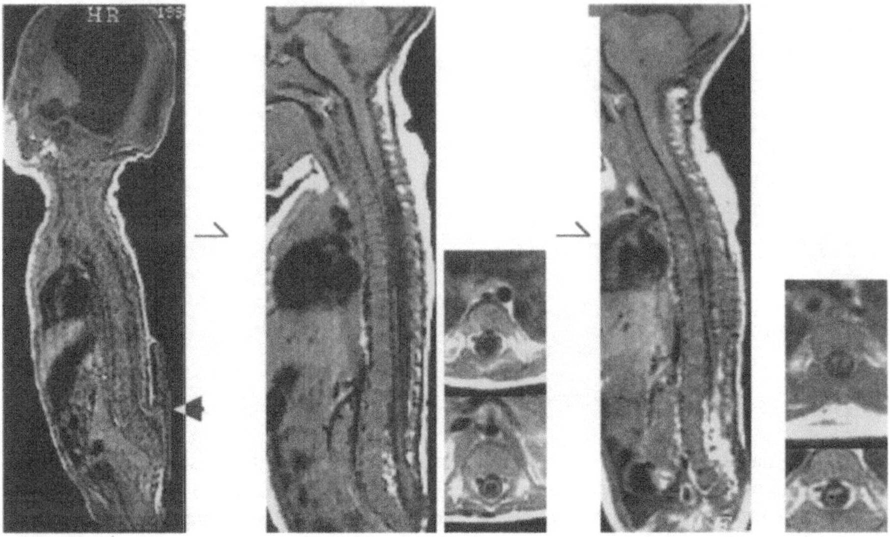

FIG. 7. Hypoplastic spinal cord that resulted from the successfully collapsed syrinx. In this premature baby, born at 32 gestational weeks, hydromyelia at birth progressed after repair of myeloschisis (*arrowhead*) at birth and VP shunting at the corrected age of 34 gestational weeks. At corrected postnatal age of 6 weeks, large syrinx changed to holocord syrinx (*center*). Osseous craniocervical decompression (CCD) followed by SS shunting successfully collapsed the syrinx within a week. However, the resulting cord was hypoplastic. The spinal cord remained thin, and a worsened motor deficit was noticed at assessment at the age of 2 years. She is the youngest hydromyelia with MMC treated by SS shunt reported in the literature

Other than the dynamic alteration after repairing of MMC and VP shunting for hydrocephalus, large size (8/12) was another feature of neonatal hydromyelia on MRI. Clinical findings suggested a correlation between associated hydromyelia and higher motor deficits rather than the upper-level spinal defects. MRI is essential for the diagnosis of hydromyelia [8]. We showed the feasibility of a neonatal MRI survey for those with MMC, especially for those who present with a higher motor deficit than with a spinal cord level of defect.

Based on the leading hypothesis and our own findings, we have summarized the likely deteriorating factors, which were significant for planning surgical strategy in our previous report [1]. In this study, we confirmed the transobex cerebrospinal fluid (CSF) influx (VP shunt dysfunction, isolated fourth ventricle) isolated central canal: post-VP-shunted obex–Magendie stenosis, obex–Magendie adhesion, the impaired transforamen magnum CSF dynamics related to the post-VP-shunted amelioration of vermian shift, and the developmental cerebellocranial disproportion. In Chiari type II, the foramen magnum is large but tight on the transforaminal CSF dynamics. The MRI survey unequivocally discloses the tightness in the dorsal aspect of the shifted brainstem and vermis. CSF dynamics at the craniocervical junction may be influenced both by the ventricular diversion operation and by the maturation of the brain. All the shifted vermis migrated upward after VP shunting. The low incidence of hydrosyringomyelia in those with either severe or mild tonsillar shift is described in Chiari I

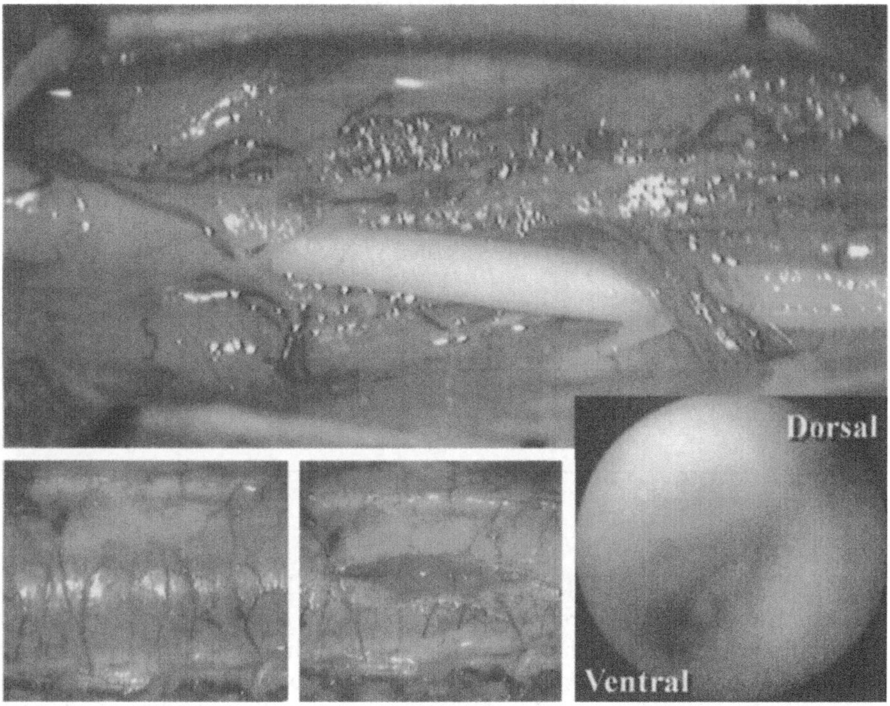

FIG. 8. Operative view and the endoscopic findings of syrinx in the patient shown in Fig. 7. SS shunt with the distal slit valve (Pudenz' infantile cardiac catheter; OD, 1.3 mm, ID, 0.7 mm) was set at Th 10. Interpedicular distance was 6.5 mm. The distal end was placed into the ample ventral subarachnoid space. SS shunting transformed the bulged-out spinal cord (*lower left*) into a flattened sheetlike cord (*upper*). The spinal cord was exposed as the cyst covered by transparent membrane (*center*). Endoscopic exploration visualized the well-preserved but flattened ventral spinal cord, the dorsally predominating bulging of the central canal, and the destructive alterations around the posterior longitudinal fissure (*lower right*)

[9]. We speculated on the role of post-VP-shunted reduction of the vermian shift in the deterioration of transforamen magnum and upper cervical CSF dynamics in the progression of hydromyelia.

Taking immaturity and invasiveness into consideration, the wait-and-see policy is the generally accepted attitude for surgical treatment. However, endoscopic findings revealed the destructive alterations of spinal cord from inside, especially in the dorsal side. The dorsally dominant changes correlate with the findings of hydromyelia in younger patients, which is centrally located and dorsally expanded [1]. Because the progression of hydromyelia was noticed within 4 months after the final surgical treatment for deteriorating factors such as shunt revision and craniocervical osseous decompression, it is considered reasonable to observe watchfully at least 4 to 6 months before planning syringospinalsubarachnoid shunting. It is believed that syrinx reduction correlates with neurological recovery [10,11]. In our study, some showed a hypoplastic cord without neurological improvement, even after successful SS shunt-

TABLE 3. Clinical outcome and resulting MRI findings of syrinx in neonatal hydromyelia and the spinal cord tethering-related hydromyelia with MMC

Outcome	Neonatal hydromyelia (*n* = 10)			Symptomatic tethered cord (*n* = 5)		
Follow-up period	3 months–6 years 4 months			2–9 years		
Age at syrinx-directed operation	3 months–1 years 11 months			3–9 years		
Signs and symptoms	Improved	Stable	Worsened	Improved	Stable	Worsened
Urodynamics	2/10	7/10	1/10	0	5/5	0
Motor DTRs	3/10	5/10	2/10	3/5	2/5	0
Scoliosis	0	2/10	2/10[a]	1/5	4/5	0
Pain		—		5/5	0	0
Syrinx						
Collapsed	3 (30%)			5 (100%)		
Hypoplastic cord	2			0		
Reduced	4 (40%)			0		
Stable	3			0		

[a] One appeared on follow-up.

ing (Fig. 7, Table 3). In neonatal hydromyelia with MMC, as is the prenatally formed holocord hydromyelia, the irreversibly damaged spinal cord as well as the hypo- or dysplastic cord, which was shown in hydromyelia with diplomyelia, may limit the neurological outcome even after achieving the collapse of hydromyelia. Limited neurological recovery is reported both in the spontaneously reduced cervicothoracic syringomyelia [12] and in the Chiari–hydrosyringomyelia complex presenting in adults with MMC [13]. We should recognize that inappropriately longer watchful observation might lead to insufficient neurological improvement.

The goal of treatment for hydromyelia is reduction of the syrinx and the amelioration of the adverse effect of the syrinx pressure, the slosh and the squeeze mechanism [14]. Deteriorating factors related to the progression of syrinx were discussed in our previous report [1]. The correction of VP shunt dysfunction and the appropriate maintenance of shunt function are absolutely prerequisite before planning the direct treatment of hydromyelia. Craniocervical osseous decompression revealed the syrinx reduction effect in some patients with symptomatic Chiari. Because the reduced posterior fossa volume is the deteriorating factor of acquired Chiari [1], early decompression is expected to prevent a further vermian shift, which may be brought about by the developmental craniocerebellar disproportion [1]. The reduction rate of syrinx by Gardner's obex plugging is reported as 67%–70% [15,16]. However, today, this procedure lost its feasibility because of the high mortality described as 7%–9% [17]. In our study, osseous CÇD improved symptomatic Chiari, which deteriorated even after appropriate VP shunting. The reduction of a huge syrinx was noticed in one. The authors believe CCD is useful for the symptomatic Chiari with large syringomyelia before planning the SS shunt for syrinx.

The syringospinal subarachnoid (SS) shunt is effective for the early reduction of syrinx without mortality. It has the advantage that it is not influenced by body growth, contrary to the syringopleural [15,18] or syringoperitoneal shunt. Some point to the high frequency of SS shunt use. However, in our cases, all but one showed SS shunt dysfunction. Including the one SS shunt-revised patient, all maintained the totally collapsed or reduced syrinx for a maximum of 10 years. The authors believe that the placement of a thin shunt catheter with a one-way valve into the ample ventrolateral spinal subarachnod space maintains the shunt function for a long period. Further follow-up is necessary to demonstrate validity. Hydromeylia is a complex pathological disorder related to diverse mechanisms [1], which requires an individualized treatment strategy [19]. Based on our study, we propose the stepwise protocol for the management of neonatal hydromeylia with MMC (see Table 1).

Conclusion

Neonatal syringomyelia is not rare, but poses difficult issues in its management. To improve therapeutic outcome, further effort is expected to clarify and ameliorate the deteriorating factors on an individual basis. MRI survey at birth and follow-up is useful for defining the clinical spectrum. Needless to say, the prematurity of this age group demands a prudent therapeutic attitude supported by a stabilized general condition. We propose a stepwise strategy as a protocol for neonatal hydromyelia with MMC.

Acknowledgment. This study was partly supported by the Research Grant for Nervous and Mental Disorders from the Japanese Ministry of Health and Welfare of Japan.

References

1. Sato H, Sato N (1999) Syringomyelia with MMC. Management with reference to its progression. In: Matsumoto S, Sato H (eds) Spina bifida. Springer, Tokyo, pp 19–22
2. Peach B (1965) The Arnold-Chiari malformation: morphogenesis. Arch Neurol 12:527–535
3. Carmel PW (1991) Congenital syringomyelia. In: Bartzdorf U (ed) Syringomyelia. Current concepts in diagnosis and treatment. Baltimore, Williams & Willkins: pp 140–150, 1991
4. Williamson MR, Glasier CM, Chadduck WM, et al (1989) MRI in the evaluation of spina bifida patients in the remote period after myelomeningocele repair. Pediatr Radiol 19:442–443
5. Caldarelli M, Di Rocco C, La Marca F (1988) Treatment of hydromyelia in spina bifida. Surg Neurol 50:411–420
6. Schwartz M, Coth D, Just M, Ermert JA (1993) Form and incidence of hydro- and syringomyelia in spinal dysraphia in MRI. Acta Neurochir (Wien) 123:178–182
7. Tamaki N (1993) Syringomyelia associated with spinal dysraphism: a cooperative study. In: Tamaki N (ed) The annual report of research for pathophysiology and treatment of syringomyelia and spina bifida. Research grant (5B-3) for nervous and mental disorders from the Ministry of Health and Welfare of Japan, Kobe, pp 139–150
8. Wolpert SM, Anderson M, Scott RM, et al (1987) Chiari II malformation: MR imaging evaluation. AJNR 149:1033–1042
9. Maser H, Oberwittler C (1993) Syringomyelia in Chiari malformation: relation to extent of cerebellar tissue herniation. Neurosurgery 33:948–949
10. Hardwidge C, Williams B (1992) Spina bifida and syringomyelia. Childs Nerv Syst 8:173

11. La Marca F, Herman MD, Grant JA, McLone DG (1997) Presentation and management of hydromyelia in children with Chiari type II malformation. Pediatr Neurosurg 26:57–67
12. Sudo K, Doi S, Maruo Y, Tashiro K, Terae S, Miyasaka K, Isu T (1980) Syringomyelia with spontaneous resolution. Letters to Editor. J Neurol Neurosurg Psychiatry 53:437–438
13. Craig JJ, Gray WJ, McCann JP (1999) The Chiari/hydrosyringomyelia complex presenting in adults with myelomeningocele: an indication for early intervention. Spinal Cord 37:275–278
14. Williams B (1980) On the pathogenesis of syringomyelia: a review. J R Soc Med 73:798–806
15. Hoffman HJ, Neil J, Crone KR, et al (1987) Hydrosyringomyelia and its management in childhood. Neurosurgery 21:347–351
16. Suzuki M, Davis C, Symon L, Gentili F (1985) Syringoperitoneal shunt for treatment of cord cavitation. J Neurol Neurosurg Psychiatry 48:620–627
17. Matsumoto T, Symon L (1989) Surgical management of syringomyelia: current results. Surg Neurol 32:258–265
18. Wisoff JH, Epstein F (1989) Management of hydromyelia. Neurosurgery 25:562–571
19. Milhorat TH, Johnson WD, Miller JI, et al (1992) Surgical treatment of syringomyelia based on magnetic resonance criteria. Neurosurgery 31:231–245

6. Syringomyelia Associated with Tethered Cord and Other Disorders

Syringomyelia Associated with Tethered Cord Syndrome

SHOKEI YAMADA, DAVID S. KNIERIM, DANIEL J. WON, and ANTHONY G. HADDEN

Summary. The pathogenesis and dynamic pathophysiology of syringomyelia are not fully understood. Pathogenetically, syringomyelia is categorized as either a communicating syrinx (hydromyelia) or a noncommunicating syrinx. The latter category includes those caused by (1) contusion, (2) compression, (3) traction, (4) arachnoiditis, (5) tumors, and (6) ischemia. Syringomyelia located in the lumbosacral cord is likely derived from the same types of pathogenesis. The signs and symptoms of lumbosacral syringomyelia are similar to those of tethered cord syndrome (TCS), caused by the lesion being in the central portion of the spinal cord. Neurological deficits in these disorders are motor and sensory deficits in the lower limbs, incontinence, and musculoskeletal deformities. Syringomyelia associated with TCS is a unique combination and difficult to correlate because TCS is a metabolic functional disorder and syringomyelia is an anatomic functional criterion. The authors divided a series of syrinx patients into three groups: (1) those with lumbosacral syringomyelia associated with tethered spinal cord, in which the spinal cord is anchored by an inelastic filum; (2) those with low thoracic and lumbar syringomyelia associated with TCS, in which a lipoma, lipomyelomeningocele, or meningocele manqué is the mechanical cause of tethering; and (3) those with a syrinx in the lower thoracic and lumbosacral cord without evidence of a tethered cord. The syrinxes in the patients in all three groups were considered to be isolated from the fourth ventricle cord. The authors' observations include: (1) The incidence of lumbosacral syrinx in tethered spinal cord patients is much lower than that in TCS patients; (2) The group 1 patients have milder neurological symptomatology than do the group 2 patients. The degree of improvement in the neurological conditions and physical activities are much greater in group 1 than in group 2 patients; (3) Group 3 patients tend to have more serious neurological deficits associated with hydrocephalus and severe musculoskeletal deformities. Based on these facts, the authors postulate that syrinxes should be drained in cases in which the signs and symptoms suggest that the neurological deficits are more significant than those for TCS alone.

Key words. Syringomyelia, Lumbar spine, Tethered spinal cord, Tethered cord syndrome, Occult spinal dysraphism

---

Loma Linda University School of Medicine, 11234 Anderson Street, Loma Linda, CA 92350, USA

Introduction

Syringomyelia is an anatomic term coined by Olliver d'Angers [1] to describe a cavity in the spinal cord found at autopsy. Over the years, pathologists and clinicians have studied the signs and symptoms of this disorder and correlated them with the syrinx location [2]. The syrinx in the cervicothoracic cord, in particular, is typically associated with burning pain in the suspended area of analgesia in the neck, arms, and upper chest, along with atrophy of the hand muscles. Since the advent of magnetic resonance imaging (MRI), syrinxes have been found more easily and accurately, and also incidentally in asymptomatic individuals.

Syringomyelia, thus, tends to be regarded as an anatomic criterion. In contrast, tethered cord syndrome (TCS) is a disorder based on stretch-induced neuronal dysfunction without histological damage. Together, syringomyelia and TCS comprise a unique combination of anatomic and functional disorders.

Because of this combination, correlating syringomyelia with TCS is not an easy task. Several authors have combined syringomyelia with spinal dysraphism, both being anatomic criteria [3–5]. In this chapter, the authors endeavor to correlate TCS, a neuronal functional disorder, and syringomyelia, an anatomic, partly hydrodynamic abnormality, based on their work with a series of patients treated at Loma Linda University Medical Center, Loma Linda, CA, and Valley Children's Hospital, Madera, CA, USA.

Material and Methods

In this series, the patients have been divided into three groups: (1) those with tethered spinal cord (TSpC) and lumbosacral syrinxes; (2) those with TCS and lumbosacral syrinxes; and (3) patients with lumbosacral syrinxes alone. The third group was included for comparison with the other two groups.

For clarification, the reader is reminded of the definitions for TSpC and TCS. The tethered spinal cord (TSpC) was defined by Hoffman et al. [6] as an elongated spinal cord attached to a thick filum terminale, causing dysfunction of the lumbosacral cord segments. Tethered cord syndrome (TCS) was defined by Yamada et al. [7–9] as a disorder characterized by impaired oxidative metabolism resulting from excessive tension within the spinal cord, anchored by an inelastic structure, such as a myelomeningocele, lipomyelomeningocele, tumor, or scar formation, in addition to a thick filum.

Additional specifications regarding the three groups of patients are as follows:

1. The spinal cord anchored by a thin fibrous filum terminale is included in group 1 (TSpC with lumbosacral syrinxes).
2. Group 2 is restricted to patients with TCS associated with occult spinal dysraphism, such as a lipoma, lipomyelomeningocele, or meningocele manqué. The myelomeningocele was excluded because of its complexity in presentation; many of these patients had signs and symptoms related to neuronal agenesis and scar formations.
3. The L1–S5 cord segments are normally located between the T10 and L2 vertebral bodies (Fig. 1). Therefore, in cases of an elongated spinal cord, the cord levels were carefully evaluated relative to the vertebral level.

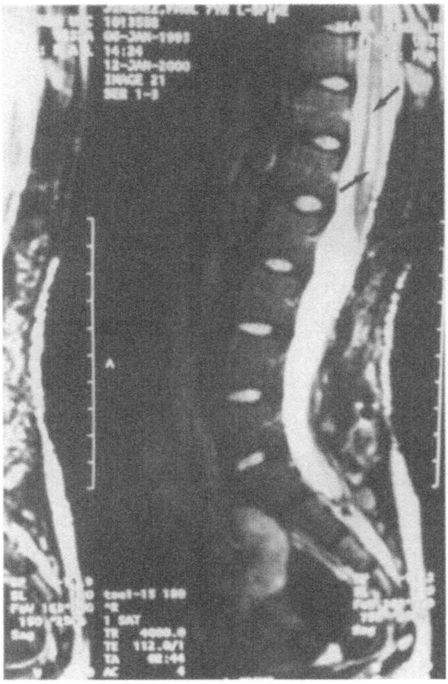

FIG. 1. Magnetic resonance imaging (MRI) of the syrinx demonstrated in one of the group 1 patients that is associated with tethered spinal cord (TSpC). The syrinx (*arrows*) extends from the T11 vertebral level to the middle of L2 vertebral level, located in the lumbosacral segment of the spinal cord with a normal length. Posterior displacement of the conus and apparently of the filum are noted

Case Analysis

Syringomyelia was found in 8 of the 145 patients (5.5%), with TSpC in the lumbosacral cord (group 1); and in 11 of 50 patients (22%) with TCS in the low thoracic and lumbosacral cord (group 2). The incidence of the latter is similar to that previously reported for syringomyelia and spinal dysraphism [3–5].

Of the eight patients who presented with TSpC and isolated lumbosacral syrinxes, three were males and five were females, with ages ranging from 1 to 14 years. The presenting signs and symptoms included weakness of some muscles in the lower extremities in seven cases, gait disturbance in six, complaint of pain in five, sensory deficit in two, incontinence in three, abnormal deep tendon reflexes in five (hypoactive in four and hyperactive in one), foot deformity in three, easily noticeable scoliosis (greater than 20°) in three, and an association with Chiari I malformation in three. Table 1 compares these incidences to the statistics for signs and symptoms of TCS in general, including an inelastic filum as well as related spinal dysraphism. Weakness in the lower extremities was found in more than 90% of the patients in all age groups. The pain complaint increases as patients grow older; sensory deficit is low in young children. Other signs are evenly distributed throughout all age groups.

Group 2 comprised 11 patients who presented with TCS associated with occult dysraphism and isolated lumbosacral or lower thoracic and lumbosacral syrinxes. The ages of the patients ranged from 1 to 19 years, with 1 patient aged 39 years; 5 were males and 6 were females. The signs and symptoms were similar to those in group 1: weakness in 11 patients, gait disturbance in 10 (4 of them in wheelchair), pain in 6,

TABLE 1. Statistics for tethered spinal cord (TSpC), lumbo sacral syringomyelia, and tethered cord syindrome (TCS) patients

TSpC and lumbosacral syringomyelia group 1 (8 patients):			
Age range:	1–14 years		
Gender:	3 males, 5 females		
Signs and symptoms:			
Muscle weakness	7		
Gait disturbance	6		
Pain	5		
Sensory deficit	2		
Incontinence	3		
Abnomal DTR	5		
Foot deformity	2		
TCS in general: 187 cases (1988–1999)			
Age groups (years):	0–9	10–19	>20
Signs and symptoms (%):			
Muscle weakness	96	90	90
Pain	7	50	98
Gait disturbance	81	70	70
Sensory deficit	48	90	93
Incontinence	61	50	73
Hyporeflexia	92	80	85
Leg deformity	74	80	75
Scoliosis	100	100	100

sensory change in 9 (2 with suspended analgesia), incontinence in 8, foot deformity in 9, and marked scoliosis in 4. However, 6 of these cases had some degree of permanent deficit, apparently resulting from congenital neuronal dysgenesis. Chiari I malformation was found in 6 and Chiari II in 1 patient.

The authors have also managed eight patients who presented with a syrinx in the thoracic and lumbosacral cord without associated TSpC or TCS (group 3). Signs and symptoms include motor deficit in eight patients, gait disturbance in eight, pain in eight (belt like pain in the lower trunk in two), sensory deficit in eight (suspended analgesia in three), incontinence in six, hyperreflexia with long tract signs in three, marked scoliosis in four, and wheelchair requirement in four (one of them stands by himself). Although the presenting symptoms were similar to those of groups 1 and 2, there were definite differences between this group and the first two:

1. The patients with syrinx alone had a higher incidence of burning or tingling pain in a beltlike distribution in two; long tract signs, thus tending to have more severe neurological deficit, in four; and severe scoliosis.
2. In contrast, TCS patients in general showed a patchy distribution of sensory changes and nonmyotomal motor deficit, as previously described [7–10].
3. Chiari malformations were found in all cases.

Imaging Studies

Magnetic resonance imaging (MRI) was the most reliable diagnostic imaging tool. However, in the early years of the diagnostic studies for this series (before MRI), metrizamide myelography was performed. This diagnostic study had the advantage of detecting the contrast material in the syrinx several hours after instillation, suggesting absorption of this material through the spinal cord substance. All the cases in the current series had definitive demonstration of the syrinx.

In group 1, TSpC was diagnosed by identifying a thick filum terminale or adipose filum attached to an elongated spinal cord or to a spinal cord of normal length. If the spinal cord was not elongated and the filum was not thick, a posteriorly displaced conus and filum and fat tissue in the filum tip were diagnostic for this category. In such cases, imaging was closely correlated to neurological signs and symptoms (mainly in adults), and the inelastic filum was confirmed at operation. In group 2, a lipoma, lipomyelomeningocele, or meningocele manqué was demonstrated by MRI. The myelomeningocele case was excluded from group 2 because of complex anomalies, including those of the cord, nerves and membranous covering, and connective tissue. In group 3, the syrinx was found to be isolated in the thoracic and lumbosacral cord, without evidence of cord tethering.

Surgical Techniques

Syringomyelia

Surgical techniques for promoting safe drainage of syrinxes have been described by Yamada [11]. Regardless of the size of the syrinx, it is reached via a posterior midline incision. After laminectomy of appropriate levels, the dura is opened. A short (less than 5 mm) arachnoid opening reveals a fine vertical midline in the dorsal surface of the cord. However, the midline can be easily lost after coagulating venous channels, particularly in the lower lumbar and sacral cord, which is crowded with venous channels on its dorsal surface. It is important to keep watching for small arterioles and venules approaching laterally toward the midline. These small (50-μm) vessels make a 90° turn vertically, cephalad or caudad, for a short distance and then disappear into the dorsal median sulcus (Fig. 2). Several of these landmarks allow determination of the exact midline.

Using a Beaver blade knife, the pia mater is incised in the midline. Rhoton's spatulas are used to separate the right and left posterior columns without damaging these long tracts until the syrinx is reached. Several arachnoid trabeculations are cut under the arachnoid membrane, and one end of the tube is inserted into the syrinx cavity and the other end into the subarachnoid space. After arachnoid closure with 8-0 nylon sutures (Fig. 3), unsectioned trabeculations surrounding the tube will hold it snugly, preventing its movement. No posterior column signs develop. This approach is similar to the technique used for anterior commissurotomy for pain control, except that no further sectioning is done anterior to the central canal, and is useful in preventing posterior column damage.

A translucent shunt tube (outer diameter, 2.5 mm) is impregnated with a radiopaque substance, which will help identify the location of the tube on plain x-ray films at any time after surgery.

Group 1: Tethered Spinal Cord

In group 1 patients, the prominent operative findings are that the filum terminale is fibrous or fibroadipose and resists stretching. In a normal individual, the filum can

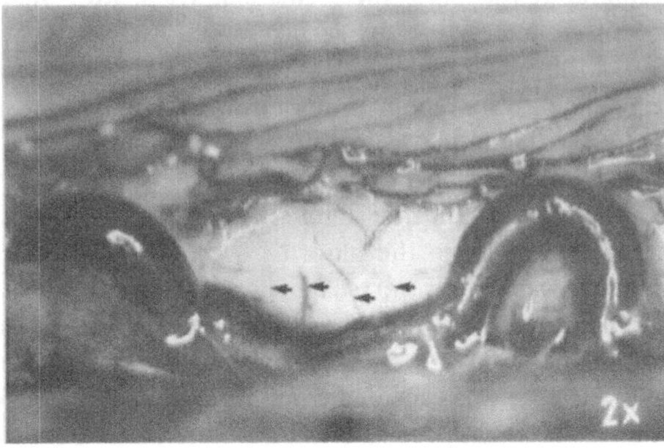

Fig. 2. The dorsal midline can be seen in this operative field, after the crowded larger veins are isolated from the dorsal surface of the lower lumbar and sacral cord. Four of the lateral arterioles and venules, less than 50 μm in diameter, are indicated by *arrows* on the left side of the midline. On reaching the midline, these tiny vessels turn 90° vertically cephalad or caudad, and then disappear into the dorsal median fissure. The midline is thus accurately determined

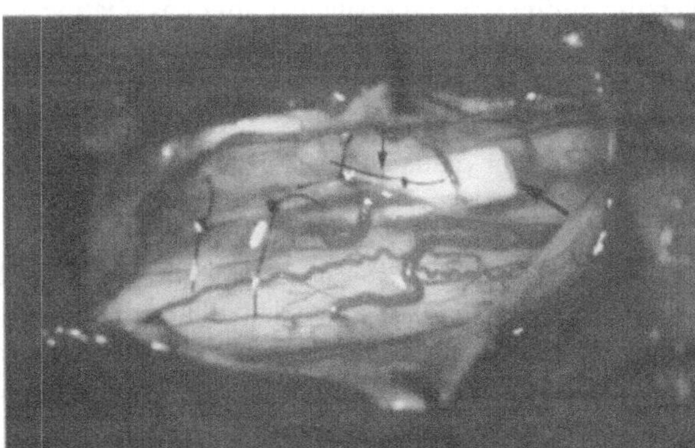

Fig. 3. After insertion of the shunt tube into the syrinx, the other end of the tube is passed into the subarachnoid space between the unsectioned arachnoid trabeculations. The five sutures placed through the arachnoid membrane secure watertight closure of the subarachnoid space, and the arachnoid trabeculations snugly hold the subarachonoid portion of the shunt tube. The *small arrow* points to the tube insertion through the dorsal midline into the syrinx, and the *large arrow* indicates the subrachnoid end of the tube. A 1.5-cm-long Sylastic tube 2.5 mm in diameter, cut off from the Lumboperitoneal Shunt T-tube (44520; PS-Medical, Goleta, CA, USA) was used

stretch to a length of at least 50% greater than the original length, but TSpC patients show filum elongation of less than 10% [12]. After resectioning the filum, the spinal cord jumps cephalad, usually 1 cm or more, due to the elasticity of the spinal cord. The oxidative metabolism can be evaluated by measuring the reduction:oxidation ratio (redox) of cytochrome a,a_3. This cytochrome is reduced before untethering but is reoxidized after the untethering. Reoxidation is a favorable sign for postoperative neurological improvement.

The surgical procedure includes a midline incision, laminectomy of an appropriate level, opening of the meninges, resection of a short segment of the filum for untethering of the spinal cord, and closure of the wound. Laminectomy levels are chosen to adequately cover the area where the tip of the filum is considered to be located. If the cord is located in the normal position, L2 and L3 laminectomy may be selected. A 2-cm incision in the midline of the dura mater is performed, followed by a 1-cm incision of the arachnoid membrane. The filum is found immediately underneath the arachnoid membrane. The filum is grasped at two points with the forceps, and pulled in opposite directions, i.e., one forceps caudad and the other cephalad [12]. Elongation less than 10% confirms the lack of elasticity. A 1-cm length of the filum may be resected. This distance between the sectioned ends prevents their postoperative reconnection. It is important to determine the exit of the lowest coccygeal nerve root, which is usually 100 μm in diameter under the microscope; this is the authors' strict rule for determining the border between the cord and the filum to prevent cord damage. The arachnoid and dura, although two separate layers, may be sutured together for watertight closure.

Group 2: Tethered Cord Syndrome

The basic techniques for untethering the tethered cord associated with a lipoma, lipomyelomeningocele, or meningocele manqué have been previously described [13] and are similar to those for treating the group 1 patients. After a midline skin incision or a vertical elliptical incision around the underlying fat tissue is made, laminectomy is performed one level above and one level below the spina bifida, and the normal dura is exposed. The fat tissue protruding through the pia arachnoid and dura mater is dissected from these membranes.

1. The caudal type. The fibroadipose tissue is transected through or immediately caudal to the lipoma–cord interface. The transection through the dura is, however, performed cephalad to the fusion of the dura and arachnoid to the fibroadipose tissue. This technique allows tight closure of the arachnoid and dura.
2. The dorsal type. The lipoma is removed from the spinal cord tissue. The plane of the lipoma dissection should be flush with the junction of the lipoma and surrounding cord tissue.
3. The transitional type. Transection through or slightly caudal to the lipoma–cord interface is performed first. The lipoma extending to the dorsal surface of the spinal cord is then dissected from the spinal cord. If a tight filum is found in the sac of a lipomyelomeningocele as an extension of the ventral end of the spinal cord, the filum should be resected as for the caudal type.

When the surgical procedure for Group 2 patients is complicated by a lipoma surrounding or extending into the spinal cord, it is important to limit lipoma resection to the degree of adequate untethering. In the transitional form of lipomyelomeningocele, the tight filum terminale must also be sectioned. The dermoid tumor must be removed completely; otherwise, it may regrow rapidly and cause chemical meningitis and scar formation around the spinal cord. It is emphasized that at least two layers of the pia arachnoid, dura mater, and reflected fascia be used to secure formation of the membrane covering the spinal cord and to maintain the subarachnoid space.

Results of Surgical Treatment

Group 1: Tethered Spinal Cord

All eight patients in group 1 underwent untethering procedures; four also underwent syrinx drainage at the time of the untethering procedure, three with a subarachnoid shunt and one with a midline dorsal myelotomy. All signs and symptoms were alleviated in all patients immediately after surgical treatment (after the untethering procedure alone in four patients and after the untethering procedure and drainage in four patients). One unshunted patient showed recurrent signs and symptoms 5 years after the untethering procedure. A lumbosacral syrinx was found on MRI and was shunted into the subarachnoid space; the patient's neurological condition then improved. Two patients who were not treated with shunting had small syrinxes that were considered unrelated to the signs and symptoms. All eight patients are ambulatory; six of them are walking normally and the other two have a mild degree of foot instability. One patient was found to have Chiari I malformation without related symptoms.

Group 2: Tethered Cord Syndrome

The results of surgical treatment for all group 2 patients were similar to those for the group 1 patients except for some associated symptoms of congenital origin (neuronal agenesis). Six of 11 patients had shunt drainage at the time of untethering: 4 with a subarachnoid shunt, 1 with a peritoneal shunt, and 1 with myelotomy. One additional patient underwent syrinx drainage 7 years after the untethering procedure. Three patients did not have shunt drainage because the syrinx was considered noncontributory to the neurological problems. The signs and symptoms were alleviated in all 8 patients after untethering and shunt drainage and in all 3 patients after untethering only. Three patients with preoperative wheelchair dependency became ambulatory with crutches. Three patients continue to require the use of a wheelchair, although motor function improved in the lower extremities in 2 of these patients. Chiari I malformation was found in 2 patients and Chiari II in 1 patient.

Illustrative Case

This 2.5-year-old boy presented with difficulty in walking; he demonstrated inversion of the left foot due to weakness of the peroneus longus muscle. An elongated split spinal cord was found buckled in an occult meningocele and reunited caudally. In addition, fixation of the spinal cord was found at two levels: at the L3 vertebral level cephalically and at the S1 level caudally, anchored by the fibroadipose filum. After the untethering procedure, he regained a normal gait. However, 7 years later, the family noted that his foot turned in when he walked rapidly. A syrinx was found at the L1 and L2 vertebral levels on MRI, i.e., in the lumbar segments of the elongated spinal cord. Motor and sensory deficits were exactly the same as before the untethering procedure 7 years previously. A 5-mm-diameter tense syrinx was drained via a subarachnoid shunt. The left foot regained normal function. At this operation, the lumbosacral cord was found to be straight (no longer buckled or stretched). This history describes the symptoms caused by functional abnormalities in the gray matter of the spinal cord that are common to both TCS and syringomyelia.

Group 3: Syrinx Only

Two of the eight group 3 patients (with syrinx alone) were treated with placement of a subarachnoid shunt, three with a peritoneal shunt and two with a pleural shunt. In one patient, no shunt was placed. After surgery, signs and symptoms were alleviated in five patients, and the three other patients continue to use a wheelchair although motor function improved.

Histological Findings

Each small biopsy specimen of the syrinx wall taken from 10 cases (from groups 1, 2, and 3) was examined with hematoxylin and eosin stain. Only fibrous tissue resembling the archnoid membrane was found, but no ependymal tissue was detected. These syrinxes were not strictly terminal ventricle (unless ependymal cells were hidden in the corner of the syrinx), and probably an extension of the syrinxes derived from the central canal but isolated from it.

Discussion

Group 1: Syringomyelia and Tethered Spinal Cord

Developmental processes can explain the low incidence of syrinxes associated with TSpC. Kunitomo [14] established that the primitive spinal cord fills the entire spinal canal by the 9th week of gestation. At the 11th week, the coccygeal medullary vestige is isolated from the newly formed permanent spinal cord and filum. The caudal end of the primitive spinal cord is surrounded by mesodermal tissue, in which the vestige remains immersed after its separation (Fig. 4). Therefore, it is postulated that if at this stage the embryo fails to separate the coccygeal medullary vestige, fibrous tissue continues to grow to replace ependymal tissue in the filum, which consequently loses its elasticity [14]. The amount of fibrous tissue that grows may be variable, forming a thick, thin, or fibroadipose filum.

The terminal ventricle is formed at the 6th to 7th gestational week, much earlier than the separation of the coccygeal medullary vestige [14]. It is unlikely that fibrosis of the filum contributes to the formation of the syrinx, which is closely related to the terminal ventricle.

Group 2: Syringomyelia and Tethered Cord Syndrome

It is natural that the incidence of syrinxes associated with spinal dysraphism is higher, because the neurulation process is already involved in central canal formation at 4 to

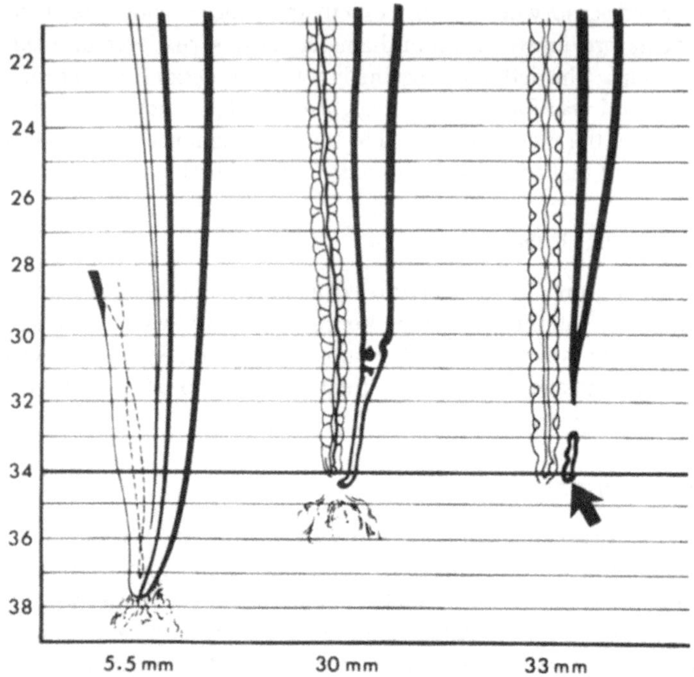

FIG. 4. Diagrammatic illustrations of the spinal cord in the developing embryo. The two images on the *left* show the mesodermal tissue surrounding the caudal end of the primitive spinal cord. On the *right*, the coccygeal medullary vestige is shown to be separated from the newly formed permanent filum and spinal cord (at 11 weeks). The vestige remains immersed in the mesodermal environment (*arrow*) as the permanent filum is freed from the mesodermal tissue. (Reproduced by permission from [24])

5 weeks of gestation. The ventriculus terminalis derives from the caudal part of the cephalic central canal at 6–7 weeks of gestation whereas the caudal part of the central canal becomes atrophic at 5 weeks. The lumbosacral syrinxes are either the remnant of the ventriculus terminalis or extension (or expansion) of the central canal.

Correlation of Pathophysiology with Symptomatology

Tethered cord syndrome is a unique diagnostic category that requires explanations for pathophysiology, symptomatology, and treatment. When the vertebral column grows faster than the spinal cord or when the spine is forcibly flexed or extended, the tension within the spinal cord increases beyond its tolerance. Strain develops between the attachment of the lowest pair of dentate ligaments and the caudal end of the spinal cord, which is anchored by an inelastic structure. Therefore, the symptomatology of TCS never extends to the thoracic or cervical cord, unless additional pathology exists in these cord levels.

The following should be considered when diagnosing patients with TCS or TSpC and syringomyelia.

1. The diagnosis of TCS is based on functional impairment of spinal cord neurons. This nomenclature is different from the anatomically based diagnosis of Chiari malformation, which is characterized by descension of the cerebellum and brainstem but lacks explicit correlation with symptomatology.
2. The diagnosis of TSpC relies heavily on a combination of an elongated spinal cord and a thick filum. These abnormalities are not essential for the diagnosis of TCS in many adults.
3. Tethered cord syndrome is a gray matter disease. If any long tract sign is found, neuronal dysgenesis or additional trauma to the tethered cord must be considered.

Infants with TCS present with dribbling of urine early in life. It is important to tell parents to observe diapers every 15 min for a few hours a day. If there is no dry period, they should consult a physician. Skin stigmata include a dimple, a tuft of hair, fatty swelling, and a dermal sinus in the lumbar or sacral area. Foot deformity, pes equinus, and different sizes of feet are common. Any degree of spinal dysraphism should be recognized [8,15]. Young children with TCS show progression of the following symptoms: (1) beginning to stumble after walking normally; (2) beginning to dribble urine after successful toilet training; (3) foot drop; (4) a painless sore; and (5) scoliosis. These symptoms must be quickly detected for prompt surgical treatment.

The spinal cord has its own viscoelasticity, and glial tissue protects neurons from distortion and stretching to maintain proper neuronal function. There are certain rules that regulate the elongation rate and traction weight applied to the spinal cord [7–9]:

1. The greater the weight, the greater the elongation.
2. The lower and thinner the spinal cord, the greater the elongation.
3. Elongation of the filum terminale is far greater than that of any cord segments. Therefore, the filum functions as a buffer to protect the spinal cord from overstretching. This conclusion is supported by another experiment: placing a ligature at the caudal end of the spinal cord. Each spinal cord segment was elongated much more than when tractioned with a ligature on the filum.

Before elongation studies, oxidative metabolism was evaluated by measuring cytochrome a,a_3 in vivo by reflectance spectrophotometry. Consistent results were obtained:

1. The greater the traction weight, the more reduced the cytochrome a,a_3 in spinal cord mitochondria.
2. The higher the reduction, the more impaired the oxidative metabolism and the lesser the energy production.
3. The lower the cord segment, the more reduced the cytochrome a,a_3; This explains the high incidence of incontinence.

There is a parallelism between the elongation rate, oxidative metabolism impairment, and evoked potential deterioration. The latter indicates that increases in neurological dysfunction are correlated with worsening of these factors. After release of high-grade weight traction, the cord length, oxidation metabolism, and evoked potentials slowly return to normal, whereas after low-grade or medium traction, these return to normal immediately. These findings correspond to the better surgical results when untethering procedures are done in the early stages of TCS.

Regardless of weight increases, no histological changes were noted on light microscopy [7–9,11]. Electron microscopy showed only wrinkles of cell membranes after release of traction. Stretching membranes during traction may explain the basis for metabolic and physiological changes. Horseradish peroxidase transport studies have shown no prolongation in axonal transport under traction with any weight.

Older children and adults complain of moderate to severe back and leg pain, which is aggravated by exercise, particularly those involving flexion–extension of the spine, and by lifting a weight. Weakness is found either in small muscles only (e.g., the extensor hallucis longus) or extensively in the lower limbs without corresponding to a myotomal pattern [8,9,12]. In some patients, weakness of these muscles is found only when the patient lowers the heels or the balls of the feet or shows inversion or eversion of feet on tiptoe or heel walking. Reflexes are hypoactive in at least one of the knee or ankle tendons corresponding to gray matter lesions. Sensory deficits are usually patchy in a wide distribution, frequently in the dorsum of the feet, around the perianal area, and anywhere in the lower extremities, but not above the L1 dermatomes.

Differential diagnoses includes nervous system, skeletal or disk, and vascular system disorders:

1. Spinal cord lesions: intramedullary lesions, such as gliomas, syringomyelia, arteriovenous malformation, and poliomyelitis; and extramedullary lesions, i.e., epidural or intradural tumors
2. Peripheral neuropathy, Friedreich's ataxia, Charcot-Marie-Tooth disease, familial diplegia
3. Incomplete paraplegia of any type, birth injury, or accident-related spinal injury (recovery period)
4. Scoliosis (e.g., tumor bearing or congenital)
5. Neurofibromatosis
6. Disk hernia
7. Spondylolysis or spondylolisthesis
8. Osteoarthritic spondylosis
9. Multiple sclerosis

The differential diagnoses of disk hernia, spondylolysis or spondylolisthesis, osteoarthritic spondylosis, and multiple sclerosis are particularly important to consider in adult patients.

Hydrodynamic Aspect of Isolated Syringomyelia

An understanding of the pathogenesis and hydrodynamics are important for treating syrinxes, which have been clearly explained by other authors [16–20]. It may be equally important to understand another mechanism involved in enlargement of an isolated lumbosacral syrinx.

Signs and symptoms of syringomyelia have been previously described [17,21–23]; these are due to cavitation of the central spinal cord, often destroying the secondary pain fibers in and near the anterior white commissure and anterior horn cells. The expansion of the syrinx and its increased internal pressure are often the causes of aggravation of these signs. It is the general opinion that decompression of the syrinx fluid is effective in alleviating the signs and symptoms or preventing their progression [3–5,22]. Burning and tingling pain in the totally analgesic area, associated with preservation of other sensory modalities, is often relieved after syrinx decompression.

The mechanism is probably an osmotic one, as the following explanation may demonstrate. In CT myelography, metrizamide instilled into the lumbar subarachnoid space is also demonstrated in the syrinx. In other cases, metrizamide has been found to fill the syrinx 4–5h after instilling the agent into the subarachnoid space [16]. It is probable that metrizamide is absorbed from the subarachnoid space into the bloodstream, circulates through the spinal cord, and later diffuses into the syrinx through its fibrous wall (which the authors observed in the biopsy specimens). This effect results in high osmotic pressure, and the syrinx imbibes water from the surrounding tissue. Thus, the pressure in the syrinx continues to increase and the syrinx enlarges. Any small molecular material, such as metrizamide (molecular weight, 789), can act as an osmotic agent.

Imaging Studies

The MRI findings were described earlier. Metrizamide myelography was found to be valuable for finding noncommunicating syringomyelia, as discussed next. Imaging studies are also important in diagnosing TSpC or TCS.

Interpretation of the Surgical Results

The patients with lumbosacral syrinx and TSpC (group 1) presented with mild or, less frequently, moderate neurological dysfunction. Six of the eight patients in this group regained normal or nearly normal function after untethering and syrinx drainage. These results are similar to the surgical results of untethering in the patients with TSpC only. Untethering and syrinx drainage in the patients with TSpC appears to be the most appropriate treatment, particularly for those who have dermatomal sensory deficit to pain stimulus and pain complaint in the analgesic area. These signs and symptoms are clearly different from those caused by TCS in general, as described in the symptomatology section.

The patient with a lower thoracic and lumbosacral syrinx can develop rapidly progressive neurological deficits. Although congenital neuronal agenesis can be one of the factors, a tethered spinal cord and syrinx must be seriously considered as the causes of the neurological deficits. Decision making for performing untethering and syrinx drainage in acute cases requires an understanding of the basic neurological problems correlated with imaging studies.

The patient with a thoracic and lumbosacral syrinx without associated TCS may be treated by various methods, including decompressive suboccipital craniectomy for correction of cerebrospinal fluid (CSF) flow impairment related to the Chiari malformation.

Syringomyelia and Spinal Dysraphism

There is a general agreement among authors who published articles on the combination of lower thoracic and lumbosacral syringomyelia and spinal dysraphism that shunting syrinxes of a significant size is of benefit to alleviate or prevent the progression of neurological signs and symptoms [3–5]. The combination of syringomyelia, when discussed as an anatomic abnormality, and TCS, as a functional disorder, is difficult to analyze. From the authors' experience with a limited number of cases with a combination of syringomyelia and TCS, they have observed that group 1 patients with TSpC are less in number (5.5%) than group 2 patients with TCS associated with occult spinal dysraphism (22%). The group 1 patients also tend to have milder neurological deficit and better postoperative neurological improvement than the group 2 patients. In addition, the incidence of postoperative complications in group 1 patients, such as adhesion of the spinal cord to the surrounding tissue, is less than that in the group 2 patients. Untethering of the spinal cord by resection of an inelastic filum or adequate removal of the lipoma and drainage of a syrinx of significant size (3 mm or greater) with insertion of a syringosubarachoid shunt tube result in neurological improvement. The authors agree with anatomic correction of the isolated lumbosacral syrinx, as advocated by other authors [3–5].

At this time, no clear-cut distinction exists between the indication for syrinx draining of a large versus a smaller syrinx. The authors rely on the symptomatology when making the decision about whether shunt drainage should be performed. The hydrodynamics of the syrinx and compliance of surrounding cord tissue are crucial to the efficacy of shunting procedures. This situation is similar to placing a ventricular shunt for hydrocephalus. The purpose of a ventriculoperitoneal shunt is to normalize abnormally high CSF pressure. However, neurological improvement in ventricular shunt patients is not always associated with a decrease in the ventricular size to normal, and a large ventricle is not always associated with increased pressure (normal pressure hydrocephalus).

Unfortunately, intrasyrinx pressure is difficult to measure, mainly because the volume of the syrinx fluid is so small. The purpose of drainage of a large syrinx is not only to normalize the pressure, but also, and more importantly, to relieve or prevent hydrodynamic stress caused by an imbalance between the positional changes, as discussed previously [16–20]. For this reason, a syringosubarachnoid shunt for an isolated lower thoracic and lumbosacral syrinx is more effective than a shunt to the extraspinal space (such as a pleural or peritoneal shunt) in constantly maintaining the pressure balance between the syrinx and the subarachnoid space, even with postural changes, lying, sitting, standing, or the Trendelenburg position.

As in the early phase of hydrocephalus, a small syrinx may have increased internal pressure. The next case is an example of a small syrinx that was treated effectively by drainage of the syrinx, which was found isolated from the fourth ventricle by obex inspection.

Illustrative Case

This 47-year-old woman presented with typical signs of isolated cervical syringomyelia (as described in the Introduction). However, the myelogram with instillation of contrast as well as air showed a normal-sized spinal cord. (The studies were performed before the availability of computed tomography [CT] and MRI.) At the 2-year follow-up, symptomatic worsening was clearly indicated. The patient underwent cervical laminectomy and dural opening; no swelling or atrophy of the spinal cord was noted. However, a dorsal midline myelotomy approach toward the central canal allowed the exposure of a syrinx only 2–3 mm wide. After a 1-cm myelotomy, the patient was relieved of pain, with improvement in motor and sensory functions and return to normal activity for another 10 years until she died of an unrelated disease.

Erkan et al. [5] reported a provocative cases of terminal syringomyelia in association with TCS and included an exhaustive clinical analysis. Several authors critiqued the analysis, stating that the number of cases was not large enough to make statistically based conclusions This criticism is particularly true regarding the difference between the results of patients with cord untethering only and those with both cord untethering and syrinx. We have found that the percentage of each neurological symptoms and signs that Erkan et al. observed is significantly less than those observed in our group 1 and 2 patients. It is conceivable that if the examiners look for subtle changes that occur in TCS, minimal neurological defects may be found in a larger number of cases. The division of syringomyelia cases into three groups provides clear differences between the syrinx patients with TSpC and those with TCS (associated with lipoma, lipomyelomeningocele, or meingocele manqué with occult spinal dysraphism), and further between these two groups and patients with syrinx at the thoracolumbosacral level.

Conclusions

Patients with a syrinx associated with TSpC have a good outcome when untethering and syrinx drainage procedures are done. If signs and symptoms are significant for syringeal signs, such as suspended analgesia or burning pain, the syrinx should be drained. It is preferable to shunt into the subarachnoid space for a syrinx of 3 mm or greater in horizontal diameter, and to perform a midline myelotomy for the syrinx of less than 3 mm. In cases of expanded, tense syrinxes associated with occult dysraphic TCS, one should consider placing a syringosubarachnoid shunt. A syringoperitoneal or pleural shunt should be selected if the subarachnoid space is occluded with adhesions.

Signs and symptoms caused by tethered cord and those by syrinx are often indistinguishable. Subarachnoid shunting is the most logical draining procedure because the equilibrium of syrinx pressure and CSF pressure is optimally maintained regardless of any positional changes or respiratory pressure fluctuation.

References

1. Oliver d'Angers CP (1824) De la Moelle Epiniere et de ses Maladies. Chez Crevot, Paris
2. Foster JB (1991) Neurology of syringomyelia. In: Batzdorf U (ed) Syringomyelia: Current concepts in diagnosis and treatment. Williams & Wilkins, Baltimore, pp 91–115

3. Iskandar BJ, Oakes WJ, McLaughlin C, et al (1994) Terminal syringomyelia and occult spinal dysraphism. J Neurosurg 81:513–519
4. Koyanagi I, Iwasaki Y, Hida K, et al (1997) Surgical treatment of syringomyelia associated with dysraphism. Childs Nerv Syst 13:194–200
5. Erkan K, Unal F, Kiris T (1999) Syringomyelia in association with the tethered cord syndrome. Neurosurgery 45:1351–1360
6. Hoffman HJ, Hendrick EB, Humphreys RP (1976) The tethered cord: its protean manifestations, diagnosis and surgical implications. Childs Brain 2:145–155
7. Yamada S, Zinke DE, Sanders DC (1981) Pathophysiology of "tethered cord syndrome." J Neurosurg 54:494–503
8. Yamada S, Iacono RP, Andrade T, et al (1995) Pathophysiology of tethered cord syndrome. Neurosurg Clin N Am 6:311–323
9. Yamada S, Iacono RP, Yamada BS (1996) Pathophysiology of tethered cord syndrome. In: Yamada S (ed) Tethered cord syndrome. American Association of Neurological Surgeons, Park Ridge, IL, pp 29–48
10. McLone DG, Dauser RC (1996) The tethered cervical spinal cord. In: Yamada S (ed) Tethered cord syndrome. American Association of Neurological Surgeons, Park Ridge, IL, pp 99–102
11. Yamada S (1983) Microsurgery: syringomyelia, section X. In: Austin GM (ed) The spinal cord. Igaku Shoin, Tokyo, pp 413–444
12. Yamada S, Iacono RP, Morgese V, et al (1996) Tethered cord syndrome in adults. In: Menezes AH, Sonntag VH (eds) Principles of spinal surgery. McGraw-Hill, New York, pp 433–445
13. Yamada S, Lonser RR, Yamada SM, et al (1996) Tethered cord syndrome associated with myelomeningoceles and lipomyelomeningoceles. In: Yamada S (ed) Tethered cord syndrome. American Association of Neurological Surgery. Park Ridge, IL, pp 103–123
14. Kunitomo K (1918) The development and reduction of the caudal end of the spinal cord. Contrib Embryol Carnegie Inst 8:161–198
15. Pang D (1986) Tethered cord syndrome. In: Hoffman HJ (ed) Advances in pediatric neurosurgery. Hanley & Belfus, Philadelphia, pp 45–80
16. Heiss JD, Patronas N, DeVroom HL, et al (1999) Elucidating the pathophysiology of syringomyelia. J Neurosurg 91:553–562
17. Batzdorf U, Klepkamp J, Johnson JP (1998) A critical appraisal of syrinx cavity shunting procedures. J Neurosurg 89:382–388
18. Menezes A (2000) Indication for fusion of the craniovertebral junction. Lecture at the 16th annual meeting, section on disorders of the spine and peripheral nerves of the American Association of Neurological Surgeons and Congress of Neurological Surgeons, Indian Hills, CA, February 23–26, 2000
19. Milhorat TH, Kotzen RM, Anzil AP (1994) Stenosis of central canal of spinal cord in man: incidence and pathological finding: cases. J Neurosurg 80:716–722
20. Milhorat TH, Johnson WD, Miller JI, et al (1992) Surgical treatment of syringomyelia based on magnetic resonance imaging criteria. Neurosurgery 31:231–245
21. Barnett HJM, Jousse AT, Ball MJ (1973) Syringomyelia. Saunders, London, pp 179–219
22. Barnett HJM (1973) Syringomyelia. Saunders, London, pp 179–219
23. Gardner WJ (1965) Hydrodynamic mechanism of syringomyelia: its relationship to myelocele. J Neurol Neurosurg Psychiatry 28:247–259
24. Yamada S, Iacono R (1995) 10. Tethered cord syndrome. In: Pang D (ed) Disorders of the pediatric spine. Raven, New York

Surgical Management of Syringomyelia with Craniosynostosis

Yasuko Yoshida, Reizo Shirane, and Takashi Yoshimoto

Summary. Chronic tonsillar herniation (CTH) is a relatively frequent finding by magnetic resonance (MR) imaging studies in patients with craniosynostosis. Formation of a syrinx is also sometimes recognized by MR imaging. This study evaluated the appropriate surgical approach. Cranial reconstructive surgery was performed in 29 pediatric patients with craniosynostosis from 1989 to 1999. All patients underwent MR imaging before operation. Three patients with Crouzon's syndrome had CTH and syringomyelia; in 2, the formation of CTH and syringomyelia was observed during the follow-up period after the diagnosis of craniosynostosis. Supratentorial cranial decompression surgery resulted in disappearance of their symptoms and reduction of the syrinx in 1 patient and no change in another patient. Formation of syrinx with CTH in craniosynostosis may be caused by increased supratentorial intracranial pressure with a small posterior fossa. We propose that decompression of the supratentorial cranium is the first choice of surgical treatment.

Key words. Syrinx, Craniosynostosis, Chronic tonsillar herniation

Introduction

Chronic tonsillar herniation (CTH) is relatively frequently demonstrated by magnetic resonance (MR) imaging in patients with craniosynostosis. Formation of a syrinx is also sometimes recognized by MR imaging. This study investigated the pathophysiology and appropriate surgical management of this disease.

Materials and Methods

Cranial reconstructive surgery was performed in 29 pediatric patients with craniosynostosis, 10 girls and 19 boys aged from 1 month to 11 years, from 1989 to 1999. The diagnosis of craniosynostosis was based on skull radiography and brain computed tomography (CT) (Table 1). All patients also underwent craniospinal MR imaging and cine-MR imaging flow analysis before and after surgery.

Department of Neurosurgery, Tohoku University, School of Medicine, 1-1-1 Seiryo-cho, Aoba-ku, Sendai 980-8574, Japan

TABLE 1. Patients with syringomyelia and craniosynostosis

Syndromic craniosynostosis	
Crouzon's syndrome	3/8 (cases)
Apert's syndrome	0/1
Nonsyndromic craniosynostosis	
Scaphocephaly	0/6
Brachycephaly	0/3
Trigonocephaly	0/2
Oxycephaly	0/3
Plagiocephaly	0/4
Complex	0/2

TABLE 2. Summary of patients with craniosynostosis and chronic tonsillar herniation

Case no.	Age at discovery of: Craniosynostosis	Chronic tonsillar herniation	Hydrocephalus	Syringomyelia	Symptoms
1	9 months	10 months	9 months	6 years	Dyspnea
2	2 years	7 years	7 years	7 years	Headache, vomiting
3	At birth	11 years	At birth	11 years	Scoliosis, muscle atrophy, trunkal ataxia, hypesthesia of bilateral C4-Th6

TABLE 3. Summary of surgical treatment

Case no.	Surgical treatment: First operation	Second operation	Outcome
1	Biparietal skull morcellation, VP shunt	Frontal advancement and biparietal skull morecellation	Improvement, syrinx reduced
2	Frontal advancement and VP shunt	Suboccipital decompression, C1 laminectomy	Improvement, syrinx unchanged
3	Foramen magnum decompression	—	Improvement, but died after 5 months

VP, ventriculo peritoneal.

Results

Three patients had CTH and three patients had symptomatic syrinx with CTH and hydrocephalus with Crouzon's syndrome (Table 2). The process of formation of CTH was observed during the follow-up period after the diagnosis of craniosynostosis in two of these latter three patients.

Supratentorial cranial decompression surgery was performed first (Table 3), followed by frontal advancement for case 1, and foramen magnum decompression and ventriculoperitoneal (VP) shunting for case 2. Additional surgical procedures were selected after craniospinal MR imaging. The symptoms disappeared and the syrinx was reduced in case 1 and unchanged in case 2. Foramen magnum decompression and C1 laminectomy were first performed in an 11-year-old boy with a symptomatic holocord syrinx (case 3). His symptoms were all improved after surgery and he went home, but he died at home suddenly at dinner 3 months after surgery.

Illustrative Case

Case 1 was a 6-year-old girl with Crouzon's syndrome underwent frontal advancement and VP shunt at age 1 year. She developed uneventfully until age 6 years, when she experienced respiratory and gait disorder, soon followed by respiratory arrest that required tracheotomy. She also suffered sleep apnea, when her O_2 saturation decreased to 60%. T_2-weighted MR imaging showed slight ventriculomegaly and little subarachnoid space on the brain surface. Despite shunt revision, her status did not change. MR imaging revealed tonsillar herniation and syringobulbia, which were not recognized in infancy. We considered that this pathophysiology was not the same as a Chiari malformation. CTH and syringomyelia in Crouzon's syndrome may be caused by elevation of intracranial pressure, which results from closure of the coronal and lambdoid sutures. Foramen magnum decompression in the presence of increased intracranial supratentorial pressure would lead to further herniation of the posterior fossa contents. Therefore, we performed frontal advancement and biparietal skull morcellation to reduce the supratentorial pressure. Postoperatively, her syrinx, syringobulbia, and tonsillar herniations were improved and the respiratory arrest and sleep apnea disappeared. She continues to be in good condition at age 11 years.

Discussion

CTH associated with craniosynostosis was first reported in 5 patients, all with Crouzon's syndrome, in 1992 [1]. The incidence of CTH was 72.7% in 44 patients with Crouzon's syndrome and 1.9% in 51 patients with Apert's syndrome [2]. The high incidence of CTH in patients with Crouzon's syndrome may be related to the premature synostosis of the lambdoid suture in the first 24 months of life. All patients in the series with Crouzon's syndrome and progressive hydrocephalus had CTH [2]. The association of hydrocephalus and craniosynostosis has been well documented and reported [3,4]. This retrospective study of 1727 cases found hydrocephalus was present before surgery in 12 cases and developed after surgery in 10 cases with Crouzon's syndrome.

Abnormal cerebrospinal fluid hydrodynamics may occur in Crouzon's syndrome as a complex succession of events takes place in the first 2 years of life. Early closure of the lambdoid sutures causing crowding in the posterior fossa may increase venous outflow resistance by compressing the sigmoid sinus, and hindbrain herniation may increase cerebrospinal fluid outflow resistance [5]. Therefore, CTH may be caused by closure of the coronal and lambdoid sutures. We propose that the narrowing of the supratentorial cranium between the coronal and lambdoid closed sutures occurs first. A small posterior fossa and hydrocephalus may be involved in the formation of CTH and syringomyelia. We propose that expansive skull plasty covering the coronal and lambdoid closed sutures should be the first surgical treatment for patients with CTH and Crouzon's syndrome. Foramen magnum decompression alone may cause further hindbrain herniation.

Conclusion

Syringomyelia with craniosynostosis associated with hydrocephalus and CTH is caused by the early closure of the lambdoid sutures, resulting in crowding in the posterior fossa in Crouzon's syndrome. We propose expansive skull plasty covering the coronal and lambdoid closed sutures as the first surgical treatment for patients with CTH and Crouzon's syndrome. Foramen magnum decompression alone may cause further hindbrain herniation. We recommend staged surgical treatment with VP shunting or suboccipital decompression and foramen magnum decompression for patients with progressive hydrocephalus or syringomyelia who show no improvements in their symptoms.

References

1. Francis PM, Beals S, Rekate HL, et al (1992) Chronic tonsillar herniation and Crouzon's syndrome. Pediatr Neurosurg 18:202–206
2. Cinalli G, Renier D, Sebag G, et al (1995) Chronic tonsillar herniation in Crouzon's and Apert's syndromes: the role of premature synostosis of the lambdoid suture. J Neurosurg 83:575–582
3. Hayward R, Harkness W, Kendall B, et al (1992) Magnetic resonance imaging in the assessment of craniosynostosis. Scand J Plast Reconstr Hand Surg 26:293–299
4. Cinalli G, Sainte-Rose C, Kollar EM, et al (1998) Hydrocephalus and craniosynostosis. J Neurosurg 88:209–214
5. Rollins N, Booth T, Shapiro K (2000) MR venography in children with complex craniosynostosis. Pediatr Neurosurg 32:308–315

Pathophysiology and Treatment of Syringomyelia Associated with Tuberculous Meningitis

Tatsuya Nagashima, Kazuki Yamamoto, Shogo Tamura, Mitsugu Nakamura, Abesh Kumar Bhattacharjee, Kanak Kanti Barua, and Norihiko Tamaki

Summary. Syringomyelia associated with tuberculous meningitis tends to be intractable because of its complex pathophysiology. There is almost always a long interval between the diagnosis of tuberculous meningitis and the onset of syringomyelia. Magnetic resonance imaging (MRI) findings, hydrodynamics, pathophysiology, and treatment of this difficult condition were analyzed. We treated five cases of syringomyelia associated with tuberculous meningitis with an age distribution from 35 to 72 years old. Syringomyelia developed 6 months to 30 years after tuberculous meningitis. All patients showed incomplete or total paraplegia, sensory deficit below the thoracic level, and ascending sensory-motor disturbance of the upper extremities. All were examined with MRI. Cine-MRI and computed tomography (CT) myelography were useful for assessing patency of the subarachnoid space. When the cranial subarachnoid space was intact, a syringosubarachnoid (SS) shunt was selected, but when it was obliterated, a syringoperitoneal (SP) shunt was selected. Three patients underwent an SP shunt and one underwent an SS shunt. A flexible endoscope helped with accurate placement of the shunt tube in the subarachnoid space. Local arachnoid adhesion was dissected, and expansive dural plasty was performed with an artificial dural patch to prevent postoperative adhesion. In two cases, arachnoid adhesion was so diffuse that aggressive dissection could not be performed. The surgically treated patients were neurologically stable after the last operation. Careful dissection of arachnoid adhesion and reestablishment of normal cerebrospinal fluid (CSF) hydrodynamics is essential. For diffuse arachnoid adhesion, an SP shunt should be used.

Key words. Syringomyelia, Arachnoiditis, MRI, Tuberculous meningitis

Introduction

Despite effective chemotherapy, syringomyelia may develop following tuberculous meningitis (TM). Surgical treatment of the syringomyelia associated with TM has been difficult and often results in deterioration. We present the results of a surgical treatment procedure for this complicated condition.

Department of Neurosurgery, Kobe University, Graduate School of Medicine, 7-5-1 Kusunoki-cho, Chuo-ku, Kobe 650-0017, Japan

Materials and Methods

Five cases of syringomyelia subsequent to TM were studied with magnetic resonance imaging (MRI). The three women and two men ranged in age from 35 to 75 years old. Typical clinical presentation was increasing atrophy, weakness, and sensory disturbance of upper limbs following long-term paraparesis caused by tuberculous meningomyelitis. The interval between initial symptoms and surgical treatments ranged from 2 to 10 years (mean, 5.8 years). Four of the cases were surgically treated, one with arachnoid dissection and a syringosubarachnoid (SS) shunt, two with a syringoperitoneal (SP) shunt, and one with a syringopleural shunt following the initial SS shunt and arachnoid dissection. One patient was treated conservatively because the syrinx was too small for placement of a shunt tube.

Results

All surgical cases showed improvement in terms of ascending neurological signs. Three of four patients did not undergo dissection of the arachnoid adhesion, but have maintained a stable neurological condition and collapse of the syrinx as seen on MRI. Two cases showed no recurrence of syrinx 5, 6, and 9 years after the operations, while one suffered recurrence of the syrinx due to SS shunt obstruction 1 year after the operation despite extensive dissection of the arachnoid adhesion. The patient who did not undergo any surgical treatment showed gradual deterioration and became wheelchair-bound 3 years after the onset of syringomyelic symptoms.

Case Reports

Case 1

A 35-year-old male patient gradually developed paraparesis 6 months after he suffered tuberculous meningitis. The patient underwent an SS shunt and a revision of the procedure at another hospital 2 years after meningitis. Two years after the second shunting operation, the patient complained of increasing weakness, sensory disturbance, pain, and muscle atrophy of the upper extremities. He was then transferred to our department. On admission, the patient showed paraplegia and muscle atrophy of the right hand. MRI showed a tuberculoma with calcification in the T6 spinal cord, an ascending thin syrinx up to the C4 spinal cord, and a descending large syrinx in the thoracolumbar spinal cord (Fig. 1). Myelography revealed complete blockage at the level of the tuberculoma. Brain computed tomography (CT) showed no hydrocephalus.

At the operation, a diffuse and thick arachnoid adhesion was observed around the spinal cord. The tuberculoma was removed by sharp dissection, and after syringostomy an SP shunt was performed. The arachnoid adhesion was so severe that arachnoid lysis was not attempted in this case.

After the operation, pain in the upper extremities improved. Muscle atrophy in the hand improved 2 years after the operation. The patient's neurological condition has been stable for 7 years since the operation. The postoperative MRI showed decreased syrinx in the cervical spinal cord.

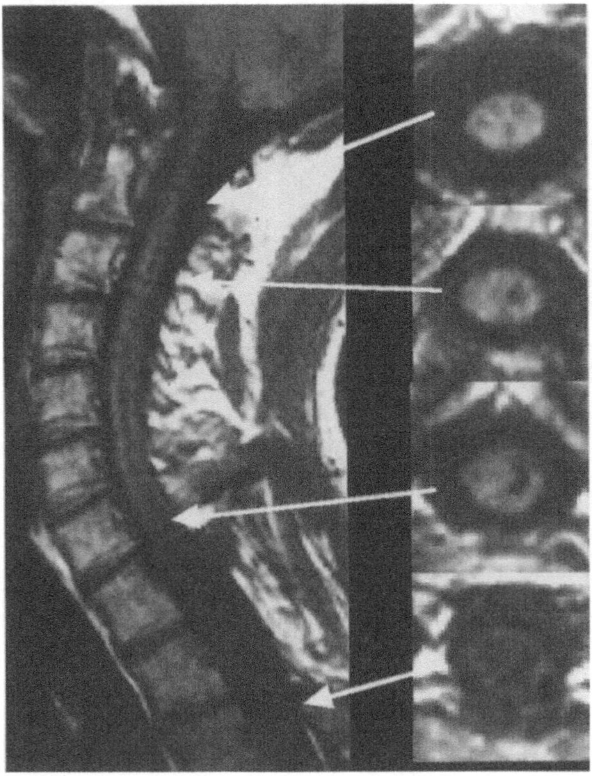

FIG. 1. Case 1. T_1-weighted magnetic resonance imaging (MRI) of the cervical spinal cord shows a small syrinx ascending to the C3 level. A large syrinx is seen in the thoracic spinal cord (*arrows*). A tuberculoma, which is not shown in this figure, was located in the midthoracic spinal cord

Case 2

A 49-year-old woman began to feel weakness in the bilateral lower extremities 27 years after she suffered tuberculous meningitis. She then began to complain of pain and weakness in the right upper extremity. Neurological examination at admission revealed weakness of the right upper extremity and paraparesis. Deep tendon reflex of the right upper and lower extremities and the left lower extremity had increased, but that of the left upper extremity had decreased. The bilateral Babinski reflex was positive. MRI revealed a large syrinx in the cervicothoracic spinal cord that extended up to the C5 level (Fig. 2). Cine-MRI showed no pulsatile movement of the fluid in the syrinx and subarachnoid space, which indicated diffuse adhesion of the subarachnoid space (Fig. 3). An SP shunt was placed at the most dilated part of the syrinx. The syrinx decreased in size postoperatively, and neurological symptoms of the upper extremities improved (Fig. 4). The size of the syrinx has remained unchanged for 4 years, and the patient's neurological condition has remained stable. Paraparesis has not improved.

Discussion

Despite effective chemotherapy for tuberculous meningitis, late complications such as hydrocephalus, syringomyelia, cranial nerve palsy, myelopathy, and vascular obstruction may occur. Appleby et al. reported that two of six cases of syringomyelia

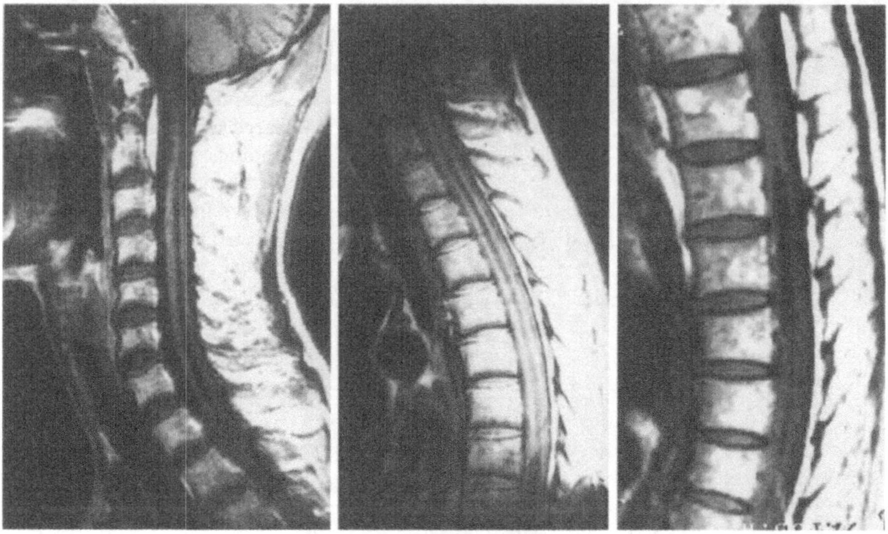

FIG. 2. Case 2. T_1-weighted MRI of the cervical spinal cord revealed a small syrinx ascending to the T2 level. A large syrinx is seen below the midthoracic level

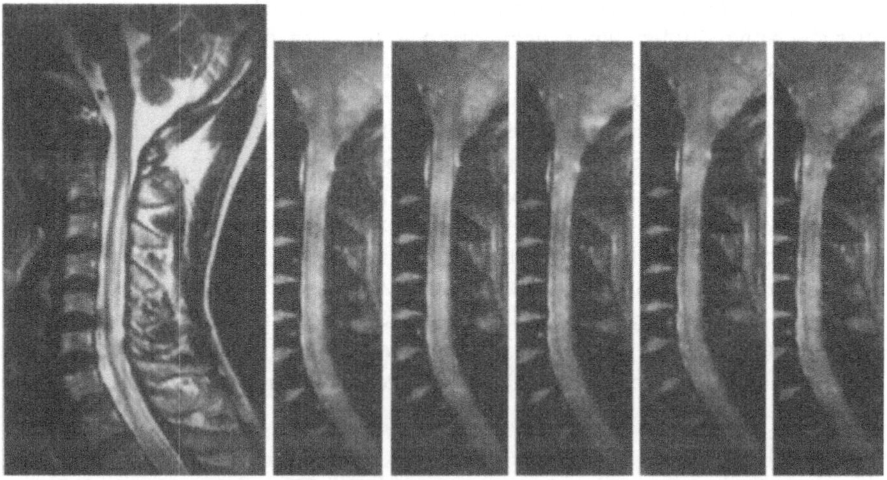

FIG. 3. Case 2. Cine-MRI demonstrates absence of subarachnoid flow void, which indicates diffuse obstruction of the subarachnoid space

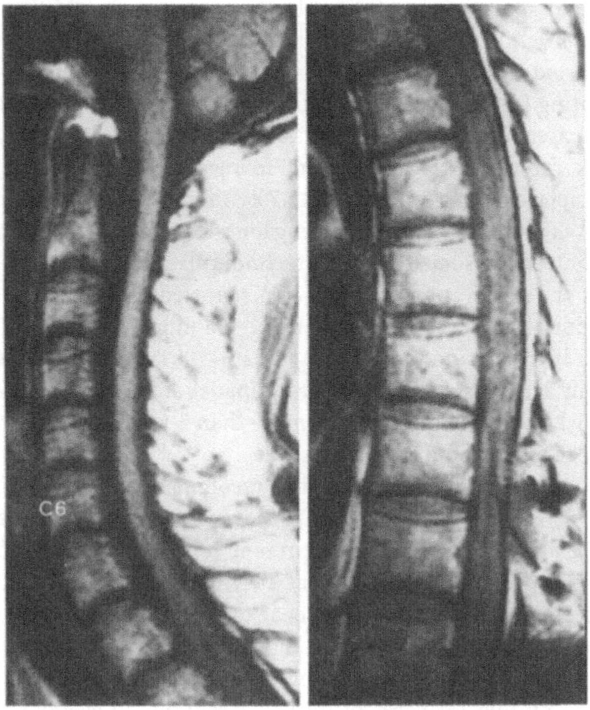

FIG. 4. Case 2. Postoperative T_1-weighted MRI showing disappearance of the cervical syrinx. A syringoperitoneal tube was placed in the large syrinx at the midthoracic spinal cord

associated with arachnoid adhesion at the foramen magnum were of tuberculous origin [1]. The average interval between the occurrence of tuberculous meningitis and the onset of syringomyelia is reported to be 12.2 years (6 months to 36 years). Our study also revealed a long interval before the onset of syringomyelia. In exceptional cases, syringomyelia may develop during acute tuberculous meningitis. In cases of tuberculous meningitis, hydrocephalus frequently develops because of disturbance of cerebrospinal fluid (CSF) circulation by diffuse obstruction of the basal subarachnoid space. Foster and Hudgson reported that syringomyelia due to basal arachnoiditis was frequently accompanied by hydrocephalus [2]. One characteristic of the cases presented here is that there was no evidence of accompanying hydrocephalus. This finding indicates that the arachnoiditis was localized at the spinal subarachnoid space in these cases. Cine-MRI demonstrated diffuse obstruction of the subarachnoid space in two cases and localized obstruction in the other cases. The mechanism of formation of syringomyelia associated with spinal arachnoiditis is not yet well understood. Caplan et al. indicated two possible mechanisms: vascular change and localized abnormality of CSF circulation due to arachnoid adhesion [3]. The factors that make syringomyelia resistant to treatment are the long period of suffering, irreversible change in the spinal cord parenchyma, and severe arachnoid adhesion.

In the study presented here, an SS or SP shunt was used with dissection of the arachnoid adhesion. As diffuse obstruction was confirmed by cine-MRI or myelography, an SP shunt was selected for one case and an SS shunt was selected for two cases as the patent cranial subarachnoid space was confirmed by preoperative cine-MRI or intraoperative endoscopic observation.

Sgouros and Williams reported a 10-year follow-up study of 73 cases who underwent any kind of syrinx shunting [4]. About one-half of the patients who underwent syringo-pleural shunting (56 cases) or syringosubarachnoid (SS) shunting (14 cases) experienced deterioration as determined by long-term follow-up. Fatal bleeding, infection, and shunt tube displacement occurred in 15.7%. In cases of traumatic syringomyelia, 12 cases (35%) showed deterioration during long-term follow-up. Most of the patients with syringomyelia associated with arachnoiditis who underwent syrinx shunting showed signs of deterioration. Batzdorf et al. reported a 50% obstruction rate of syrinx shunting during a long-term follow-up of 106 months on average [5]. Klekamp et al. reported a high obstruction rate, up to 92%–100%, in 78 cases of syringomyelia who underwent syringosubarachnoid or syringoabdominal shunting [6]. In our study, three cases who were followed up for more than 3 years showed no neurological deterioration or reexpansion of the syrinx.

Regarding the method of surgical treatment, Klekamp recommended dissection of the arachnoid adhesion instead of syrinx shunting. However, syrinx shunting is inevitable in cases of diffuse arachnoid adhesion. At present, it is recommended to avoid contamination of the shunt tube by blood, unnecessary use of the shunt bulb to reduce resistance, and placement of the shunt tube near the arachnoid adhesion. It is still controversial whether arachnoid dissection alone is sufficient for cases with localized arachnoid adhesion. Under the present circumstances, we recommend syringoabdominal or pleural shunting for cases of diffuse arachnoid adhesion. On the other hand, arachnoid dissection, syringosubarachnoid shunting, and expansive dural plasty with a Gore-Tex membrane are recommended for localized arachnoid adhesion. Endoscopic observation during the operation is useful for assessing the patency of cranial subarachnoid space and to confirm proper placement of the subarachnoid tube.

References

1. Appleby A, Bradley WG, Foster JB, et al (1969) Syringomyelia due to chronic arachnoiditis at the foramen magnum. J Neurol Sci 8:451–464
2. Foster JB, Hudgson P (1973) Basal arachnoiditis. In: Barnett HJM, Foster JB, Hudgson P (eds) Syringomyelia. Saunders, London, pp 30–49
3. Caplan LR, Noro AB, Amico LL (1990) Syringomyelia and arachnoiditis. J Neurol Neurosurg Psychiatry 53:106–113
4. Sgouros S, Williams B (1995) A critical appraisal of drainage in syringomyelia. J Neurosurg 82:1–10
5. Batzdorf U, Klekamp J, Johnson JP (1998) A critical appraisal of syrinx cavity shunting procedures. J Neurosurg 89:382–388
6. Klekamp J, Batzdorf U, Samii M, Bothe HW (1997) Treatment of syringomyelia associated with arachnoid scarring caused by arachnoiditis or trauma. J Neurosurg 86:233–240

Subject Index

GPSR Compliance

The European Union's (EU) General Product Safety Regulation (GPSR) is a set of rules that requires consumer products to be safe and our obligations to ensure this.

If you have any concerns about our products, you can contact us on ProductSafety@springernature.com

In case Publisher is established outside the EU, the EU authorized representative is:

Springer Nature Customer Service Center GmbH
Europaplatz 3
69115 Heidelberg, Germany

Batch number: 10682213

Printed by Printforce, the Netherlands